HEMATOLOGIES

HEMATOLOGIES

The Political Life of Blood in India

**Jacob Copeman and
Dwaipayan Banerjee**

CORNELL UNIVERSITY PRESS   ITHACA AND LONDON

First published 2019 by Cornell University Press

Library of Congress Cataloging-in-Publication Data

Names: Copeman, Jacob, author. | Banerjee, Dwaipayan, 1983–author.
Title: Hematologies : the political life of blood in India / by Jacob Copeman and Dwaipayan Banerjee.
Description: Ithaca : Cornell University Press, 2019. | Includes bibliographical references and index. | Summary: "Hematologies examines how the giving and receiving of blood has shaped social and political life in north India in the twentieth and twenty-first centuries"— Provided by publisher.
Identifiers: LCCN 2019020871 (print) | LCCN 2019981063 (ebook) | ISBN 9781501745096 (cloth) | ISBN 9781501745119 (epub) | ISBN 9781501745102 (pdf)
Subjects: LCSH: Blood—Social aspects—India, North. | Blood—Collection and preservation—India, North. | Blood donors—India, North.
Classification: LCC GT498.B55 C66 2019 (print) | LCC GT498.B55 (ebook) | DDC 306.4—dc23
LC record available at https://lccn.loc.gov/2019020871
LC ebook record available at https://lccn.loc.gov/2019981063

Contents

Acknowledgments

"Perhaps anthropologists bleed pure context like saints excorporate pure blood" (L. Cohen 2013, 321). Our contexts of bleeding in this work have been many, and correlatively so have been the contributions of all those whose support has helped us carry through the research reported here. It is a pleasure to acknowledge these many kindnesses and salutary to notice just how numerous they are.

We thank the innumerable people who took time to talk with us and explain things to us. In particular, we thank Debabrata Ray and Subrata Ray from the Association of Voluntary Blood Donors, West Bengal. It was thrilling to spend time with you and to experience the pedagogy of fieldwork at its highest pitch. In Delhi, the consideration and companionship of Neera Bawa and Tim Bray led to the richest of fieldwork experiences. Thanks also to the International Campaign for Justice in Bhopal for the wonderful opportunity to work alongside you and learn from your decades of powerful activism.

Dwaipayan was fortunate to have the support of a Social Science Research Council (DPDF) grant and a fellowship at the Humanities Center at NYU while researching this project. Jane Tylus and Gwynneth Malin, along with a marvelous cohort of fellows, made the experience an intellectual and personal pleasure. Much of the writing unfolded with the support of a Mellon Humanities Postdoctoral Fellowship at Dartmouth College. Thank you to my wonderful colleagues in the anthropology department at Dartmouth, and particularly to Sienna Craig and Laura Ogden for your guidance and invaluable conversations about writing. Thanks also to Doug Haynes and William Elison for an opportunity to workshop early versions of the work that appears here. A special thanks to Kerry Jessup for her unflinching support through New York, Hanover, and Boston.

Jacob benefited from several visiting fellowships. The first was at Minpaku, the National Museum of Ethnology in Osaka. Thank you to everyone who made me so welcome there, to Mizuho Matsuo for being the perfect host, and to Aya Ikegame and Crispin Bates for your comradeship, hospitality, and practical help. I am also immensely grateful to everyone at Le Centre d'Études de l'Inde et de l'Asie du Sud in Paris for their warm hospitality and intellectual generosity, but in particular Aminah Mohammad-Arif, Caterina Guenzi, Raphaël Voix, Ines Zupanov, and Catherine Clémentin-Ojha.

We are grateful for stimulating discussion with and encouragement from Deepa Reddy, Kriti Kapila, Maria Olejaz Tellerup, Prasannanshu, Rachel Douglas-Jones,

Susan Bayly, Olivier Allard, Adam Reed, Frédéric Keck, Satish Kumar Jha, Tulasi Srinivas, Nikolai Ssorin-Chaikov, Carlo Caduff, Mathangi Krishnamurthy, Marika Vicziany, John Zavos, Johannes Quack, Marilyn Strathern, Nate Roberts, Ed Anderson, Aditi Saraf, Moyukh Chatterjee, Hemangini Gupta, Sandipto Dasgupta, Debashree Mukherjee, Anand Vaidya, Jyothi Natarajan, Poulami Roychowdhury, Brandon Hamilton, Nishita Trisal, Ishani Saraf, William Stafford, Durba Mitra, Ram Natarajan, Gabriela Soto Laveaga, Projit Mukharji, Bharat Venkat, Amit Prasad, Prakash Kumar, Banu Subramaniam, Brian Mooney, Bridget Hanna, Aquene Freechild, Raghu Karnad, Priyanka Pruthi, Kareem Khubchandani, Gowri Vijayakumar, Josh Williams, Anirudh Nair, Ernesto de Carvalho, Danielle Carr, Saiba Varma, Rita Brara, Lily Defriend, Yana Stainova, Vijayanka Nair, Anand Vivek Taneja, Sunayana Ganguly, Martin Lin, and Sophia Powers. John Hagström, Aya Ikegame, Yosuke Shimazono, Heid Jerstad, Ashley Lebner, and Sandra Bärnreuther read parts of the manuscript and offered many helpful interventions. Thank you. Arkotong Longkumer has been with this project every step of the way, providing exceptionally helpful close readings of the text and sustenance both intellectual and vinous. We also owe large debts of gratitude to Klaus Hoeyer, Boel Berner and Johannes Quack—not only for the stimulus of their exemplary work but also for invitations to speak in Copenhagen, Lund, and Zurich, respectively, which together constituted the intellectual beginnings of this project. We also acknowledge the kind invitation from Filippo Osella and Sumathi Ramaswamy to contribute to their edited collection "Charity and Philanthropy in South Asia" (Osella and Ramaswamy 2018)—our very first experience of writing together and a key first step toward this book.

We thank our friends, mentors, and colleagues at NYU, MIT, and Edinburgh who have provided support, advice, and insight. We mention in particular Neil Thin, Janet Carsten, Toby Kelly, Stefan Ecks, Tricia Jeffery, Heid Jerstad, Lotte Hoek, John Harries, Hannah Lesshafft, Crispin Bates, Hugo Gorringe, Diego Malara, Laura Jeffery, Delwar Hussain, Lydie Fialova, Roger Jeffery, Morteza Hashemi, Jon Bialecki, Emily Martin, Tejaswini Ganti, Rayna Rapp, Faye Ginsburg, Helena Hansen, Julie Livingston, Bruce Grant, Fred Myers, Bambi Schieffelin, Noelle Stout, Allen Feldman, Kate Brown, William Deringer, John Durant, Michael Fischer, Deborah Fitzgerald, Graham Jones, David Kaiser, Jennifer Light, Clapperton Mavhunga, Amy Moran-Thomas, Heather Paxson, Robin Scheffler, Merrit Roe Smith, Sherry Turkle, Christine Walley, and Rosalind Williams. Thanks also to the flawless academic and administrative staff at MIT: Karen Gardner, Judith Spitzer, Gus Zahariadis, Carolyn Carlson, and Paree Pinkney. The intellectual debts, roots, and inspirations of this book are too many to enumerate, but deserving of special mention in that regard are Joseph Alter, Deepak

Mehta, Sarah Pinto, Ann Stoler, Laura Bear, Lawrence Cohen, Stefan Helmreich, Veena Das, Alberto Corsín Jiménez, and Ajay Skaria.

Parts of this book have been presented before audiences in Tokyo, Osaka, Paris, Copenhagen, Durham, London, Minneapolis, Lund, St. Andrews, UCL, Sussex, Edinburgh, Boston, San Diego, and Dartmouth. We are grateful for the invitations and thank the audiences for their very helpful suggestions.

Fieldwork was supported by the UK's Economic and Social Research Council, and the School of Social and Political Science at the University of Edinburgh.

The text reviews some of the publishing pasts of its authors, albeit in reinvented form. Those previously published works are "Ungiven: Philanthropy as Critique" (D. Banerjee and Copeman 2018), "The Art of Bleeding: Memory, Martyrdom, and Portraits in Blood" (Copeman 2013a), "Writing the Disaster: Substance Activism after Bhopal" (D. Banerjee 2013), "Portraits of Substance: Image, Text, and Intervention in India's Sanguinary Politics" (Copeman 2013b), and "The Mimetic Guru: Tracing the Real in Sikh-Dera Sacha Sauda Relations" (Copeman 2012). We are grateful to their initial publishers for permission to reprint them here in substantially revised form, and to their initial peer reviewers. Those reviewers, and in particular the two manuscript reviewers for Cornell University Press, gave us tools to immeasurably enrich and refine the final outcome. Thank you. We are grateful to Jim Lance at Cornell University Press for his strong support of this project and his expert guidance, and to everyone involved at the press. It has been a real pleasure working with you.

To our families (including our cats), thank you for your love and support. The book is for you.

HEMATOLOGIES

BLOODSCAPE OF DIFFERENCE

In October 2013, a medic from the Archana Pathology Lab and Diagnostic Center posted a Hindi poem on the company Facebook page. Titled "Story of Blood," the poem was written in the voice of blood itself ("*Rakt kahe apni kahani swam ki zubani*—Blood tells its own tale by its own tongue").

> *Hindu ho ya musalmaan, nirbal ho ya pehalwan.*
> *Sikh ho ya isai, moulvi ho ya kasai.*
> *Khojte hi reh jaayenge, Par mujme fark na kar payenge.*
> *Koi sarhad mujhe rok sake aisa kisi mein dam nahi, mein kisi bhi mulk*
>   *mein rahun mujhe koi gam nahi.*
> *Bush ya Obama, Chahe jo le lo naam, Rang bhed se pare hun raktva-*
>   *hiniya mera dham.*
> *Mujh par rajneeti karne ki, mat karna tum bhul, bas insaan ki rago mein*
>   *behna, yahi mera usool.*
> *Samaj ke rakhwalon se karta hun apeal, Mera vyapar kar ke, Mat karo*
>   *mujhe zaleel.*
> *Jati dharm aur warg se bana raha pehchaan, Kitna chota ho gaya lahu*
>   *bech insaan.*
> *Noton ke iss khel mein rehna chahtahun azad, Kash! ki meri soch ka, Ho*
>   *pata anuwad.*
> *Jeevan mein karna ho, yadi kaam mahaan, To niyamit karte rahen*
>   *swam raktdaan.*

Whether a Hindu or a Muslim, weak or strong.
Sikh or Christian, Mullah or butcher.
They'll keep searching, but won't be able to find any difference in me.
No political borders are strong enough to stop me. I can reside in any
country, I don't mind.
Bush or Obama—whichever name you take, I am above racial
differences, arteries are my only destination.
Do not make the mistake of dragging me into politics. To flow in
humans' veins, that is my only essence.
I appeal to people with intelligence, don't abase me by transacting me
in business.
Mired in caste, religion and *varna*, how man has diminished himself
by selling blood.
I want to be free from this game of money, I wish that this thought of
mine could find voice.
If you truly aspire to do something great in life, then you must yourself
donate blood regularly.[1]

"Do not make the mistake of dragging me into politics," says blood. This book
concerns the many manifestations of that "mistake" as found in a variety of North
Indian contexts or sanguinary scenes.

"Where blood was, there politics shall be," says Gil Anidjar (2011). There is
an apt sense of pursuit in Anidjar's remark: politics seems to pursue a path that
blood seeks to evade, that abases its essence. All it wants, in the words of the poem,
is to "flow in humans' veins."

On 9 January 2017, Hindi daily *Dainik Times* reported the following: "Though
Prime Minister Narendra Modi remains a target of the Congress and other opposition parties, those impressed by Modi's policies are *ready to do anything for him
(kuch bhi kar guzarna)*. . . . One young resident of Baghpat made a painting of the
PM with his blood. . . . Nitin Tyagi, in order to make this painting, drew his blood
with a syringe and filled the painting with the color of his hopes (*umeed ke rang*)"
(emphasis added). Tyagi is reported to have said, "Our current PM is the first
leader I have seen who has a unique style of functioning, be it demonetization or
surgical strike.[2] He has taken some bold steps for the benefit of the nation. Drawing a portrait of Modi is my way of paying tribute to his leadership."[3] The poem
and the portrait congeal the themes of this book. Blood flows both away from and
toward politics. It has various destinations: other bodies, certainly, but also letters,
petitions, and portraits of politicians that represent not just their subjects but the
artists' willingness "to do anything" for them. This book explores the relation

between the substance's multidirectional flows and unpredictable clotting, often utopic, sometimes cynical, but always enmeshed in sociopolitical aesthetics.

The political hematology we trace is one in which the "p" in "politics" figures in both the upper and lower cases.[4] In the domain of overt big-P politics (which is to say in situations defined by their own actors as belonging to the domain of the political [Spencer 1997, 4]), contestations take place *through* the use of extracted blood. Blood flows in acts of violence or national solidarity, into syringes, art brushes, and pens, all in order to compel actions and persuade imaginations. Here our area of inquiry is that of hematology as a sort of political style.[5] How and why did publicly enacted blood extractions—principally political rallies, memorials, protests in the form of petitions or paintings in blood—become such a noteworthy form of political enunciation in India? Complementing this approach is a counterpart focus on less overt, small-P politics, which we gloss as the domain of contestations *about* blood and its use. Exploration of this domain takes us into hospitals, blood banks, and campaigns aimed at getting people to understand and use the substance "correctly." What are contested here are definitions, economies, and practices of blood, both inside and outside human bodies.

The chapters in this book reveal a productive and dynamic relation between overtly political blood flows and an imaginary of blood as an aspiration to transcend politics. We find that new ways to take the politics out of blood are constantly discovered, yet each attempt ends in a kind of failure; the "amoral" world of the political inexorably tarnishes the secular and technoscientific utopias imagined through the substance.[6] It is, as a substance, laden with hopes, wishes, and possibility, but also with the twin poisons of politics and violence. We shall argue that blood is the exemplary subjunctive substance, but in as much a negative as a positive sense, where its sense of possibility always includes the dangerous threat of its future spillage.

A recent newspaper report headlined "Hindu Activists Paint Lord Rama with Blood to Protest against Sethu Samundram Project" shows how bloodshed in the present may be used to preview just such a future spillage. The report states that the use of blood as a medium is intended to show the anguish of the Hindu community: "We have expressed the pain we have felt regarding Ram Sethu [a chain of limestone shoals which featured prominently in the famous Hindu mythological text the Ramayana and was believed to have been threatened by a government project to dredge a channel between India and Sri Lanka]. If one can give blood [for the cause] he can shed it as well." In addition to being an ascetic demonstration of bodily commitment to the cause, the article reports a threat of further bloodshed: "'This is a message to those who are opposed to [the Hindu god and king] Ram and the ones concerned with the project that they should relinquish the idea of destructing the bridge or they will have to face the consequences,' said a leader of [Hindu right activist organization] the Bajrang Dal."[7] The blood portrait is thus a kind of premonitory bloodshed, a sanguinary forewarning. There is a staging of analogical connection: blood extraction, in such instances, is ostensibly for the nonviolent purpose of devotional image-construction. But it points forward toward future violent bloodshed, should the image-as-warning go unheeded. The image seems to both intimate and prefigure future violent bloodshed.

The present-tense bloodshed of the portrait may be made to form analogies with past bloodshed or future bloodshed (as with the Bajrang Dal). Exploring this problematic in chapter 2, we enter a neglected corner of Gandhi's political thought—his preoccupation with blood—as it indexed a past and present colonial violence, as well as the future possibility for an ascetic transcendence of both politics and the body. In the same chapter, we go on to discuss how past, present, and future bloodsheds are evoked simultaneously in the iconography of fallen freedom-fighter martyrs. In this genre, heroes of India's independence struggle who shed their blood for the nation are depicted in portraits composed of human blood in the present, the aim of which is to inspire others to willingness to shed their blood, and that of others, in the future for the nation.

Similar temporal dynamics unfold in protests by activists that deploy blood as a medium of writing. For example, in chapter 3 we describe the work of feminist activists who use menstrual blood and writing on sanitary pads to evoke and critique the violence of sexual assault and gender segregation. Unlike right-wing Hindu visions, these activists appraise the past critically rather than nostalgically: for them, the past is a time of the religiously mandated discrimination against women who bleed. In the same chapter, we examine the work of activists that have emerged in the wake of the Bhopal gas disaster who write with blood to evidence the durability of toxicity in the present. And through the force of blood as a medium, they seek to enforce a relation of duress upon political figures to demand a more habitable future. Thus, we shall be concerned to show how political blood extractions and displays such as these act as both mnemonic devices that review past violence at the same time as they serve as templates for future action and change. Blood, we argue, is a transtemporal hinge (Pedersen and Nielsen 2013) that flows between times, connecting and separating them.

The book further explores ways in which blood is considered to transcend differences, as in the words of the poem, even as it marks and accentuates them. To return to our opening poem: in order to "not do business with [it]" anymore (paid donation is now officially banned in the country), new bodily understandings must be communicated to a new voluntary donor constituency in order to persuade them to do "something that is great in life [and] donate blood regularly." We find that these new, utopic imaginations of a disinterested, secular giving constantly come into friction with durable conceptions of bodily integrity, religious practice, and even astral reckonings. Further, campaigners must topple existing understandings according to which one's lifeblood subsists as a finite store. A new antisacrificial hematological economy must be made convincing. We follow the work of these campaigners as they try to make persuasive a new imagination of hematological exchange, one that reckons with past and present conceptions of giving and receiving blood simultaneously. Relatedly, what of the legal status of blood as a drug? This does not accord well with campaigners' hematological humanism. The contested economy of the blood bank is also at issue: How do medical reformers seek to persuade recalcitrant medics to prescribe blood transfusions with due care (economy)? The matter of temporal economy is also vital; rather than one-time family-replacement blood donations, the ideal voluntary blood donor gives repeatedly, every three months, over time. How to secure such a hematic economy of repetition? Contests with blood and campaigns about blood are thus the constituent ingredients of India's hematic political economy.

Broadly, then, the first half of the book concerns contestations with blood: protests, public spectacles, campaigns, and art that employ the substance as political media (blood as a big-P political substance). The second half focuses on contestations about the substance, as it flows inside and outside of bodies, within and outside biomedical discourses (blood as a small-P micropolitical substance). At the same time, we should note here that our "with blood-"/ "about blood-" division is merely a heuristic for navigating the themes of the book. There is no hard and fast binary between the hematological modes; contestations *with* blood inform and affect contestations *about* it, and vice versa—blood is a "recursive" political substance in this sense due to the dynamic relation between the way it forms both the subject of political arguments and a liquid infrastructure through which such arguments can be made (Kelty 2008; Corsín Jiménez and Estalella 2016). But if differences between activism *with* and *about* blood blur at the edges of practice, we retain the distinction here as an organizational heuristic that allows us to see how they have such a relation. We further elaborate the intermingling of the two modes of hematological contestation at the end of this introductory chapter.

Juxtapositional Ethnography

Although we carried out our respective stretches of fieldwork in North India independently, in order to avoid unnecessary distraction we do not differentiate between ourselves when presenting ethnography in this work. Jacob's first main stretch of fieldwork on blood donation took place in Delhi, Kolkata, and elsewhere in North India from 2003 to 2005 and has continued intermittently since that time. Dwaipayan's fieldwork presented in this book took place in Bhopal and Delhi in 2009, and discontinuously until 2011. Interviews with significant figures in India's political hematology continued into 2012.

We present an ethnography composed of disparate materials—"a juxtapositional ethnography of sorts" (L. Cohen 1998). Anthropologists in the 1980s took to reevaluating the discipline's ability to comprehend the complex flow of global processes, paving the way for experiments with research methods and widening the domains of legitimate inquiry (Clifford and Marcus 1986). Anthropological examinations of global biotechnology have been particularly enlivened by this upheaval of methods and objects (Dumit 2012; Ong and Collier 2005; Petryna, Lakoff, and Kleinman 2006). As Sunder Rajan (2006) has suggested, following processes of biotechnology requires attentiveness not only to shifting scales but also to temporal uncertainties. Possible biotech futures are filled with promissory hype for some populations, while others are experimented upon and sacrificed—as they remain durably embedded within histories of inequality. In a similar spirit, we follow how transactions in blood promise aspirational technoscientific futures that transcend class, caste, and religion. At the same time, we discover older vocabularies of blood-based difference, purity, and hierarchy reanimated within contemporary worlds.

While grounded in sustained, long-term fieldwork in Delhi in medical and activist contexts, this kind of inquiry requires us to shift temporal and spatial scales. We draw promiscuously on historical materials, newspaper articles, Facebook entries, exhibition visitor-book entries, related poetry, and other materials, interested—as we are—in discursive constructions of what goes on and of what should and should not go on, as well as in what actually goes on. None of these are isolates, but rather they inform one another in intimate and complex ways.[8] This book shows that *imagination* of blood economies—noetic spaces of blood's own voice (as in our opening poem), of "as if" blood units and donations, of possible future blood flows—is a key part of the story of the economic and political life of blood in India. Therefore our consideration of written accounts of hematic extractions in a wide range of contexts—both literary and otherwise—was for us an important component of fieldwork. If analysis of poetry, fiction, and other media borrows from literary criticism, such texts also comprise people's own reflexive ethnographies of themselves (Barber 2007); one engages, then, with other people's engagement with their own social circumstances.[9] Particularly in the anthropology of biomedical and scientific worlds, anthropologists have understood the vitality of examining "reflexive social institutions within which medical, environmental, informational, and other technosciences must increasingly operate" (Fischer 2009).

In Delhi, we accompanied blood bank teams—small teams composed of medics, technicians, and a "social worker," or donor recruiter, who campaigns to attract donors and who liaises with local institutions to set up collection events— as they took "donor beds to donors," a key strategy for promoting the voluntary mode of donation throughout India and elsewhere.[10] We set off each morning in a dedicated "blood mobile" to conduct the day's blood donation "camps" (or in Hindi, *shibir*). Mostly we accompanied the Red Cross team, an affiliation that was sought (and kindly granted) due to its central place within the capital's campaign to promote voluntary blood donation, which affords it a larger reach; it is the most prolific collector of voluntarily donated blood in the city. Its destinations are diverse: they may be broadly categorized as corporate, educational, devotional, and political, but each of these is in turn internally diverse. Corporate camp locations run the gamut from shabby dilapidated offices to corporate social responsibility initiatives in gleaming new shopping malls. "Religious" camps, too, are multidimensional: churches, *gurudwaras*, temples, and a variety of *satsang bhavans* associated with specific gurus all form camp locations.

Blood donation camps, as we encountered them in Delhi, crosscut the two main public arenas identified by Partha Chatterjee (1998, 57–69): state and civil society on the one hand (the legal and formal apparatuses of governance through which interests are negotiated), and political society on the other (the more chaotic space of interaction between state and population as mediated by political parties and other more informal networks). These included collaborative endeavors between state or NGO-run medical institutions, and a mixed assortment of associations and *samitis* of primarily religious, corporate, educational, and political provenance. Quickly, we discovered that state ventures of medical provision were always entangled with the divergent priorities and imperatives of an array of informal networks and competitive-minded groupings, some of which enlisted the camp as a medium for their agonistic relations with one another. To borrow a term from Jonathan Spencer (2007, 151), blood banks and donor recruitment organizations employ "pluralizing strategies" in their attempt to form viable blood donor communities. The "great muddle of the plural," which characterizes Indian civil and political society, is treated as a resource to be harnessed. The quest for donor communities leads to blood banks operating within and courtesy of an array of associations that bestride civil and political society, with donation camps organized in conjunction both with Rotary clubs and student bodies (in other words, in the realm of the "properly constituted" civil society of the urban elites [Chatterjee 1998, 64]), but also with devotional sects and political parties seeking, through their largesse, to outdo other sects and political parties (this is the realm "built around the framework of modern political associations" but that "spills over its limits" such that it is "not always consistent with the principles of association in civil society" [64]).[11]

We have written about devotional blood donation elsewhere.[12] Guru-led organizations, in particular, have developed into a significant resource for bodies such as the Red Cross and others tasked with promoting the voluntary mode of collection. The Sant Nirankaris, a devotional movement that we shall encounter at several points in this book, account for as much as 20 percent of Delhi's voluntarily donated blood. Most recently, we have suggested the term bi-instrumentalism to acknowledge the processes by which "religion" may be mobilized as a toollike resource, but also to acknowledge that such mobilizations may be marked by instability and disjunctions so that it is not always clear who is "using" whom.[13] In turning to overt politics in this book, the intention is not to downplay the political nature of the devotional modes of collection we have discussed elsewhere; donated blood was the very stuff of contestation between devotional orders. Yet the particular focus of those works—what their ethnography revealed—is how gurus and their devotees themselves instrumentalize the Red Cross and others in employing blood donation to define themselves and their internal struggles in becoming new kinds of devotional subjects. In this work, we move away from blood donation theologies to consider other modes of hematic instrumentalization.[14] The form of the camp remains central as we shift to consider blood donation in the domain of overt politics, but we also consider here nondonative scenes of extraction, such as portraits, petitions, and letters in blood (chapters 2 and 3), seeking to lay the foundations for a political genealogy of blood in India (chapter 2), before considering contestation *about* the substance (chapters 4–6) and the modes of economy it demands and that enfold it. We do not cease to consider blood donor devotionalism in this work, but train our sights on its overtly political and conflictual manifestations.

During the initial Delhi fieldwork, we attended roughly thirty "political" camps (mainly organized by the two largest Indian political parties, the Bharatiya Janata Party and the Congress Party) on the birthdays of current leaders and death anniversaries of former leaders.[15] Subsequent to that initial fieldwork, we conducted archival research on camps conducted by the Samajwadi and Shiv Sena political parties, and we also conducted *post hoc* interviews with attendees of those camps: donors, activists, organizers, and medical teams.

What is a "political" blood donation event like? The first we ever attended was a camp organized by the Youth Congress in conjunction with the Red Cross in 2003 on the birthday of then–party leader Sonia Gandhi.[16] In this camp, situated in central Delhi's Talkatora stadium grounds, activists and supporters were bled beneath a colorful marriage tent, as is the case in most outdoor camps. Even as they donated their blood, activists signed an anticorruption pledge, joined hands with other activists standing near the donor beds, and chanted "Sonia Gandhi *zindabad*" ("Long live Sonia Gandhi"). The chant was fervent enough to intermittently drown out the Rajasthan steel band playing beside a giant poster of Sonia Gandhi, and the words "To all people, let's join together and finish corruption. We will begin a new, fresh India." Over a loudspeaker a local leader encouraged everyone to donate their blood, declaring that it is a safe thing to do: "It comes back again in forty-eight hours only." Speaking with us later, he referred to the party's recent humiliating losses in the states of Madhya Pradesh and Rajasthan; the camp formed part of an effort to raise the spirits of party workers. Activists framed their donations as gift-sacrifices to the party leader: "Giving blood is a sign—we are ready to work and do anything for Sonia Gandhiji and our party." "We are making a sacrifice of one unit, but she sacrificed her family." "We dedicate ourselves to Soniaji on this auspicious day—we are showing our love and affection for her." "We are the only party which gives its blood. Giving blood in these camps is not only Congress-support, it is nation-support." "Donating our blood today shows that we are Soniaji's *Fedayeen* (self-sacrificing fighters)—we are the soldiers of Soniaji and we want to give her homage and show our commitment both to Soniaji and the Congress."[17]

But we must emphasize that by no means are all political camps so carnivalesque. We attended one organized around then–BJP leader Atal Bihari Vajpayee's birthday that involved virtually no donors at all. On such occasions, blood bank teams understandably mutter about donation camps wasting everyone's time. There was brief enthusiasm when the local BJP MLA (Member of the Legislative Assembly) arrived to inaugurate the event, and a flurry of activity as local workers queued to donate in his presence. But after he left, they too quickly departed. In Kolkata, where political camps are more routine than anywhere else, there is little fanfare—just a few exhortations by local leaders and one or two garlanded portraits of the politician being remembered or celebrated. The party's temporary taking of ownership of the road—as frequently happens for camps but also for many other reasons—may cause minor local controversy, but this is also quite routine.[18] Sometimes on death anniversaries, such camps may be genuinely somber occasions.

As we became more and more intrigued by both the prevalence and differential nature of modes of hemo-political expressionism, we conducted participant observation with Bhopali activists, whose use of their own blood as a political substance, and other body imagery, has been prominent as they continue to seek redress and support so long after the devastating gas disaster of 1984. This fieldwork too continued the "para-ethnographic" orientation of our work, as the term describes fieldwork conducted alongside subjects that are themselves engaged in reflecting upon the force and meaning of their bodily practices (Holmes and Marcus 2008).

The Bhopal activist network comprises of several subgroups that come under a broader conglomerate organization: the International Campaign for Justice in Bhopal (ICJB).[19] In several spells between 2009 and 2012, we conducted ethnographic fieldwork alongside the ICJB across Delhi, Bhopal, and New York. In this book, we pay particular attention to a sustained activist campaign in 2009, when the ICJB gathered about fifty survivors and activists and set out on foot from Bhopal to Delhi. We spent several weeks with the activists here, as they encamped at Jantar Mantar—an oddly shaped eighteenth-century observatory in the capital city. In the present, the observatory plays a different role: the streets around it have been designated by the city administration as the space within which groups of civil dissent can make public displays and be observed by the police. Here we observed and recorded—both for this book and for the organization—campaigns that mobilized blood and metaphors of other bodily substances, particularly hearts, to shame and make claims upon the national and state governments. At the same time, we continued to conduct interviews with various political actors and artists who employ their blood as an artistic medium on research visits into 2012. Fieldwork conducted in Kolkata in 2004 and 2008 with a prominent voluntary blood donor organization, which we introduce fully later in the book, informs chapters 4 and 5 on the political economy of blood and efforts to reform prevalent popular and medical understandings of the substance.

We have anticipated already how we understand blood as a transtemporal hinge. We have also gestured to why we are attracted to studying the substance—namely, for its generative ability to flow spatially and congeal in unpredictable forms and arenas. In what follows in this chapter, we first lay out the conceptual and contextual ground in relation to which the figures of extraction and donation that we describe take shape. As throughout the book, we tack between the domains of overt nationalist and party politics, as well as a subtler politics of biomedical transactions.

Political Style

How did political involvement in blood donation activities begin? India's first prime minister—Jawaharlal Nehru—was himself known to donate blood, and central and state government ministers donated blood in front of the media at the time of China's invasion in 1962 (Naipaul 1964, 79). But from the perspective of the present, when senior blood bank employees speak about their memories of political involvement in blood donation, it is Sanjay Gandhi's name that is most often invoked. In recounting Indira Gandhi's youngest son's role in campaigns to boost voluntary blood donation, a donor recruitment specialist at Delhi's Red Cross blood bank (situated across the road from the national parliament) revealed her intimate knowledge of the blood groups of Indian political leaders:[20] "Sanjay Gandhi started the movement of voluntary donation in politics. He made it his mission. He gave blood himself to start it off. Indira Gandhi was O negative. We took two units of this type every 15 days to [her residence at] Safdarjung Road and exchanged it for the previous units in her fridge (we had a special refrigerator). Rajiv Gandhi was B negative, and when he was PM we had to take the blood to Race Course Road [the location of the prime ministerial residence]."

Another blood bank recruitment specialist recalled to us, "Sanjay gave the youth a four-point program: (1) blood donation, (2) tree plantation, (3) dowry abolition, and (4) family planning, and Rajiv also donated blood before he was PM. There is none like [Sanjay Gandhi] now." In fact, blood donation did not form a part of Sanjay Gandhi's youth program. Though Sanjay Gandhi did indeed put forward a program of promoting literacy, birth control, and planting trees at the time of the Emergency in 1976, blood donation was not among these priorities.[21] However, even though blood donation was not a part of the official program, it is significant that it is remembered to have been (and not only by this recruitment specialist), and it was most certainly a key focus of Sanjay Gandhi's activities at various points in his political career (as one of his "pet themes").[22] For example, blood donation was particularly prominent during his tenure as leader of the Youth Congress.[23] It was probably at blood donation events organized by the Youth Congress that being seen to donate blood became so prized as a means to gain advancement. (The Youth Congress was described more recently as a "rag-tag bunch of petty wheeler-dealers and politically ambitious wannabes"—a label befitting the earlier incarnation as well, even if in the 1970s it had far more clout.)[24] If fasting and spinning were the iconic practical compulsions Mohandas Gandhi had imposed on the Congress in its early years, Sanjay Gandhi supplemented this demonstration of bodily commitment with the donation of blood. As a result, it became a key means for political parties to display their *seva* (service) of a generalized *janata* (people, public) to the media—a generalization well afforded by anonymous blood donation.

A little higher up the political food chain, organizing (as well as donating at) such events became a means of getting noticed and is still marked in bold letters upon political CVs. Sanjay Gandhi's association with blood donation was such that Rajiv Gandhi himself is reported to have donated blood at a meeting held in memory of his younger brother (Siddiqui 1982, 271).[25] It is also worth noting that

Sanjay Gandhi's systematic promotion of blood (and eye) donation among Youth Congress workers was done at a time when he was promising to "donate new energetic blood [to] old senile Congress" (J. Singh 1977, x)—that is, to produce a new generation of leaders, for "in any revolution, reconstruction or rejuvenation, cultural, social or political, young blood of the nation plays a major and decisive role" (28). His camps were part of his constructive program for invigorating the Congress, and there is a sense in which they also sought to transfuse the nation with youthfulness, the literal and symbolic exchanging their properties. Unlike the "forcible deal" (Tarlo 2003) of Emergency-era mass sterilizations, there was no suggestion here of forced blood donations (though there have been accusations of forced political blood donations in other periods, discussed elsewhere in this book). Yet Youth Congress blood donations certainly formed part of the mood music of the Emergency and have ever since formed a template for mass political communication: internally in respect of the observing leader, and externally in respect of the observing public.

Most blood bank professionals in Delhi have little positive to say about collaboration with political parties. One former blood bank director we spoke with was repelled enough by the spectacle to want to put an end to such camps:

> Political camps are terrible. When I was [employed] at [a Delhi government hospital] I said, "Let's stop going for these—but we can't stop because they're so powerful—because they call everyone and when the VIP comes, whether it's Sonia Gandhi or Sanjay Gandhi or whoever, they make such a big noise. And the moment he or she goes, that's it—they've all gone. We don't need such camps. There's no other motivating factor other than "I'm trying to please the leader." I hate all these things. I find them so disgusting. But those are the realities.

Another blood bank director—a pragmatist prepared to enter the "dirty" world of politics if it means replenishing his always-fragile stocks—recounted one such political blood donation camp:

> Last year I got a call in the evening: "There is some political leader who wants a camp to be held." After great difficulty I reached that place—I met those people—totally, totally disorganized. But they wanted a camp tomorrow. Next day when I reach there with my team, we organize everything, and then a girl is brought who happens to be the daughter of that political leader for whom the blood donation camp is being held, and the political leader is behind bars, and he is fighting an election from jail. Now to give an emotional backup to vote in his favor, the daughter is brought and they say we are to weigh the daughter against the blood.

It is an election point. Now the daughter is weighing 48 kg. And they asked me to translate it into blood. So I roughly translated that this is the amount of bags, and he said, "No problem, we'll provide you with more than that." And believe me, he was the only person who won as the independent candidate. His followers wanted to take advantage and make it an emotional upheaval to draw the sympathy of the voters—wanted to draw advantage out of the situation. The votes were to be cast on that day. It is a *tamasha* [show-off, spectacle], but I just took the blood. Blood is blood.

These two quotations underline that the importance of display at these events is twofold: the political party makes visible its committed *seva* (service to society), while—as was suggested in the first quotation—the activist may donate in order to be seen by the leader they wish to impress.[26] The political camp aims to rejuvenate an ailing political class through demonstrating a renewed political commitment to a generalized *janata* (public). The political camp thus entangles an abstract *janata* with particular, political self-interest. The figural tie between party-activists and leader is enacted as *seva* even as the party performs *seva* to the *janata*. Blood bank officials resent overt politicking; blood donation as pristine service, or *seva*, is considered by them to be beyond politics, or to belong to the sublime (i.e., not the dirty, competitive, profane) dimension of politics.[27] But beggars can't be choosers. As a Kolkata-based donor recruitment specialist put it: "Actually, we do not consider political donation to be strictly voluntary—there is a political compulsion. They use us [i.e., the voluntary blood donation movement] to get votes on the basis of the consciousness *we* created among the public. They utilize this to get votes: 'Look how much we contributed in giving blood.' They have never done it. Making people conscious was done by us. They are reaping the harvest."

The director of a blood bank run by an internationally known NGO in Chennai recalled to us a Congress-organized camp at the very site, twenty-five miles from the city, at which Rajiv Gandhi was assassinated: "This was on May 21 [his death anniversary], and we received eight donors. Two hundred people were there for the photos, and then they went." For this doctor, that was the final straw. He no longer conducts "political" camps. A blood bank technician at a Delhi government hospital recounted a similar experience:

One camp I attended, most probably it was for Rajiv Gandhi—you will not believe—there was a corridor full of refreshments: all sorts of bananas and apples. There were about twenty-five beds. The workers were waiting for the VIP, Sonia Gandhi, to enter. Then Sonia came and about fifty people rushed and pushed into the tent; they all occupied one bed each. Their leader came. Only then would they let us prick, and they took photographs, and the moment she left they gobbled the refreshments and ran away. I have seen this with my own eyes. So I feel it's nothing to do with doing good deeds on someone's death anniversary. Because when you do something like this you should do it very quietly, not with so many cameras around.

Similarly, we heard several complaints from doctors about last-minute cancellations of blood donation camps scheduled by different parties after it was announced that the party leader was unable to attend.

We are particularly concerned here with what we have called the "truth-force" of substances (D. Banerjee 2013, 240). Throughout this book, we will witness a variety of episodes in which excorporation of substance is held up (more and less convincingly) as the stuff of communicative truth: blood donation as the truth of one's political convictions and self-constancy; extracted human blood as a substance of the real, so to speak, in contestations over "genuine" and "fake" gurus. Excorporated blood objectifies and thereby provides evidence of commitment and sentiment in making them available for inspection. Such extractions set up vital and powerful analogies with other spillages of substances across space and time. In providing an account of the different ways in which blood extractions as forms of political statement generate enunciative force, the present work joins studies by Bernard Bate (2002; 2009) and Michael Carrithers (2010) to show how present-day forms of Indian political rhetoric, though creative and novel, draw heavily on earlier conventions of political iconography. Indian hemo-politics often refer to a Gandhian tradition of austerity and restraint, which at the same time is also a politics of notable "semiotic excess" (Spencer 2007, 15) belying the austerity it had seemed to suggest.

Discussing artistic style, Alfred Gell (1998, 157) equates psychological saliency with "the capacity, possessed only by painters with a developed personal style, to so engage the spectator's attention that the aesthetically significant aspects of the work of art are the ones which actually do attract our notice." For the present analysis, such saliency refers to the effects the organizers or "donors" hope or expect to achieve in the viewer by way of such a style. But there is also a more prosaic sense in which we employ the term "style," for the expression also refers, of course, to "those characteristics of an artist's work by reference to which we assign works to him" (Wollheim 1987, 197). In this sense, the use of blood in mass political milieus constitutes a distinct style of political expressionism. This book seeks both to define the genre and to discern reasons for its saliency for those who perform and witness it.

Of course, blood extraction is not one representation but a protean family of representations.[28] Political parties compete to collect the most donated blood in

Bengal; antisuperstition campaigners and the followers of a maligned guru each organize letter-writing campaigns in their blood; blood may be donated to mark pledges to build a corruption-free nation; underage schoolchildren are "forced" to donate their blood by Congress Party functionaries on the birth anniversary of slain former prime minister Rajiv Gandhi; blood is donated in protest at "political" attacks on it by devotees of a controversial devotional movement with ambiguous ties to Sikhism (see chapter 6).[29] In the Indian context, blood has proved an extremely productive material and medium of political communication—hence our effort here to describe a diverse and disparate Indian political hematology.

The examples discussed so far have featured blood donation camps conducted by political parties in which the transactional form at stake is "voluntary" (anonymous, non-remunerated) blood donation. However, this has not always been the case, as the following critical episode in the history of political blood donations makes clear. A Supreme Court order banning payment for blood came into effect in January 1998. Prior to that, as much as a third of all blood donations in India came from paid "professional" blood donors (Mudur 1998, 172). While paid donors are stigmatized by voluntary donor recruiters and in public discourse more generally as drug-addicted rickshaw drivers who place others at risk, on occasion various kinds of political and social activists have sought to define a "social" model of paid blood donation, according to which the cash that is generated is immediately transferred to a particular cause.[30] So it was perfectly legal when in 1988, the Communist Party of India (Marxist) (CPI(M)) in West Bengal lined up its activists to sell their blood to raise funds for the building of the Bakreswar power plant. The CPI(M) was not the first outfit to encourage its members to sell their blood "for a cause." For instance, activists belonging to the organization that later became the Association of Voluntary Blood Donors, West Bengal (AVBDWB, see chapters 4 and 5) in 1970s Kolkata sold their blood explicitly in order to financially support a funds-starved student medical institution. In instances such as these that figure throughout this book, the literal and the metaphorical properties of blood exchange places: "We founded a mobile medical unit *with our blood*," an AVBDWB volunteer told us, while the CPI(M)'s slogan at the time was "*Rokto diye Bakreswar gorbo*" ("We shall build Bakreswar *with our blood*").[31]

The CPI(M) in West Bengal had then been embroiled in a dispute with Rajiv Gandhi's administration in Delhi, whom it accused of restricting funds for what had become a centerpiece of the party's industrial strategy: "The Bakreswar Thermal Project initially faced serious problems, specially resource crunch. The then rulers of the Central Government took this issue in a political way" (Bhaṭṭācārya, Biśvāsa, and Bhaṭṭācārya 1997, 224). In a spin upon what is probably the most famous hematic political rallying cry in Indian history—Netaji Subhash Chandra Bose's "Give me your blood and I will give you freedom" (see chapter 2)—the CPI(M)'s clarion call became "Give us blood and we will give you Bakreswar power plant."[32]

An official party history recalls that the agitation caused "literally [the party to have] a blood-relation with the people of the State" (Bhaṭṭācārya, Biśvāsa, and Bhaṭṭācārya 1997, 224). In a column of the CPI(M)'s online news magazine headlined "People of the State Made Bakreswar by Donating Blood," the episode is remembered thus:

> The whole Left Strength of Bengal then in 1988 had taken oath to build Bakreswar project by donating blood. So it was not just a thermal project to have been established, it was rather a history of Bengal's real political will. Jyoti Basu finally laid the foundation stone in 1988 and the Thermal Power Plant started production in 1999. A thermal power plant is a sign of progression. But Bakreswar Thermal Power Plant is not just another power plant. The then State Government's blueprints were moulded by the thousands of students, young men and women, working class beings, labourers, farmers of the state. To stop the Rajiv Gandhi-led Central Government's conspiracy the people of West Bengal gave blood to build the Bakreswar Thermal Power Plant. The present chief minister of Bengal being an [sic] Congress MP, helped Rajiv Gandhi in every possible way to stop the Left Front Government. A section of media also joined in to a crack a laugh about the passion of the people. But the crowd had spoken out to them in that matter.[33]

In addition to enabling the party to (claim to) form a substantial political relation with the people of Bengal (see also the discussion of Shiv Sena blood donation camps in chapter 3), there is also the striking similarity between activists' blood offerings for the building of the plant and the role of blood sacrifice, or *bali dan*, at foundation ceremonies. "You can't have a foundation ceremony," as a Saurashtra Brahman told David Pocock (1973, 73), "without a blood sacrifice, it's essential and that's that." And as Jonathan Parry's Bhilai informants put it to him, "There is hardly a bridge, a dam or an irrigation canal within a hundred kilometres of Bhilai which can have been constructed without a real bali [sacrifice]" (2015, 15). Moreover, it is a longstanding idea that the victim is often human. "Rulers properly make sacrifices *on behalf of* their subjects," suggests Parry, "but [this] often turns out to mean offering their subjects *as sacrifices*" (14).[34] Similarly, when a ruling party's activists donate their blood—especially where there is the understanding that an irreversible depletion will result (see discussion in chapter 4)—then the boundary between sacrificing *on behalf of* and offering subjects *as* sacrifices is blurred. Substances of the civic (blood for medical transfusion, steam and electricity for nation-building) intersect with the substance of the *bali dan* (sacrificial blood). While the selling of blood makes the Bakreswar case unique in the history of India's political hematology, its sacrificial dimension is not in the least exceptional—as we shall see in chapters 2–4.

It is difficult to quantify the number of units for transfusion that political blood donation events provide. Such events are less frequent than student or corporate organized ones, certainly in Delhi. And there seem to be fewer in Delhi than in Bengal, where local political rivalries are more frequently expressed through the medium of competitive blood donation camps, with different activist groups attempting to out-donate each other. That political camps do form a significant resource for blood banks, however, was made clear during a shortage experienced in Bengal in 2016, when the leader of the West Bengal Voluntary Blood Donors Forum, Apurba Ghosh, directly attributed the shortage to a concurrent state legislative assembly election:

> The situation has turned from bad to worse as the Election Commission [EC] has issued notification imposing a ban on political parties to hold blood donation camps till the election is over. The election will start on April 4 and continue till May 5. The results will be out on May 19. Then there will be swearing in ceremony of the government. Things will become normal and blood donation camps can once again be held in July. Ghosh has requested the EC to allow blood donation camps to be held without banners or symbols of a political party. The state requires 60,000 to 70,000 units of blood per month which means around 9 lakh units are required per year. Kolkata alone requires around 4.5 lakh units per year. But as camps cannot be held since the code of conduct came into force, the collection of blood has dropped sharply.[35]

Epoch Sanguinis

Of course, the liveliness of blood as a substance of political imagination and mediation is not unique to India.[36] In fact, in his work on the relation between (predominantly Christian) blood and politics, Gil Anidjar makes an ambitious claim: "All significant concepts of the modern theory of the state are liquidated theological concepts" (Anidjar 2011, 2).[37] Anidjar's work is an insightful rejection of conventional periodizations of European political history that posit that "archaic" blood ties have come to be replaced by "modern" contractual political relations. In other words, Anidjar's account of political hematology rejects the characterization of contemporary politics as the transcendence of blood ties drawn around religion, descent, family, and so on. Instead, he argues, while blood itself does not rise to the status of an operative political concept, its (absented) presence fundamentally animates our contemporary political vocabularies. It is incumbent upon us then to offer a few remarks on how we situate our analysis of political hematology in India within broader scholarly characterizations of the relation between blood and politics elsewhere in the world.

For historians and anthropologists of science and medicine, this absented-presence of blood is at its most evident in the continuing dependence on Foucauldian vocabulary to understand the relation between bodies and politics. Famously, blood appears in Foucault's analysis as a hinge to periodize European history: his delineation of the epoch sanguinis (Strong 2009, 187). His remarks on blood in volume 1 of his *History of Sexuality*, while criticized, continue to generate the conceptual vocabularies with which historians and anthropologists describe the relation between life and politics (Foucault 1978). For example, terms such as biopolitics, biopower, biocapital, biological citizenship, and biosociality rest on his characterization of our contemporary epoch in relation to its priors characterized by bloodshed. To elaborate, Foucault suggests that in a historically prior epoch—categorized by an unquestioned sovereign command over life and death—blood constituted a fundamental value. In other words, in that "thanatopolitical" society where death was always imminent, blood tended to play a material and symbolic role: the sovereign threatened bloodshed, society was divided along bloodlines of descent, and the precarious subject risked shedding blood. Crucially then, in anthropological description of our present epoch—shot through with biopower and biopolitics—blood is that which is transcended. In our contemporary epoch, as many anthropological accounts have it, political sovereignty founds itself on more complex contractual forms of making life, sustaining bodies and managing well-being (Rabinow 1992; Rose and Novas 2005; Rose 2007).

Importantly, however, anthropologists critical of Foucault's periodization argue that the old order of blood did not entirely disappear within the new. Contemporary invocations of concepts such as "thanatopolitics" and "necropolitics" highlight precisely the generativity of death as a sovereign strategy and effect (Bear 2012; Caple James 2012; Mbembé 2003; Murray 2006; Stevenson 2012). More pertinent to our focus on blood, Thomas Strong (2009, 187) questions the antonym blood/sex in an important discussion of how gay men in numerous contemporary global settings are required "to examine themselves as sexual subjects" in blood donation clinics—learning precisely "the social meaning of their sexuality *through connection to their blood*" (187, emphasis in original).[38] Consonantly, while some anthropologists contest Foucault's periodization, Ann Stoler asks whether that periodization is a fair representation of Foucault's thought. She finds that his analysis never postulates cleans breaks between periods, but rather shows the "re-animation" and "conversion" of old languages, techniques, and representations in the new (Stoler 2016). This is explicitly laid out in his lectures, where he states quite clearly that "there is not a legal age, then disciplinary age, and then the age of security" (Foucault 2007, 8). Stoler thus convincingly demonstrates that Foucault does not propose a clean transition from a "pre-modern symbolics of blood" to a modern "analytics of sexuality." Instead, Foucault's own thinking proposes a recursive analytic that urges us to attend to co-temporalities and temporal overlays—where blood and sexuality (and consonantly, the sovereign power over death and the biopolitical impulse to regulate life) run in concurrence (30). In that spirit, this book examines the complex timescapes of the Indian political present, as it is enlivened by past, present, and future metaphors and flows of blood. Particularly, following Stoler, we are attentive to the "re-animations" and "conversions" of past anticolonial deployment of blood as a political metaphor in the present; as such metaphors are awakened, distorted, and reconfigured by contemporary forms of divisive religious nationalism.

One might ask at the outset: What constitutes India's epoch sanguinis? Surely it is different from the history of premodern Europe that concerns Foucault? We argue that any answer to that question requires overturning the clear presence (and concomitant absence) of a historical period (and not others) marked by a political concern for the flow and shedding of blood. While anthropologists of India recognize the provisionality of the temporally successive categories of the colonial, early postcolonial, and contemporary, we are too often drawn into their seductively neat analytical divisions. Instead, our attempt here to think historically and anthropologically is true to Foucault's commitment to genealogical analysis. Foucault's explication of the genealogical method—a dissociative glance toward the past that disperses elements previously held together by traditional history mired in teleology and universals—is only too well known. However, that Foucault explicitly links his genealogical method to genealogical science—the less fashionable study of blood ties—is easily forgotten: "The analysis of descent permits the dissociation of the self, its recognition and displacement as an empty synthesis, in liberating a profusion of lost events" (1977, 145–46). The genealogical method is attractive to Foucault, and indeed to us in this book, because blood-ties and bodies are attached to each other—in the nervous system, in diets, in respiration and debilitation. Blood-ties and bodies are fragile in precisely the ways histories based on origin and evolution are not. They carry the "stigmata" of past errors, breakdowns, and failures, eschewing clean breaks between colonial pasts and postcolonial presents. They exceed proper lines, extending uneasily across time and space, confounding the best hopes of those invested in racial, familial, and corporeal purity.

For this same reason, we are attracted to blood as the hinge of our analysis. Through the substance, we are drawn into peculiar histories of bodies, and their reanimations and operationalizations in the present. For instance, we follow how contemporary middle-class actors invoke the blood sacrifices of anticolonial nationalism. In these invocations, the violent materiality of blood is offered as a corrective to a "secular" historiography they perceive to be biased toward Gandhian nonviolence and the Indian National Congress. Present-day bleeding under the sign of anticolonialism then becomes a way of sustaining the vitality of a prior epoch, with all its connotations of affective and divisive nationalist plenitude. We are also drawn into a new reading of Gandhi that reveals his obsession with blood for its ability to transcend politics and community. Our point is that the epoch sanguinis is an *indiscrete* period of time. Blood marks time, but it also facilitates ruptures in it. This is one of the reasons why we describe blood donation as a transtemporal hinge, for it is an action "imbued with the capacity for bringing together phenomena that are otherwise distributed across disparate moments in time. . . . Similar to an ordinary physical hinge between, say, a door and its frame, the trans-temporal hinge holds together otherwise disparate elements (certain past, present, and future events)" (Pedersen and Nielsen 2013, 123–24). Drawing on Laura Bear's (2014a; 2016a) work on modern social time, we extend this idea, including within our sense of blood donation as a transtemporal hinge, not just differently positioned durational moments but all the disparate and conflictual rhythms, representations, and effects of time held together in and by blood donation and transfusion practices (see chapters 6 and 7).

If blood donation events have the potential to "re-sanguinize" the present, they also serve as markers of relative archaism (absence of blood bank technologies, persistence of the paid and replacement donation forms) and development (presence of recent technologies and of the voluntary form of donation). Not being willing to donate voluntarily for *anyone*—that is, in a way that is considered both moral and modern—is the occasion for journalistic clichés about the juxtaposition of the medieval and the modern in India.[39] Indian news reports on campaigns to promote blood donation turn up references to "superstitions, taboos, obscure ideas of bygone centuries [that] stand in the way of progress," "inherent prejudices and religious taboos," "poor people with religious biases," and the need by way of blood donation to "rid [the country] of superstition."[40] The state of a nation's blood service constitutes an important indicator of development (Simpson 2009, 105)—of where it sits in time. In seeming confirmation of this, the Indian government provides state-by-state figures on the percentage of total blood collection voluntarily donated. Bengal's 85.7 percent renders abject Uttar

Pradesh's 17.3 percent.[41] What is widely perceived as the latter state's "feudal rot" is indicated in its figure of voluntary collection.[42] But it is not only in India that blood donation appears as a measure or indicator of civility, and of the state of nations and projects of "modernity." With the country's electricity cut off and inflation standing at 8,000 percent, the inability of Zimbabwe's National Blood Transfusion Service to test the donated blood in its possession was reported in late 2007 as further proof of national catastrophe. Similarly, it was reported in 2005 that "Iraqis desperate for cash are selling their blood via private brokers who supply orders from people whose relatives are in urgent need of transfusions as a result of ongoing violence and the chronic shortage caused by the war." Sarcastically observing that burgeoning blood brokerage is proof of the United States delivering on its pledge to create jobs in the region, the report concludes, "Yes, half a pint goes for $10 and is sold on for $50, as Adam Smith's *Wealth of Nations* gets itself an inspirational Operation Iraqi Freedom makeover."[43] Again, blood donation practices are used as a gauge, a kind of measure, of the state of nations—a market in blood being indicative of the perversions consequent on a mismanaged war. Blood has been, and remains, a temporally charged and effective substance. Most obviously, representations of its historicity may act to naturalize systems of domination in ways that crosscut kinship, race, ethnicity, and nation (Williams 1995).

Such a temporal charge is amplified in a "biotechnological time" that also "mixes frames and registers," so that "the now" can appear simultaneously as "then" (Strong 2009, 187). Particularly, anthropologists of biotechnology have paid a great deal of attention to the future-producing ability of biotech infrastructures, discourses, and practices. For instance, in studying global genomics, Kaushik Sunder Rajan argues that all biotechnology is "a game that is constantly played in the future in order to generate the present that enables that future" (Sunder Rajan 2006, 34). Crucially, this anthropological attention to speculation and hype has led to calls to pay attention to the "infrastructural firewalls, speed bumps, accountability mechanisms" that provide friction to future-producing industries, as the future is not ceded but is continuously negotiated and contested by diverse groups of social actors (Fischer 2009, 113).

As another response, anthropologists ask: What might it mean to refuse anticipation, or to charge ourselves as responsible for anticipation (Adams, Erwin, and Le 2009, 260)? Our work here is in agreement with the anthropological caution about promissory futures via the hype of "cutting edge" biotechnological interventions. Yet we develop this anthropological charge in a different direction. We practice something akin to a "creative sabotage of the future" (Cooper 2006, 129) in moving away from the global imbrication of venture capital and financial markets in biotechnology and dwelling on an "older" biological material that (mostly) escapes this particular form of hype: blood.[44] Blood science, donation, and transfusions do not rely on new technologies of genetic recombination and large capital investments. At the same time, the circulation of blood engages in abducting time, juxtaposing archaic pasts with promised futures—some divisive, some integrative. As much as new kinds of life-forms entangle nature and culture in ways that disrupt prior meanings of either term (Rabinow 1992), blood—as biological material—flows, separates, and congeals, beckoning collectivities in unpredictable ways. Indeed, as Kath Weston shows, it is impossible to think of our present political economy without the hydraulics of blood: "liquidity," "life-blood," "cash flow" are some of its guiding metaphors. From William Harvey to Adam Smith and from Karl Marx to contemporary discourses surrounding finance capital, somatic metaphors of "blood" have consistently guided analysis of the circulation of money (Weston 2013a). In our work here then, we develop the idea of blood as a transtemporal hinge as a way of seeking to ground the heterochrony—the diversity of temporal activities and understandings—of blood in India. We begin by paying attention to blood metaphors in anticolonial politics, transitioning into the deployment of these varied metaphors in contemporary national politics, finally arriving at articulations of activist and biomedical hopes of a promissory future—all through somatic metaphors concerning blood. Thus, we argue, richly complex timescapes appear as powerfully in contestations around mundane biomaterial substances such as blood as they do when newly bioengineered life-forms assert the malleability and artificiality of nature and culture (Rabinow 1992).

Blood and/as "Other" Substances

Having gestured toward broader relations between blood, temporality, and politics, we return now to the political life of the substance in India, and in particular its relation to other politically charged biomaterials. It should already be clear that blood donation as a political tool finds one of its primary purposes in making certain commitments demonstrable. In their work on the politics of gift-giving, Nikolai Ssorin-Chaikov and Olga Sosnina (2004) downplay the anthropological problematic of reciprocity, emphasizing instead the ability of gifts to demonstrate facts: "matters of fact" are demonstrated through the giving of "facts of matter." While Indian political party activists certainly donate blood with the hope of reciprocity in the form of their own political advancement, Ssorin-Chaikov and Sosnina's demonstration of the irreducibility of giving to reciprocity helps illuminate a second dynamic at play. Through blood donation, Indian politicians and political party activists also seek to underscore an association between themselves

and the national good through the witnessed offering of their blood; their donations are "material reports" of their embodied commitment to and service of the
nation. We explore the political function of the apparent verifiability of such biomaterial giving in India's hall-of-mirrors politics in chapter 3. In the same chapter, we encounter the paradox that appears when such political spectacles meet
the biomedical norm of anonymous, voluntary donation—namely, that anonymity enables political parties, devotional orders, and other mass camp organizers
to claim that self-serving public performances of blood donation really conform
to the highest principles of disinterested *seva* (see Mayer 1981 on politicians and
the expectation of *seva*).

Blood is not, of course, the only politically charged biomaterial in the region.
In particular, semen is just as much a political substance as blood, even if it is so in
a very different way. Two prominent nationalists, Swami Vivekananda and Mohandas Gandhi, notably—although quite differently—reinterpreted the traditional vow of *brahmacharya* (including the practice of celibacy) as a way to achieve
perfect self-control and their own versions of Indian masculinity. Classical Hindu
texts define *brahmacharya* as the first stage of the fourfold ideal life cycle, the stage
of initiated studentship, which marks the ritual initiation of second birth for high-
caste, twice-born boys. Combined with South Asian ideas of seminal discharge as
a loss of vital energy, modern nationalists developed the concept of *brahmacharya*
in opposition to Western masculinity (Alter 1994a, 49; Chowdhury 2001). While
Western masculinity was based on physical strength, its Eastern counterpart was
viewed as an embodiment of spiritual strength deriving from control over bodily
desires and especially retention of semen. Semen, then, was central to political
struggle while also embodying the promise of a future hypermasculine and self-
contained nation. Such connotations make all the more intriguing the present-
day matter of sperm donation in the subcontinent, as explored for instance by
Aditya Bharadwaj (2003) and Sandra Bärnreuther (2015; 2018a). Semen-
distributive (L. Cohen 1995a, 401) assisted reproductive technologies (ARTs) apparently demand a fluidic incontinence quite at odds with the semen-retentive
antipornography of Indian nationalism. Perhaps the retentive fast, which stakes
verifiable political truth on the depletion of food and flesh, was the mode of political contestation fit for an age when "modernity" was seen to "deplete a man's
vigour" (L. Cohen 1995a, 400). As Sanjay Srivastava puts it, "The discourse on
semen-conservation and that on 'nation-building' were conjoined and represented an aspect of the overall schema of frugality and saving that was characteristic of the planning ethos" (2007, 151). But a newer scholarly focus on non-
Gandhian sexuality in an age presided over by the commodity form (Srivastava
2001), coupled with the remarkably meager exchange value of semen vis-à-vis
third-party donations in the domain of ARTs—which dramatically contrasts with

the value placed on the substance in other times and contexts (Bärnreuther 2015)—suggests the apparent appropriateness of a shift in contestatory style from the retentive fast to the extractive/distributive excorporation of blood as mass political form, even while both modes enact a kind of corporeal emptying and physical self-subjection that would, in excess, result in death. Indeed, the political excorporation of blood draws power from its depletive similarity with fasting, even as it departs from that form (extending the body into the world instead of withdrawing the body from it).[45] Further, and to return explicitly to the political publicity of excorporated blood, semen (Alter 1994a; Skaria 2010) and breast milk (Saha 2017) may have an array of nationalist connotations, but one cannot imagine an MLA (Member of the Legislative Assembly) publicly donating either of *those* bodily substances in service of the nation in quite the same way as blood.

But we must be very careful in forming these kinds of contrastive definitions, for blood, critically, is an "indiscrete" substance. To look at blood is not necessarily to see only the blood before one's eyes. We have already noted the propensity of blood-flows to form analogies across space and time. Excorporation of blood in medical contexts such as for transfusion or diagnostic or DNA testing is often brought into analogy with blood in other contexts and other modes of excorporation: bloodshed in war, blood sacrifice, menstruation, blood ties of kinship, and so on. This can be for the purpose of encouraging blood donor motivation—for example, blood donors may be asked to bleed for others like India's freedom fighters bled for the nation (see chapter 2)—but also to stimulate reform of "wasteful" or "inappropriate" blood excorporations such as those found in animal sacrifice, as in the promotion by animal rights organizations of blood donation in place of animal sacrifice at the time of Kali Puja: "If you want to offer blood to the Goddess Kali, give your own, and help to save a human life."[46] But it is not only the analogizing capacity of a given blood-flow vis-à-vis "other" blood-flows that is of critical importance here; it is also the transitivity and convertibility of blood vis-à-vis "other" substances: milk, food, and semen are often understood to be particular variants of one another, as well as of blood. Stefan Ecks (2014, 89), whose main focus is digestion, describes the substantial imbrication of transformation and movement: "The model of the progressive metamorphosis of food into semen is about the transformation of one 'juice' into another. . . . The body is a container in which substances are carried from one place to another." Such understandings of imbricated flow and change are not unique to India (see Carsten 2013) but are pronounced enough there to make it necessary that we qualify our contrastive depiction of "public" blood donations versus "private" transactions of milk and semen. Indeed, what you see when you see blood is not necessarily only blood but also its past and future manifestations

BLOODSCAPE OF DIFFERENCE   25

as milk, semen, food, or another substance. One cannot imagine MLAs or activists publicly donating their own milk or semen in the form of conventional semen or milk donations (a witnessed expressing or ejaculation), but one can imagine them donating these substances publicly through their witnessed excorporation of blood as a substance that may have been or later may become one or more of those "other" substances. Equally, but in reverse, once we recognize the salience of understandings of substantial convertibility, we see that fasting, too, may be considered a kind of blood donation.

A further key point proceeds from this acknowledgment, which is that as far as South Asia is concerned, it is important to resist the conventional distinction made in the literature between "reproductive gifts" (e.g., ova, sperm, embryos) and other biomaterial donations that do not engender new life but help sustain an existing life (e.g., hearts, kidneys, corneas). At first glance, donated blood would seem to fall into the latter category of sustenance rather than the former of reproduction. But such a classification would be mistaken, for blood, as we have already explained, is an "indiscrete" substance; in donating it, one may be donating "other" (reproductive) substances besides. It is common across the subcontinent for kinship ties to be figured in terms of both breast milk and blood as substantive variations of one another (Lambert 2000; Pande 2009): "After all milk comes from blood and blood from food" (Sujatha 2007). It is a woman's condensed blood, according to the South Indian understanding, that produces breast milk (Fruzzetti, Östör, and Barnett 1982, 162–63), and in Bengal breast milk may be referred to as "breast blood" (*buker rokto*) (Aparna Rao 2000, 107).[47] In Delhi's ART techno-economy, too, donors may conceptualize their egg cells as a form of blood (Bärnreuther 2018a). The gift of blood, it follows, is not straightforwardly a gift of *only* blood; conversely, nonhematic gifts of substance are not *not*-gifts of blood.

Such understandings of transubstantiation are informed by the central tenet of Ayurvedic medicine that is concerned with digestion, or "cooking." Here, "digested food . . . becomes *dhatu* [body tissues] of the chyle variety. The *pitta* in the body, what allopathy understands as stomach acid, transforms the *chyle* first into blood, then into flesh and into all of the other forms of *dhatu* until the food finally becomes semen. This also explains the transformation of food into *mala* [waste products], including sweat, urine and mucus" (Berger 2013, 27). Two key points follow. First, there is the continuing importance of bloodletting (*raktmoksan*) in *pancakarma* (purification practices), as highlighted in Jean Langford's (2002) work on contemporary Ayurveda practices (cf. Ecks 2014, 101). Skin complaints, for instance, may be treated with leeches. Elsewhere, we have considered how local purgative understandings of blood donation demonstrate ways in which Ayurvedic logics inform conceptions of an otherwise iconically "biomedical" blood donation.[48] We revisit the matter in chapter 4, in which we find a resonant purgative logic in the attempts of clinical activists to persuade Bengalis that the human body contains a surplus portion of blood that can be safely donated. Blood donation, once again, is presented as a kind of evacuative therapy at the same time as it functions as a gift. Second, we find our analytic of material and conceptual blood-flows echoed in Ayurvedic conceptualization of the body as "a series of tubes through which the *dosas* flow to the various *dhatu*. Propelling them is *ojas*, energy, which is the source of strength for all bodily functions" (Berger 2013, 27).[49] If *nadis* both stand for and channel flow (Mukharji 2016, 82), *vaids* (Ayurvedic practitioners) seek to locate and lift problematic "'flow blockages' in the *srotas* that transport blood and waste products"—blockages that cause "life processes [to] stagnate" (Bode 2012, 72). The balances and flows of Ayurveda have been described as "functions of time" (Alter 2008a, 184). Our work here shows that the excorporable body substances of biomedicine, too, may be thought of in terms of temporal relations—"a step on the way from having been part of a body to not being so anymore" (Hoeyer 2013, 7). Substances that flow within the body and substances that flow without it flow *in time*, as much temporal relations as entities. The hemato-temporal ebbs and flows that interest us in this book—particularly in chapters 6 and 7—do not, of course, map neatly onto the flows of Ayurveda. What we will see, however, is how allopathic blood-flows, just as much as those of *dosa* and *dhatu*, "are processes happening over time, not [only] objects in space" (Langford 2002, 34).

Of particular significance here is that *vaids* have sometimes employed the relative hematic propensities of Ayurvedic medicine (figured as Hindu) to delegitimize Unani traditions (figured as Islamic). Rachel Berger considers the case of the influential *pandit* and *vaid* Shaligram Shastri, whose 1931 report for United Provinces government officials described Unani in macabre terms as preoccupied with hemorrhaging or bloodletting—practices considered to be wholly unsuited for "Hindu" bodies, even if they may be appropriate to "foreign" (i.e., Islamic) ones (Berger 2013, 89). In his work on a Muslim weaver community of Uttar Pradesh, Deepak Mehta (2000) similarly shows how attitudes toward bloodshed are used to mark community distinctions. He shows also how Muslims might in fact accede to Shastri's hematic binary categorization while reversing the moral terms. The ritual wound that Muslim males bear—which is both of and exceeds the body—engenders pain and blood. Hindus, on the other hand, only get cut in hospital, but there is no spirituality in that (92). Indeed, they lack purity precisely "because they are afraid of shedding their blood" (92–93). The question of masculinity is front and center here. Male Muslims, explains Mehta, "say they only become male and Muslim when circumcised" (81). To be an adequate male, indeed, is defined as "having enough blood to reproduce" (81).

This helpfully points us to the critical duplexity of understandings of the masculinity of bloodshed in the region: if people do not donate the substance because they feel they have too little of it (*khuun ki kami*), or because they believe it to be irrecoverable (i.e., because it is like donating a kidney), or because it will render them infertile or impotent, then enacted donation of blood potentially forms a masculine demonstration of substantial abundance—that is, *one has enough of the substance to donate it and to reproduce.*[50] So while on the one hand the act is figured as emasculating—"I can't donate, as I'm getting married next month"— on the other it can demonstrate precisely one's copiously substantive masculinity, if one nonetheless goes ahead and donates. In this way, the donation of blood is capable of carrying representations of both depleting and demonstrating masculine vigor. The Facebook page of a Jalandhar-based blood donors association is indicative of this aspect of the masculinity of blood donation, albeit in its most explicit form.[51] It consists of photographs glorifying individual blood donors as they donate. Every donor depicted is male, and each photograph contains the words "Blood Commando" emblazoned over the donating figure. In several of the photographs, the donor poses to flex his muscles even as his blood departs from them. A local gym advertises on the page: blood donors get fifteen days free. Here the number of times one has given blood is the gauge of one's masculinity (see also chapters 5–7 on the numeracy of blood donation), precisely a mark of vigor rather than its exhaustion. In particular motivational contexts, blood donation has been depicted as fortifying.[52] But far more pervasive is the belief in its dramatically weakening effects. That these "blood commandos" donate in spite of this serves to demonstrate their excessive manliness—that they have enough masculine substance to spare.

This gendering of blood, coupled with a prevalent association of female blood with breast milk, helps explain why we found many male hospital patients specifying that the units of blood for their transfusion originate from male donors. Such requests almost always occasion homilies from attendant staff about there being no distinctions in blood (the discourse of transcendence that we discuss below and in chapters 2 and 4). Indeed, it is striking that we found requests along the axis of gender, and not religion or caste, to be more prevalent (though this may be partly due to growing illegitimacy concerning public expressions of caste allegiance).[53] (On the other hand, as Bärnreuther [2015] explains, in contexts of semen and egg donation the categories of caste and religion almost always, and unequivocally, do matter. These biological exchange modes have evidently not been enrolled into the brand of social reformism that equates blood donation and typing precisely with the possibility of the transcendence of caste, which we explore below.) Further, at blood donation events we attended in Delhi and Jawaharlal Nehru universities, there were often minor controversies concerning the requirement for female donors to write their father's (and not mother's) name on the donor registration form. In one planned action at Jawaharlal Nehru University, about ten female students lined up to donate their blood but refused to complete the "sexist" form when it was their turn. A standoff ensued. When eventually the students agreed to complete the form and donate, the irritated blood bank director seized his chance to retaliate, declining to accept the female students' "angry" blood.

As we have written elsewhere, while one frequently witnesses a fairly equal number of men and women attempt to give blood in donation camps, this does not result in an equal level of accepted donations, since a large number of women are disqualified due to low hemoglobin levels or because of blood loss due to menstruation.[54] Official state health policy asserts, "Women donor should not donate during her menstrual cycles" (NACO 2007); on the other hand, World Health Organization policy baldly states, "Menstruation is not a reason for deferral" (WHO 2012, 46). The difference is intriguing: if Indian blood bank medics sought to explain it to us in terms of Indian females' particular tendency toward hematic depletion (which they certainly do have), we might also speculate that, even if unacknowledged, persistent understandings concerning the ritual impurity of menstrual blood remain salient here.[55] In 2008, WHO reported that just 6 percent of Indian blood donations came from women.[56] Such a drastic discrepancy results in moralizing narratives about the debt women owe to men (since most blood is donated by men and most blood is transfused into women), in obviation of the physical symptoms that cause the asymmetry in donation figures in the first place: widespread anemia and maternal health emergencies. South Asian women, once again, are "represented as passive recipients of charitable interventions" (Osella 2018, 33). But though we did not encounter this in our (mainly urban) fieldwork, it is likely that Indian women are reluctant to donate blood for reasons very similar to those discussed by Zubia Mumtaz and Adrienne Levay (2013, 264) in reference to the districts of Rawalpindi/Islamabad, Jhelum and Layyah, in Pakistan: "The primary reason women do not donate blood, nor are they expected to, is the belief that a woman's fertility, in particular the ability to give birth to sons, is determined by the volume of blood in her body (as 'measured' through the health of her physical appearance). Donating blood could render her subfertile or prone to giving birth to daughters." In our work here, however, we shift our focus from the gendered dimensions of donation to the deployment of blood as a feminist strategy. In chapter 3 we discuss Indian feminist actions—both in the diaspora and within the country—that deploy the symbolic and material medium of menstrual blood. Our focus in the discussion of menstrual activism is the polyvalence of the substance, as we track how a range of campaigns deploy the substance toward more and less radical activist claims.

Transitivity

In his powerful exploration of the liveliness of another substance—ocean water—Stefan Helmreich (2009) makes the case that our newfound biotechnological capability to reengineer life itself marks a new age, one in which culture and nature no longer stand in relation as figure to ground. Indeed, his insight is in consonance with the writings of anthropologists such as Paul Rabinow and Michael Fischer, who similarly argue that technological innovations into the very form of biological life often outpace the ability of social analysis to grasp their mutations. This leads Helmreich provocatively to suggest that "the relation between life forms and forms of life has become liquid, turbulent; one might even say that the relation of nature to culture is at sea." Helmreich suggests further that life is being pushed into "a fluid set of relations" (8). Our analysis of a different substance—blood—resonates with Helmreich's analytical maneuver in this: the fluidity of blood is certainly the object of our inquiry, but "fluidity" is equally the effect that we find the substance to exert upon social forms. In other words, much in the same way "relations" overlap as a kind of knowledge and an object of inquiry in the work of Marilyn Strathern, "fluidity" is simultaneously what we trace, and the instrument that we trace with, and our description of how the former often exceeds the formalism of the latter.

To elaborate, our contention here is that biological materials have outrun social analysis for longer than we might expect, and in different ways in different epistemological traditions. For instance, David Schneider's (1980 [1968]; 1984) work to denaturalize blood as the biological basis of American kinship helped enable feminist anthropologists to take on other, new forms of biological foundationalism—chief among them new reproductive technologies and disability. Here too, the guiding metaphor of "fluidity"—describing both analysis and object—was with the intent of deforming norms of descent, alliance, and proper social relations. But if Schneider's critique dovetailed with feminist perspectives on gender and sexuality in the United States, it left a lasting and curious impact on the anthropology and sociology of India. Schneider's South Asianist colleagues at Chicago—McKim Marriott, Ron Inden, Ralph Nicholas, and Susan Wadley chief among them—found in "American kinship" a foil against which they defined a contrasting theory of personhood in India. In Schneider's (1980) analysis, American kinship was a symbolic system resting on the two contrasting but mutually dependent elements of shared biogenetic substance (blood) and social code (contractual love that legitimated and reproduced blood ties). Contrarily, Marriott argued that in Indian kinship, "substance" (blood) did not oppose "code" (the moral, normative), but all aspects of reality were natural and moral at the same time. For instance, caste boundaries continue to be maintained through restrictions on who eats and drinks with whom. Thus, food was more than mere nourishment; it was also a flow of a coded substance with moral qualities that altered the persons who gave and received it. This led to the argument's dénouement: that if the American person—the individual ego in kinship—was constituted through a play between nature (blood) and culture (social codes), Indian personhood had only "dividuals"—temporary composites of bodies in ongoing processes of substance flows. Ethnosociology, the group's self-label of choice, has come under criticism for the inflexibility and ahistoricity of its analysis—the result of which was to mistake norm for practice. Yet the ethnosociological insight—that the flow of bodily material was central to the maintenance and transformation of social status—has survived its critique.

In the same spirit, our work here points to the lived enactment of the actual and virtual of blood, an immanent and provisional space where the work of conceptual labor and innovation about blood and the social relations it generates is never at rest. In the practices we trace, blood slips between metaphor and literal medium of political transactions—congealing ideology in material forms. It is certainly a biomoral substance, but not (only) because it draws power from religious or metaphysical sources. Rather, it is powerful because it reveals illegitimate and illicit flows, forcible extractions, gender politics, and histories of contamination. Chapter 3 in particular discusses several instances of activist deployments of blood that aim to reveal concealed histories of past violence. For example, we describe how survivors of the Bhopal gas disaster of 1984 write with blood as a means and medium of political communication. With blood, they index both the violence of the original event as well as the truth and sincerity of their contemporary activist claims upon the state. In these sets of deployments, among others that we discuss, biology and morality are fused through varied historical conjunctions of political economy—early colonial critique and anticolonial redeployments, postcolonial utopias, and contemporary dystopias. This is quite different from biomorality as imagined by the Chicago ethnosociologists, but it borrows from them as well. As a political substance, blood not only congeals evidence of extractive violence but also encodes the literal and figurative possibilities of its illegitimate flows and critical activist and feminist resistance.

In his book *Leveling Crowds*, Stanley Tambiah (1996) wrote of "divisive 'substance codes' of blood and soil" (261) in reference to South Asian mass politics and appeals to collective sentiments and entitlements. This intriguing usage hints at our own approach, which similarly sees merit in conserving but also (and necessarily) reshaping ethnosociological tools (see in particular chapters 3 and 7). We pick up where Tambiah left off, in extending the ethnosociological tool kit to questions of race and militant politics (chapter 7) and technological mediations (chapter 3), rescaling and radically extending it beyond "the Hindu world" as a necessary condition for defending it. The work of Joseph Alter is also of importance here. In his writings on wrestling in India, he takes forward the work of the ethnosociologists on dietetics and bodily science into the domain of national politics (Alter 1993). The biomoral substance that captures his attention is semen; he follows how the control, retention, and concern about the substance tracks different, often conflicting imaginations of what it means to be an Indian citizen (Alter 1994a; 1994b). In the spirit of Alter's analysis, Lawrence Cohen has similarly sought to move away from a theology-centered ethnosociology that might do the insalubrious work of pointing only to a radical difference, to focus instead on the emergence of substance-code politics in postcolonial scenarios.[57] In one remarkable commentary on Alter's work, Cohen (1997) points to a novel that links semen retention with the strength and virility of the postcolonial nation's nuclear bomb. However, it is Cohen's work on a different bodily substance—blood—that best highlights his commitment to a contextual history that pushes an ethnographic engagement with bodily substances even further into a modern, postcolonial political economy. Specifically, he has sought to resituate Marriott's "dividual" flows across older caste, gender, and generation into new flows in a postcolonial, scientific, and medicalized landscape of blood transfusions and transplantations (Cohen 2001). Cohen demonstrates how older networks articulate with the new, as modernity decodes and recodes old forms of biosociality. For instance, he writes of how blood groups replace caste-codings in a new imaginary of citizenship. Through the recurrent cinematic motif of blood transfusions across previously unbridgeable caste and class lines, this new imaginary contests an older form of sociality and suggests the possibility of a newer, more inclusive community of citizens within the nation.[58]

We take inspiration from Tambiah, Alter, and Cohen in our own rescaling of blood as a substance coded for politics.[59] In sum, it is a richer South Asian studies, and indeed a richer contemporary anthropology, that takes ethnosociological insights seriously, with all the provisos that we have mentioned. As Caroline Osella (2008, 6) has put it with particular acuity: Such a project is at once less ambitious than Marriott's "Thinking through Hindu Categories," since it is no longer an "all-encompassing key but . . . part of a wider and eclectic set of conceptual tools," but also more ambitious. It moves beyond an exclusively Hindu world to one of novel juxtapositions, reflective instrumentalizations, and mass mediatizations; its explanatory scope is widened, freshened, and made more compelling.

Hemo Economicus

If our focus here is on the transitive and transformative power of blood, what are some of the boundary-marking norms disrupted through such flows? As we have mentioned, blood donation is not the only hematic practice that concerns us in this book, but it is a central site: the one in which contemporary norms concerning proper and legitimate flows of blood come into clearest visibility. Earlier in this chapter we questioned readings of Foucault that separate a prior epoch sanguinis from a contemporary history of sexuality. In his discussion of biomoral substances—particularly semen—Joseph Alter too draws attention to the limits of this analytical frame (Alter 1997). That is, in thinking about South Asia, he rejects the relevance of Foucault's framing of a contemporary epoch of sexuality and its related concerns with self-knowledge and psychological truths. In particular, he argues that Hindu notions of sexuality are not concerned with knowledge of an abstract, reflexive self but rather with the moral control, emission, and circulation of substances. Thus, if according to Foucault concern about sexuality is a hermeneutic process through which the self is made into a subject unto itself, Alter contends that in Hindu practices the truth of the self is embodied in somatic rather than psychological terms. While we do not think that the distinctions between the two modes of truth are necessarily regionally demarcated, our work on blood as a political substance builds on Alter's emphasis on the need to pay attention to somatic and substance-based modes of truth and personhood. A somatic problematization of sexuality raises the question, then, of flows that highlight obvious connections between sex and blood—namely, HIV/AIDS and other blood-based diseases that are transmitted sexually. While a detailed discussion of HIV/AIDS in South Asia lies beyond the scope of this work, we must acknowledge its critical connection with blood-borne diseases, in that the modes of blood-based political giving that we discuss, and the voluntary modes of donation that enable them, were introduced and promoted precisely as a result of the transmission of disease that outdated modes of (paid and replacement) blood collection were understood to have been responsible for and accelerated (e.g., paying donors is said to provide an incentive to conceal disqualifying factors such as HIV/AIDS).[60] The focus of chapter 5 is a branch of medical activism that aims to educate physicians about the acute pathogenic dangers involved in overprescribing blood for transfusion. But where existing literature on HIV/AIDS and other blood-borne diseases in South Asia has focused on formal control strategies and technology transfer (Vicziany 2001), on activism and "prevention markets" (Qureshi 2018), on treatment regimes and kin-based commitments (Venkat 2017), and on gendered impacts and experiences of HIV/AIDS (Van Hollen 2013), our study, which takes inspiration from these works, necessarily approaches questions of blood, sexuality, and disease at a tangent. The coming of HIV/AIDS is a historical condition of the present study, but not its direct focus.

Our ethnographic descriptions of blood donation camps respond to a government move to outmode forms of blood donation such as "professional" (paid) donation and "replacement" donation, where relatives of recipients are asked to replace (in advance) the blood they require. These modes, at least officially, have been superseded by anonymous voluntary blood donation—a practice more in accord with global health standards. Paid donation, though illegal, still takes place under the sign of replacement.[61] Relatives of those requiring a transfusion—perhaps too afraid themselves to donate—often pay "professionals" to act as relatives in their place. At one of the Delhi government hospitals we regularly visited, the blood broker hid in plain sight as a *chola bhatura wala* (food seller) at the front entrance: "*Ek blood donor ka 1800 lagega, aur jitne aadmi chahiye mil jayenge*" ("One blood donor costs 1800 rupees; however many you need, we can get them for you"). This was during our first stretch of fieldwork in Delhi (2003–2005). Investigative journalists confirm the persistence of such practices in the present (A. Anand 2015), as do our own medical contacts, while also making the particularly grim discovery of a "blood farm" in Gorakhpur at which hopelessly weak "donors" were held captive and regularly bled for profit (Carney 2011).

We have written elsewhere of the dysfunction in the overall system of blood banking and transfusion, so we restrict ourselves to brief comments here.[62] Replacement (the practice of families donating a commensurate amount of blood transfused to their kin in need) is not illegal and remains the dominant collection mode, despite a government order stipulating it should be phased out by 2007. There is no central blood collection agency and barely any cooperation between blood banks (Bray and Prabhakar 2002). But the HIV epidemic coupled with a newly assertive middle class that demanded better than a second-rate blood service did eventually lead to the establishment of the National AIDS Control Organization (NACO), one of whose aims became to radically increase voluntary blood donation as a matter of safety.[63] Here NACO follows the international arbiters of health policy and funding, the World Health Organization (WHO) and the International Federation of Red Cross and Red Crescent Societies, both of which subscribe to the findings of influential British policy analyst Richard Titmuss (1970). Famously, Titmuss argued that voluntary blood donation provided the safest blood for transfusion. But statistics concerning the relative prevalence of different modes of blood collection are even murkier than usual here; nationwide figures are virtually meaningless given the variations between states and between rural and urban areas. In a further statistical sleight of hand, NACO recently began categorizing replacement donations as voluntary donations, generating the thoroughly misleading *Times of India* headline: "Voluntary Blood Donation Hits 80% Mark."[64]

In a response headlined "When Voluntary Blood Donation Percentages Go Berserk!," the voluntary organization Sankalp India stated: "This news from *Times of India* should have made all of us who work for voluntary blood donation jump in joy and distribute sweets on the streets. After all, all of us (the blood banks, the Government, the voluntary organizations, the camp organizers and the blood donors) have been working so very hard to improve voluntary blood donation. . . . But, to be frank, it does not help me feel any better."

NACO's "definition upgrade" was disturbing for Sankalp India, first because "it is incompatible with the WHO proposed definition of voluntary blood donation"; replacement involves a sense of coercion that is worlds apart from voluntary donation in ideal terms. Second, it leads to hidden payments, as detailed, undermining the actual extent of the problem: "With such false sense of having achieved what was being sought out for, the urgency and the importance that is attached to the matter will get diluted."[65] However, the so-called red market in blood is not our main focus in this book; neither are scandals concerning forced donations. In spite of much-reported setbacks, various nefarious practices, and definitional tangles, there *has* been a renewed emphasis by the state and the medical establishment on promoting anonymous voluntary blood donation, and it is this that has been the condition of possibility of the political hematology that is central to our concerns in this work.

We have written previously about how this renewed emphasis has afforded a convergence between blood donation and Indic *dana* categories of gift exchange—a convergence that lends force and meaning to the practice.[66] But equally the shift to voluntary blood donation is a shift toward modern philanthropic norms; the gift of blood is now (in theory) voluntarily given and has a moral basis. The present promotion of anonymous voluntary blood donation thus connects it to the kind of giving that is widely favored in a host of other contexts, both within and beyond India, in which anonymous, disinterested philanthropic action is considered to be both modern and moral. This kind of philanthropy promotes "idealized solidarity reigning in abstract humankind" and fosters bonds between "abstract subjects" (Godelier 1999, 5). We will see, however, that just as Oxfam and other international aid organizations personalize their exhortatory posters with pictures of needy-looking children, settings for voluntary blood donation in India undergo particular processes of repersonalization, even as efforts are redoubled to foster depersonalized voluntary donation. In this reformed mode, one no longer knows but may imagine one's recipients. This widening aligns blood donation with the idea of service and sacrifice to broader imagined communities: the nation, the abstract entity of "society," and of a "family" larger than immediate kin. We show how reformed blood donation is made congruent with a number of different social reformist agendas, with a variant of these reformist alliances found within overt political domains, with political party activists seeking access to the ethical surpluses generated by voluntary blood donation.

We do not approach surpluses and deficits in quite the same way as existing literature on biological exchange, which has tended to speak skeptically (and understandably so) of incessant demand and artificially created deficits: a "*so-called shortage of human organs*" (Lock 1996, 578; emphasis added) always necessitates increases in donor pools. In this view, the mass Indian body—teeming with "surplus" body parts—is no longer simply a burden hindering development but is resignified as valuable human capital—a developmental asset (Prasad 2009).

Excesses and shortages certainly feature in our own account—especially in chapters 4, 5, and 7—but not in ways that can be straightforwardly aligned with the practices of intensification of a "full palette capitalism" (Thrift 2006). We employ a proportional approach to blood's material political economy (MacKenzie 2017), shifting, so to speak, from "surplus populations" (Li 2010) to surplus substances, and processes of their dimensioning inside and outside of bodies. We draw in particular on an approach developed by Alberto Corsín Jiménez (2008; 2013), whose highly original work on proportionality affords social theory new ways of approaching a range of phenomena: from "well-being" to the history of science, from political thought to civil movement organizations, and from binary thinking to, in our case, the political economy of blood.[67] His project is both far-reaching and nuanced, and we cannot do justice to it here; suffice it to say that foregrounding in our analyses matters of size, measurement, and balance allows us to see the dimensioning work that goes into the creation of relations and economies. So we ask: What cultural work goes into designations of excess and shortage? How do relations of magnitude—or those between imputed parts and wholes—structure (or balance out) understandings and operations of blood economies? If proportionality has been considered in hematic contexts, it is usually fleeting references to proportional designations in histories of race, such as the "one drop rule" in the United States, according to which all persons with any black ancestry were categorized as black (e.g., Polsky 2002).[68] For us, on the other hand, it is an explicit lens. A critical proportional relation in our work—a relation that is saturated with pedagogical and political implications—is that between the given and the withheld. Obviously, the themes of excess and balance—*the proportions of the gift*—are central in Marcel Mauss's (2016 [1925]) foundational work on the gift. It is the gift as a form of criticism that we seek to draw out here. The gift as a form of criticism, we suggest, operates—is able to critique—through its proportional structure.

Drawing on the insights of economic anthropologist John Davis (1992), Cor-sín Jiménez zeroes in on partonomies in and out of balance in material exchanges, observing that "the part that we give is an indication of the whole that is not given—what you see (the gift) is what you do not get (the larger social whole). Gift-giving is thus an expression and effect of proportionality" (2008, 186). Par-tonomies are hierarchies of part-whole relationships. Though closely associated with computer science and linguistics, their role in the representation of knowl-edge should make them intrinsically interesting for scholars in the humanities and social sciences, particularly with respect to questions concerning the distribution of resources. In chapter 3, in particular, we extend these insights in order to show ways in which the given and the withheld may be made to comment on one another—often in highly critical ways. Gaps between the donated blood unit and the multitude of unpotentiated, ungiven units become the basis of critical social commentary. Partonomic relations between concrete practices of blood donation and prior failures of donation threaten the constitution of social wholes. Indeed, the ungiven blood unit as negative Other of the given is a recurrent critical-noetic figure in this work, where we understand noetic space to be that domain of the imagination which is "a specialized space for testing the limits of the possible[;] . . . successful interventions in noetic space say not simply 'things could be different,' but also encourage their listeners to . . . 'make it so'" (Belleau and Johnson 2008, 278–79).

Caste/Reform

We noted above that reform of blood donation may be made congruent with other reformist agendas. Caste is especially salient here; particularly, blood typing and donation have been engaged as potential disruptors of caste distinctions.[69] Projit Mukharji's (2014) work shows how the two—caste and blood—came to be sci-entifically linked. He demonstrates how in the early 20th century, multidisci-plinary social scientists he calls "sero-anthropologists" sought to correlate blood with particular castes and regional groups. In doing so, they ran counter to a more global scientific tendency to correlate blood with race.[70] Instead, Mukharji shows, Indian sero-anthropology postulated a "serosociality" in which blood groupings were associated with caste-based socialities of marriage rules and patterns. A later group of sero-anthropologists in the 1940s argued for region (and clustered caste groups) rather than pan-regional castes as correlative with blood groups. How-ever, according to Mukharji, this scientific interest in "serosocial identities" dis-appeared in the postindependence era, and interest in the complex social worlds from which blood was extracted diminished. Mukharji thus traces a particularly interesting, albeit fleeting, hybrid discipline that produces an imagination of blood groups as constituted by and of caste and regional sociality. However, while the scientific "serosociality" that Mukharji describes waned in the midcentury, social practices that emphasize the relation between caste and blood persist. Anthropological accounts continue to document how a caste's "purity" is held to reside specifically in members' blood—with the policing of sexual liaisons that might result in "mixed blood offspring" in order to safeguard the purity of whole castes (Fuller 2004, 21; Davis 1941), and disputes about one caste's status relative to another's continuing to take the form of arguments over whose blood is "purest" (S. Bayly 1999, 329).[71]

Ever since caste, race, and blood began to be used interchangeably in policing social boundaries, anticaste activists have imagined intermixing as a potential antidote. As early as 1936, the foremost Dalit leader of the twentieth century, B. R. Ambedkar, used ethnological accounts of regional consanguinity to argue that the caste system had come into being after Indians were already commingled in blood, and therefore to confuse caste with race was scientifically incorrect (Ambedkar 2014, 428). At the same time, he understood the symbolic power of mixing blood—particularly through intercaste marriage—as a possible answer to caste discrimination: "Fusion of blood can alone create the feeling of being kith and kin, and unless this feeling of kinship, of being kindred, becomes paramount, the separatist feeling—the feeling of being aliens—created by caste will not vanish. . . . Nothing else will serve as the solvent of caste" (Ambedkar 2014, 499).[72]

The practices of reformist blood donations in the present that we discuss in this book follow the literal letter of Ambedkar's idea of blood as a "solvent" of caste boundaries while violating its spirit. That is, in contrast to Ambedkar's desire for reform through the powerful transgression of intercaste marriage, the anonymity of voluntary (reformed) blood donation comes to be thought in terms of an almost mechanical transgression of community boundaries. Take, for example, the typical Indian Red Cross slogan: "Your blood will be used to treat patients without any distinction of caste, creed, or status." Indeed, while an insistence that blood must flow "without any distinction" is a feature of voluntary blood donation ideology worldwide, the mutating significance of caste and communal boundaries in the region lend it a particular piquancy there. The social reformist promise arising from the anonymity of reformed blood donation has lain precisely in the possibility of the transcendence of caste. We have explored elsewhere how anonymous voluntary blood donation has the capacity to buttress the Nehruvian integrative political aesthetic, even at a time when quite other forms of nationalism seem to predominate, and also the Sant Nirankari devotional movement's particular instrumentalization of what we call the "universal direc-tionality" of anonymous blood donation as a means to materially realize its own *bhakti* universalism, which likewise seeks to move beyond caste and community restrictions and distinctions.[73]

The key point that follows from this is that such performances of transgres-sion of "prior" caste and purity logics do not necessarily unravel those logics; parts of their logic may be reproduced in inverting typical patterns of restriction. Many of the middle-class blood donors we met and discussed in previous works who declaim their progressive credentials in imagining their donated blood being transfused into the bodies of any others (specifically *beyond* their own castes), meanwhile, do not inter-dine and have little day-to-day contact with people be-longing to communities other than their own. So rather than a concrete and com-plicated presence, the Other is considered abstractly in absentia, via the ab-stracted medium of blood. Donation of blood by those who harbor misgivings about contact with "unclean" caste members allows a performance of anticaste sentiment without troubling the ubiquity of caste segregation. What could be more anticaste than mixing one's substance with that of one from any conceiv-able caste? Yet this is a mixing at one remove from the donor: blood donation enables nonpolluting contact with others.[74]

This book seeks to expand and enrich our exploration of the use of blood in many kinds of reformist agendas, with all their limits and potentials for quick de-generation, in challenging caste boundaries. The work is centrally concerned with caste, but under erasure, in the sense that it gives an account of how "blood rhetorics" (Simpson 2011) are variably but consistently employed as a means of transcending caste. As several scholars of caste have noted, the postindependence emphasis on legal and governmental "caste-blindness" has encouraged and deep-ened the persistence of inequality (Deshpande and John 2010; Jodhka and Shah 2010). We suggest that insofar as the Indian blood donation and transfusion field consists of practices that appear to mechanically transgress purity and pollution protocols, they form a species of material rhetoric concerning caste-blindness, or the becoming-obsolete of caste. We will encounter numerous ways in which ex-teriorized blood is used to construct narratives of caste transcendence (e.g., in chapter 4), exploring, for instance, how this ideology was coupled with the re-formist impulse of the cinema in early postcolonial India (chapter 3). In chap-ter 2 we will discuss how, on the one hand, Mohandas Gandhi resignified the pu-rity of blood as derived from its consanguinity (rather than as an inherited index of racial or caste superiority), and on the other, interpellated blood into his re-gressive caste politics nonetheless. The utopic promise of *using blood to go beyond blood* (where caste is figured as being locatable in the blood) is thus a central motif of this book. But the work also shows how for all the "as if" potential of blood as a figure of transcendental promise, it is all too quickly liable to collapse back into regressive narratives of caste-based purity.

Let us frame this "collapsing back" in terms of reversibility: "the recurrent motif of movements between the visible and the invisible, the inside and the outside" (Corsín Jiménez 2013, 21), what we might call "seeing double" (Schaffer 2005). U.S. physician John Saunders wrote in 1972 that he "lost two fellow students in India who, while transfusing their own blood into patients in crisis, were executed by Indian attendants in the operating theatre" (Saunders 1972, 11). Though this episode is not elaborated further by Saunders, who uses it simply to demonstrate that blood has been "invested with mysterious and magical properties," it remains a dramatic instance of prohibitions in regard to the mixing of biomoral substances or qualities of persons. There would at first glance seem to have been a great change since then: now we witness political actors vying with one another to donate blood for the cause of the nation. *And yet* from across India we also come across news headlines such as "Now Available: Upper Class Blood," and "Caste Based Request for Blood Donation Causes Outrage on Twitter."[75] In a news article about high-caste refusal of treatment by Dalit medics, principally in Tamil Nadu, we meet "N. Prabhu, who operates the Uyirthuli blood donation group . . . [and who] maintains a register of blood donors for . . . emergencies." He explains: "When we get requests for a rare blood group donor, often [the] patient's relatives will ask us to determine the caste of the donor before bringing him or her to the doctor. These cases are often emergency cases, and although we deny such requests to determine the caste, there have been a couple of cases where the donor has been sent away by the patient's family."[76] The "seeing double" of caste politics in contexts of blood donation and transfusion—the kind of progressive/regressive bifocalism it embodies—is perfectly encapsulated in the activities of a Marwari caste association in Delhi. This association regularly organizes voluntary blood donation events where caste-fellows anonymously donate their blood for anyone on donor beds while positioned beside banners glorifying Marwari caste achievements. These camps vividly convey an image of both moving beyond and fortifying caste simultaneously; of the figure-ground reversibility of inner and outer, endo-praxis and exo-praxis (Lévi-Strauss 1966, 118), the "Nehruvian progressive" and "feudal rot" (L. Cohen 2007). The very same act and instant witnesses the promissory transgression of community and caste boundaries (as afforded by the anonymity of blood procurement) and a kind of inward turning and caste consolidation. Lévi-Strauss (1966, 118) was himself careful to point out that "endo-*praxis* and exo-*praxis* are never definable separately and in absolute terms," which serves as an apt description of how blood operates vis-à-vis caste in this book: both flowing across caste boundaries and clotting at their edges.

Bloodscape of Difference

Like in the poem at the beginning of this chapter, blood also has a voice in Italo Calvino's short story "Blood, Sea" (1967), in which the transiting substance conveys something of its "sensations of movement": a "general pulsation" within and outside of human bodies; different rhythms and currents, some languorous, some explosive—as when it is ejected from a driving human body in a car accident and reimmersed in the sea from whence it came, which is a return it desires. We shall see in chapter 4 how blood itself may desire to be donated.

In his arresting meditation on Calvino's story, Stefan Helmreich (2014) employs the phrase "bloodscape of difference" (52) to describe how variations in "blood waves," measured in the form of cardiogrammatic wave profiles, reveal health inequalities along axes of race and gender: "information about cardiac waves maps out a sea of difference, an ocean of blood burbling inside people and populations with different life chances" (52). In seeking to account for ways in which the giving and receiving of blood has shaped social and political life in North India in the twentieth and twenty-first centuries, we too are concerned with a bloodscape of difference. Across a range of field sites and scenes of extraction in the region, we will trace how the substance congeals political ideologies, biomedical rationalities, and activist practice. From anticolonial appeals to blood sacrifice as a political philosophy to contemporary portraits of political leaders drawn with blood, from the use of the substance by Bhopali children as activist material to biomedical anxieties and aporias about the excess and lack of donation, we hope to show how tracing a bloodscape of difference in the Indian body politic offers new entryways into thinking about politics and economy: different sovereignties, different proportions, different temporalities.

In chapters 2 and 3, our focus is on blood in the domain of overt politics. In the practices we trace, blood is both metaphor and literal medium of political transactions. Our argument in these chapters rests on this oscillation between metaphor and materiality, between symbol and substance, leading to our explanation of the pervasive power of blood as both an object and medium of politics in North India.

In chapter 2, we show how blood opened up a provocative space of thought for Gandhi, a space that he traversed through the span of his political activity and writing. We describe his political theory of blood as tripartite. First, blood for Gandhi was a substance that indexed the extractive quality of British rule; second, it was a marker signifying the consanguinity of the *satyagrahi* with the other; and third, its simultaneous control *and* spillage was the precondition for anticolonial politics. Following from this, we describe Gandhi's fascination with the hydraulic economy of his own blood, as he equated his obsessive desire to control his own bodily pressure with the success and truth of his wider vision of politics. Finally, we show how blood shows up a curious twinning in Gandhi's biopolitical thinking—namely, the eugenic tendency of his political imagination with his utopic vision of communal intermixing and solidarity.

Metaphors of blood sacrifice were famously central for another competing anticolonial figure—Subhash Chandra Bose. Our aim is not to rehearse the cliched narrative of Bose's invocation of blood as anticolonial metaphor. Rather, our interest is in what this invocation precipitates in a contemporary political world dominated by religious nationalism (Hindutva). As resurrected by Hindutva history, Bose is offered as an antidote to the effeminacy and weakness of Gandhian nonviolence and posed as a better exemplar for the Indian state in the present. In the second part of chapter 2, we describe why Bose's exhortation toward a nationalism coagulated by blood sacrifice makes him particularly appealing to contemporary Hindutva ideologues. However, building on our description of a Gandhian hemo-politics as also riven with violence, we counteract the Hindutva polarization of anticolonialism into its nonviolent and violent variants. At the same time, paying attention again to the material politics of blood, we describe our counterexplanation of a fundamental difference between Gandhian and Hindutva politics. We argue that the deep chasm dividing their politics becomes visible once we acknowledge the potent multivalence of blood as a political substance, and the contrasting political visions it reveals.

Our focus in chapter 3 is on scenes of hematological activism. These scenes constitute a historically significant genre of political performance, in relation to the ebbs and flows of other modes of activist signification. Specifically, we suggest that blood donation spectacles act as rituals of verification, in contrast to other modes of political protest such as the fast that are increasingly open to accusations of insincerity and dissembling. Blood extracted on political occasions holds an elusive promise of political transparency: it is *promissory matter*. Yet as we show, blood also exposes itself to accusations of dissembling and deception: when used by politicians perceived as corrupt, the communicative medium is drained of its material intimacy with sincerity.

Further, in our discussion of explicitly activist actions that deploy blood, we track how the promise of truth and interiority goes hand in hand with the ability of the substance to connote violence. Specifically, in our discussion of activism in the aftermath of the Bhopal disaster, we show how blood comes to materialize the violence of the long unfolding event, at the same time as it evidences the political transparency of its consequent activist mobilization. And in our related discussion of menstrual political activism, we show how blood becomes a matter of celebration that verifies a feminist politics, at the same time as it stands in as an index of sexual violence.

Through chapter 3, then, we trace this central tension in blood as political media: at the same time as the substance promises moral interiority, it simultaneously reveals the corruption and duplicity of political enunciations. And at the same time as it verifies the truth of activist claims, it exposes the violence that produces the need for an activist response in the first place. The utopic and the corrupt are joined in a dangerous, substantial proximity. The blood-gift particularly returns us to the ethnosociological imagination of "substance-code." If hematological activism responds to a series of breakdowns of the substance-code relation—a malaise at once material, biological, and political—we see how it also attempts to reflectively resituate substance and code in new confluences and juxtapositions, which show how reformist aims never escape their messy origins and how scenes of critique never cleanly detach from scenes of corruption.

Chapters 4 and 5 shift to activism about human biological substance rather than activism that employs human substance—a shift from a focus on uses of blood as a means of political engagement to a pedagogical politics of proper usage and understanding. In chapter 4, we draw on ethnographic research in Kolkata and Delhi, where we followed voluntary blood donor organizations seeking to convey to the *janata* (people) that the body produces more blood than it needs and that a portion of this excess blood can be given without the body losing anything. This is an insight at odds with conventional understandings of blood excorporation in the region as involving irrecuperable loss, understandings that inform continuing perceptions of blood donation as a sacrificial gesture. To give blood without risking irrecuperable loss would seem to fundamentally undercut the gesture of blood donation as sacrifice. An imagination of blood as excess and surplus thus involves the antisacrificial redescription of blood donation.

Such projects strive to produce a perceptual shift away from an association of blood donation with "sacrifice," articulating instead its relationship with "blood science." Yet our closer examination reveals something more complex than a simple linear shift from "sacrifice" to "science." Rather than being eliminated, sacrifice is sublated, finding new and subtle forms in the understandings and practices meant to replace it. Sacrifice as a mode of bodily practice, we suggest, is not absented but redimensioned in newer, "scientific" pedagogies of blood donation. This simultaneous enactment of surplus and sacrifice, excess and loss, has significant implications for how we understand an "Indian" biopolitics. Blood donors do not neatly disaggregate into those who sacrifice and those who can choose not to sacrifice.

Our work here goes against the grain of that portion of the existing literature on modes of biological exchange in the region that depicts bodies as being made abject by giving/donation practices. This chapter moves in a different direction in describing a project in which (Indian) bodies are depicted as precisely not needing to sacrifice. No longer abject sites of extraction in situations of constrained ethics, they are to be reconfigured into subjects of reproducible generosity.

If chapter 4 focuses on how that which is given is never enough, chapter 5 is concerned with perceptions and campaigns concerning how doctors prescribe *too much* of that which has already been given. The proportions of the transfusion, say clinical activists and others, are all wrong in Indian medicine. Once more, then, the focus is on proportionality and on educational campaigning, but here there is a different target: for if donors do not give enough because they think they have a deficit when in fact (according to the campaign) they have a surplus, doctors prescribe blood as if they have a surplus when in fact they have a deficit. The irony is obvious: in so doing, of course, they exacerbate this deficit. Once more, excess is at stake, and the different spheres of excess interlock and inform one another.

Thus in chapter 5, we track and unpack the ways in which clinical activists take on the problematic specter of doctors' "irrational" and "unscientific" blood prescription. We argue that the surplus and redistribution of donated blood can provide a novel window on debates about overprescription of drugs in the subcontinent and elsewhere. When the drug is derived from human biological matter, different questions are raised about care and hospitality for the drug that might help impede its careless disbursal. For the activists we follow in chapter 5 in particular, fidelity to the gift of blood must mean abjuring overprescribing it. Care for the gift itself takes on the form of a gift. That is, care for the sentiment underlying the original gift results in a surplus that may be gifted to an extra few *and* back to the donor, whose sentiments are honored when the gift remains animated with the spirit of its giver—what we call the *hau* of prescription. In evoking the role played by questions of therapeutic secrecy and excess, and the indeterminate numeracy of the gift, we come to see how each of these, in turn, informs the reason and form of the transfusion.

In chapters 6 and 7, we examine the different temporal registers and representations that structure and compete within the field of blood donation and transfusion in India. In chapter 6, our focus is on blood in the time of the civic— that is, blood that is donated voluntarily as a dutiful contribution to civic life, that in turn ensures the continued efficacy and productivity of transfusion medicine. These voluntary donations take place according to a seemingly simple biological time map: the biological time of cellular production determines the biomedically mandated three-month gap between donations. The time regime of the repeated voluntary donation emerges from and is mapped upon the lifetime of blood cells. This is in contrast to apparently less civic-minded blood donation modes: the potentially dangerous commercial transaction of paid blood donation and the one-time mode of "replacement" donation, performed in order to release blood for the benefit of one's immediate family member in need of transfusion. As we shall see, these modes of donation are characterized by different temporalities. A routine of dutiful repetitive bloodshed structures voluntary blood donation's time of the civic.

However, we find intersecting temporalities even at the basic level of the ideal, routinized repetition. Revealing these multiple temporalities complicates the notion of the three-monthly repetition of donation as simply a biomedical or biologically based routine. Instead, the time of the civic comes into view as being "secretly" supported by an array of temporal structures that are invisible to biomedical authority. Thus, we show how blood in the time of the civic is made possible by overlapping temporal registers and reckonings. For example, we explore the dimension of astral time as a determinant of the ideal, repeat voluntary blood donor. We also turn to inheritance and political memory as ambivalent enablers of routinized repetition in the Indian blood donation and transfusion world. Through these and other examples, we describe how a wide array of enactments of blood donation coagulates in the service of the routinized repetition of voluntary blood donation. Thus, we argue, the constitutive rhythms of astrology, politics, and religion *disruptively enable* the metarhythm of voluntary, biomedical donation.

This book presents a number of ways in which blood might be considered a substance existing in the subjunctive mood, a substance with the propensity to image shared "subjunctive . . . 'as if' or 'could be' universe[s]" (Seligman et al. 2008, 7)—for instance, soaring visions of consanguineous humanity that dethrone the antisubjunctive blood of caste—but also and equally of unfulfilled potentialities. To speak of blood's "as if" is to recognize how frequently the substance flows in bodies, tubes, and thought in states of hopeful uncertainty. Chapter 7 examines in detail the differentiated nature of hematic possibility in India.

We find in studies of biopolitics and biotechnologies a dominant rendering of biopolitical futures that picture attitudes toward them as ever more amenable to the involvement of new forms of capital and governance. Indeed, when futures are invoked in prevailing analyses of biological exchange, a certain neoliberal futurity tends to be emphasized—for instance, the forms of individualized insurance they may engender. Such accounts document how contemporary forms of biopolitical governmentality encourage individualized citizens to mitigate risk and foster an "active stance towards the future" (Rose and Novas 2005, 452). While many such accounts are persuasive, we suggest that these are not the only futures on offer. With blood donation and transfusion as longstanding technologies that, in their basic form, are no longer at the frontiers of biomedicine, we take a step back from the world of biotechnological possibility and novelty. The anticipatory logics of blood and blood donation that we trace in this book are a function of our focus on flows of blood in the margins. We will see how biopolitical imaginations of speculation and futurity may be at least as varied as impressions and durabilities of the past.

In concluding this introductory chapter, we note again that our distinction between contestations *with* blood in protests, spectacles, and political camps (which we focus on in the first half of the book), and contestations *about* blood shaped by biomedical concerns (which we focus on in the second half of the book) is heuristic. In practice, the domains of explicit politics and biomedicine both actualize shared imaginations of blood potent in the region. The relationship is "meta-material" in the sense proposed by Kath Weston: we encounter movements beyond the material to figure substance and beyond the metaphorical to enlist the material in activist projects (Weston 2013a, 37). For example, the imagination of blood as animated by its giver and sacrifice undergirds the Gandhian and activist politics in the first half of the book, at the same time as it makes biomedical injunctions about transfusion and donation persuasive in the second half. Similarly, the ability of blood to conjure visions of the past and future are as crucial for the Hindu right's political project to revise history as it is for supporting the idealized, routine time of biomedical donation. Further, a concern for restituting the moral and correct proportion of transactions drives reformist and party-political camps in the first half of the book, at the same time as it serves as a rationale for biomedical ideas and mobilizations around surplus and lack in the second half. Finally, both political and biomedical campaigns bear the weight of blood's subjunctive potential: they imagine a future through blood, where social boundaries might be transcended, even as aspirations toward transcendence through unrestricted flows harden social difference. Thus, as we shall see unfold, the differences between activism *with* and *about* blood blur at the edges of practice in bloodscapes of difference that congeal the material and the metaphorical, the biomedical and the moral.

2

SOVEREIGNTY AND BLOOD

Metaphors of blood—its extraction and sacrifice—are inescapably rife in Indian political discourse: "*Neta janata ka khuun chooste hain*—Politicians suck the people's blood." The refrain is familiar, certainly in the north of the country. At the very least, such metaphors of vampiric political extraction extend back to the early days of British colonialism. Dadabhai Naoroji, one of the founding members of the Indian National Congress, used the metaphor of blood to great effect in describing the devastating effects of colonial rule. In particular, blood and money were used interchangeably in Naoroji's writings to illustrate the extraction and flow of wealth from the colony to the metropole (S. Banerjee 2010). Of course, since Naoroji spent much of his life in Britain, the late Victorian fascination with vampires must surely have impressed itself upon his imagination, as it had upon Karl Marx and so many other contemporaries (cf. Neocleous 2003; Sugg 2016). However, Naoroji's immediate inspiration was a minute written by British prime minister and former Indian secretary of state Lord Salisbury (Salisbury 1875). Salisbury had provocatively suggested that as a matter of colonial policy, England should bleed India's resources with surgical precision, such that the lancet was applied to points of congestion among the wealthy, rather than to the rural districts that were already enfeebled by poverty. Salisbury's belabored metaphor would inform the critique not only of Naoroji but of many of the earliest Indian critics of colonial rule (Stokes 1978). Indeed, for Naoroji, the metaphor of blood helped describe the specific violence of British colonialism as qualitatively different from forms of power that came before: "An Oriental despot, when he misgoverned, acted, so to speak, like a butcher, and people were astounded and horrified; this new despotism of civilization rather resembled a murder effected by a clever but unscrupulous surgeon who drew all the blood from his victim while leaving scarcely a scar upon the skin" (Naoroji 1901). Notably, Salisbury's critics implicitly adopted his premise that made regional wealth comparable with blood quantum.[1] Decades later, in defending Naoroji's enduring belief in a lost ideal of English fairness, Gandhi would return to the blood metaphor: "It was the respected Dadabhai who taught us that the English had sucked our life-blood. What does it matter that, today, his trust is still in the English nation?" (Gandhi 1946a).

In the present, the contemporary figure of the politician-vampire resonates with the anticolonial linkage of blood and money.[2] The "material convertibility of . . . blood and money," in Street's astute formulation (2009), "relates to fears that [both] are too easily transacted." If it is people's money that is usually "sucked," the relation with blood is underscored (and literalized) in news reports of contemporary Congress activists forcibly taking the blood of underage citizens in order to make up numbers at political blood donation rallies (Mishra 2009). It finds its way into Congress vice president Rahul Gandhi's refutation of Indian prime minister Narendra Modi's claim that his strikes against "terrorists" in occupied Kashmir were "surgical": "You are a blood merchant trading and hiding behind the blood that our soldiers have sacrificed in your surgical strikes" (*Humare jawan hain, jinho ne khoon diya hai, jinho ne surgical strike kiya, unke khoon ke peeche aap chhupe huye ho, unki aap dalali kar he ho*).[3] As with Salisbury's metaphor of surgical incisions, Modi's description of military actions as surgical strikes all too easily lends itself to its own critique. In a different context, the politician-vampire figure recurs in the advertisement for a Konkani music theater CD called *Corruption*, which depicts a tube leading from a single blood bag (labeled "Mining company's vitamins") to two state politicians, while a 2012 political cartoon shows a turbaned politician receiving a transfusion made up of blood of the mangled corpses of "taxpayers." The catalogue of representations goes on.

Over the next two chapters, we unravel this tangle of blood in the domain of overt politics. On the one hand, what do such folk diagnoses of blood extraction and exchange teach us about the contemporary North Indian body politic? What political specters do such metaphors animate, and what futures do they presage? Yet, we suggest, to think here of blood as primarily a metaphor would be to do an injustice to its life as a material medium. In the practices we trace, blood is both metaphor and literal medium of political transactions. Blood as political substance congeals ideology in material forms that, in turn, circulate and shape social forms. Our argument hinges on this movement between materiality and metaphor, between symbol and substance, hazarding an explanation of the pervasive power of blood as both an object and medium of politics in North India.

Hydraulic Equilibrium

In 1910, Gandhi established the second of his series of ashrams near Johannesburg. The first had been the Phoenix settlement at Natal, inspired in part by the philosophy and writings of John Ruskin. He called this second habitational experiment Tolstoy Farm after Leo Tolstoy, with whom he had recently begun a short-lived correspondence on the question of nonviolence. At the ashram, Gandhi involved himself in the day-to-day conduct of affairs and began several experiments with manual labor, dietetics, and education (Bhana 1975). In 1911, his wife Kasturba Gandhi began to suffer from recurrent bouts of acute pain. In experimenting with a treatment regimen for her, Gandhi noticed the distinct impact of salt on her (and his own) physical condition and symptoms. Supposing that the salt had thinned her blood, he focused his attention on developing saltless diets and then imposed these diets not only on his wife but also on other willing and unwilling disciples at the ashram (Gandhi 1999).[4]

On the basis of these dietetic experiments, he ventured that the abjuration of salt could result in blood so pure that it would be immune to all kinds of poisons. This included the venom of snakes, which was a particularly pressing concern at the farm, surrounded as it was by over a thousand acres of wild land. Conversely, if the purification of blood through diet could serve as a cure to a wide array of ailments including snakebites, blood impurity as a result of bad diets, environments, or practices would manifest in an equally wide-ranging set of conditions, such as bowel dysfunctions, boils, weakness, and so on (CWG 13:29). In these last years in South Africa, Gandhi took to systematizing his nascent ideas about health in a set of essays in *Indian Opinion*—"General Knowledge about Health" (CWG 12:366). Blood began to play an increasingly key role in his understanding of a complex bodily system that integrated diet, exercise, air, water, and physical environment. To maintain such a complex system, it became necessary to separate out practices and substances that aided in or could be converted into good and pure blood. Such a system had no place for vaccinations, since the practice introduced an external infection into the blood. Gandhi's condemnation of vaccination was absolute; the "savage custom" attracted his strongest invective (CWG 13:174). Throughout his life, he remained resolute in this rejection, even while responding to recurrent outbreaks of smallpox and cholera across the country (CWG 46:218). That the British began increasingly to enforce compulsory vaccination, and that the practice was developed in part through animal vivisection (CWG 33:312), only further antagonized him.

Further, if the body possessed the capacity for self-purification, then the circulation of blood provided an index of health. (Gandhi would fix on the ideal pulse of seventy-five beats per minute [CWG 12:390].) In 1927, he tested his insistence on the self-regenerative capability of the body, as well as his trust in blood pressure as an index of well-being. Early in the year, he suffered a stroke after four months of intense, physical political activity. While recovering from this stroke, Gandhi began to measure and monitor his own blood pressure daily. Noting it to be high, he experimented with various "natural" diets and began his first forays into practicing yoga. He developed a close correspondence with Swami Kuvalay-ananda, a yoga pioneer who sought to establish the discipline's scientific creden-tials and had just founded its first journal (*Yoga Mimamsa*). Following his advice, Gandhi experimented with various *asanas* and tried to correlate each one to the rise and fall of his blood pressure (CWG 39:126). He also found that a mountain-ous climate especially ameliorated his condition, and he spent much of his recovery in the Nandi Hills of Mysore, describing them as ideal places for "blood-pressure men" (CWG 38:300). From this time in his writings, Gandhi would consistently return to blood pressure as the primary index of his well-being, as well as a mea-sure of success for his dietetic experiments. He would continuously communicate his pressure readings not only to his physician correspondents but also to his friends and family. When a doctor's reading was not to his liking, others were brought in (CWG 41:42). If that still left him unsatisfied, workers in his ashram would take and retake his pressure until it was satisfactory to him (CWG 41:40). In his later years, the measure even became the object of lighthearted competition between him and his disciples, as they strove to record the lowest measures (CWG 74:166). He would refer to blood pressure as simply present or absent (having or not having blood pressure), and to his closest correspondents, two numbers sepa-rated by a solidus were self-explanatory (e.g., CWG 73:286; CWG 80:137).

We note that such a preoccupation with "having" or "not having" blood pres-sure is not unique to a Gandhian body politics. Veena Das and Lawrence Cohen's research in North India has led them to find the measure of central narratives of health across class groups. Cohen notes that men tended to "have BP" whereas women tended to "have low BP," and that this drew upon a social semantic net-work that linked the hydraulic physiology and sociology of tensions and pressures (Cohen 1998, 195). And Das insightfully resists categorizing the (often self-diagnosed) symptom as either "folk" or "expert," instead describing its emer-gence in relation to inappropriate drug use in a context of work and cash precar-ity (Das 2015b, 45). Nor is a semantic vocabulary of blood pressure as an index of social tensions unique to India or South Asia (e.g., Garro 1988; Schoenberg and Drew 2002). But what particularly interests us here is how this hydraulic se-mantics intersects with Gandhi's anticolonial politics and subsequently with the politics of nationalism in India.

In the same set of essays in which he first systematized his thinking about bodily well-being (*Keys to Health*), Gandhi argued for a close relation of the biological body with the national body and then finally of both to the entire cosmos (CWG 12:388). This series of analogies allowed him to draw a relation between malaise in individual bodies and a broader civilizational deficit. A Sanskrit proverb that appeared in *Keys to Health* was crucial to his conceptualization of these analogies: "यथा पिण्डे तथा ब्रह्माण्डे" (*yatha pinde tatha brahmande*). The proverb recurred in Gandhi's writings, most importantly as a gloss in his translation of the Bhagavad Gita (Gandhi 1946b). In the authorized English translation of Gandhi's Gujarati reading of the Gita, Mahadev Desai translates the proverb as "As with the self, so with the universe." However, in the English translation of the *Collected Works of Mahatma Gandhi*, it appears differently: "As with the body, so with the universe." Very literally, पिण्ड approximates closer to the English word "body," as in the translation of the *Collected Works*, but Mahadev Desai's translation takes into account how the body and self were almost indistinguishable in Gandhi's thought. When the proverb appears in the original Gujarati text of *Keys to Health*, Gandhi glosses it curiously as "As with one's body, so with one's country" (when transliterated into English). This gloss, when translated into English in the *Collected Works* becomes "As with oneself, so with the country." Yet it is translated into Hindi in the *Collected Works* as "जो देहमें हैं, वही देशमे हैं," which translates literally to "As within the body, so within the country."

Ajay Skaria's powerful reading in both languages offers a persuasive account of the gaps and dissonances across Gandhi's thinking in Gujarati and English (Skaria 2016). However, our purpose in exploring the various translations of this particular proverb is to point to how the slipperiness of those translations provides a glimpse into Gandhi's imagination of the body and its relation to politics. In Gandhi's own gloss of the Sanskrit proverb into Gujarati, the cosmos/universe becomes the nation. In Mahadev Desai's translation, the body becomes the self. And in the translations by the editors of the *Collected Works*, the body and self are again shifted interchangeably. Our intention here is not to fault these expert translations but rather to appreciate that in their many betrayals, the translators underline the spirit of Gandhi's conceptualization of health—pointing to the frequent interchangeability of the body with the nation and the cosmos. The slippages in the translations are indicative of how the form of this relation is not transparent and easily disclosed in Gandhi's thought. More fundamentally, Gandhi's reliance on the "as/with" relation leaves open a productive space for exploring how he imagines the form of the relation: Is it analogical, allegorical, or metaphorical? In other words, how and on what terms are bodies, selves, nations, and the universe related? To put this more specifically, if to purify the self means a bodily regime of physical and dietetic conduct, what does it mean to purify the body politic at the level of the nation and the body politic?

Anthropologists and historians have demonstrated how Gandhi's criticism of colonialism incorporated a critique of colonial medicine. Gandhi described modern civilization itself as a disease, under the auspices of which colonialism had led to a further subordination of biological well-being for Indians. The historian David Arnold has argued that Gandhi understood colonialism as instituting a medical system of abstract dependency upon doctors and drugs upon which the sufferer had no control (Arnold 2001). Further, Joseph Alter has described how Gandhian politics links biology and morality, within which the achievement of good health goes hand in hand with decolonization (Alter 2000).[5] Fascinatingly, Alter also suggests that Gandhi anticipates some of the analytical conceptualizations of Marriott and the ethnosociologists, albeit drawing not from "Hindu" categories as they did but his own Occidentalist readings of the West (Alter 1996). We suggest here that in Gandhi's biomoral imaginary, blood purification plays a particularly crucial role. If the body, nation, and cosmos were inextricably interlinked in his thought, then the cultivation of practices that aided in the purification of blood were not only a biological concern but also a political and religious duty.[6] At the bodily level then, the injunction to the *satyagrahi* could be captured in phrases such as "Noncooperation means self-purification" (CWG 24:199), or "Swadeshi must permeate every particle of their blood" (CWG 24:405). More elaborately, Gandhi described the program of *swadeshi* and its practice of weaving as capable of generating new blood that would cure the diseased Indian industry (CWG 24:193). As for the British body politic, Gandhi mourned its diseased blood. In a letter to Mirabehn, he described New Delhi as a capital built with blood money. Consequently, Gandhi suggested, the city was in a state of meningitis since it was doubly afflicted with corrupt blood and an overly centralized circulatory system that was flooding the brain (CWG 37:450). The proper directional circulation of blood in the body politic was crucial not only to the colonial state but also to the nascent network of ashrams and local governmental institutions mobilized in the anticolonial struggle. In a speech at an ashram in the Mandvi district of Gujarat, Gandhi repeated the caution against excess blood in the brain as a result of the ashram's overdependence upon the provincial committee (CWG 38:204).

What then of his personal failure to maintain the proper circulation and pressure of blood within his body; what were the biomoral implications of his own recurring high blood pressure? Gandhi was not unaware that the strain of his political life might be the primary cause of its hypertensive predisposition. Responding to a letter from his son Ramdas, Gandhi wrote in 1937, "I believe that I am more vigilant than any other leader. This is, as I understand, the straight and simple cause of my blood-pressure. My nonattachment is less than what is meant by the *Gita*; I am full of feeling" (CWG 72:416).[7] The relationship Gandhi drew here was not only between his hypertension and his intense political practice, but also with his failure to reach the ideal of the true *satyagrahi*—nonattachment, even in the conduct of politics. For example, when against Gandhi's explicit orders, his wife and two ashram residents (including Mahadev Desai's wife) worshipped at a temple that denied entry to untouchables, he drew a direct correlation between their transgression and his own excess blood pressure. He noted that the machine recorded an alarmingly high number, but he knew his condition to be even worse, beyond the measuring capacity of the machine itself. It is not hard to imagine Mahadev Desai's consternation that he and his wife might have been the principal cause of Gandhi's present illness: "Ruthlessly I have turned out people wanting to see him, and have even interrupted talks and interviews, lest they should strain him over much and raise his blood-pressure. Fancy, therefore, my misery and my shame when I found one morning at Delang that what he considered a serious blunder on my part had raised his blood-pressure to the breaking point and might have brought about a catastrophe" (CWG 73:455).

Ajay Skaria describes Gandhi's thought and practice of *satyagraha* (a force proper to truth that resists domination) as a constant striving toward "self-ciphering," as an endeavor to turn oneself into an automaton free of desire, autonomy, and will (Skaria 2016). Going beyond prior readings of Gandhi's anticolonial politics as directed toward a recapture of bodily and political self-mastery, Skaria argues that the goal of the *satyagrahi* was not to establish a new decolonized sovereign state but rather to undo the problematic of sovereignty itself, in both its secular and religious forms. At the level of the body, this meant not bodily self-mastery but rather the abandonment of concern and feeling for the body—the body transformed into an empty, perfectly calibrated machine. It is in this sense that Gandhi strove toward the understanding of "nonattachment" he finds in the Gita, one that would turn his own body into a machine whose hydraulic pressure would be an unchanging constant. In this paradigm, the colonial state was to be faulted for establishing centers of control, both metropolitan and peripheral, that were clogging up the system. But if colonial policies were imperfect, so was the anticolonial struggle. At moments where it faltered, it too demonstrated continued attachments to sovereignty that threw the hydraulics of the machinelike body awry. When his disciples continued to visit temples that denied untouchables entry, this exemplified their continuing failure to renounce an attachment to the sovereign form of religious worship. And when Gandhi himself failed to maintain equanimity in relation to the successes and failures of the anticolonial movement, he demonstrated his own enduring attachment to an abstract political cause and his enduring commitment to establishing new sovereign relations in the place of the old colonial regime. The goal was to relinquish

such attachments to the domains of both theology and politics in their contemporary forms, thereby attaining perfect harmony and synchrony between the
circulation of blood within the body, the body politic, and an ineffable cosmos
beyond the politics of sovereignty. It is in this sense that exercise and dietetics were
a political practice and a hemo-politics; the goal—perfect hydraulic equilibrium.

The stakes of Gandhi's commitment to this particular form of bodily homeo-
stasis appeared most starkly during the outbreak of Hindu-Muslim violence
around the time of independence. Joseph Alter describes Gandhi's belief and "science" that he could mend that violent national division through a bodily practice directed at the achievement of hydraulic equilibrium (Alter 1996). While the
bodily substance we focus on here is blood, Alter's concern was with Gandhi's
preoccupation with celibacy and semen retention. He describes Gandhi's uncom-
promising insistence that an excessive loss of semen resulted in a loss in personal
and national vitality that consequently hindered the regeneration of the physical
and political body.[8] The outbreak of communal violence introduced another obstacle to the flourishing of bodily capacities: its violence violated bodily boundaries, spilling blood onto the streets. As Alter describes, this troubled Gandhi, leading him to propose a return to hydraulic equilibrium through an increased focus
on celibacy as penance for the violence of blood spilled outside the body. Extrap-
olating from Ayurvedic texts, Alter even ventures a guess at what Gandhi might
have imagined as the precise ratio between retention and spillage: one drop of
vital fluid preserved would balance every sixty drops of blood spilled.

Anticolonial Immunity

In an essay in *Navjivan* in 1920, Gandhi continued to explicitly link the biomorality of the individual body with that of the body politic: "It is a principle of medical science that so long as one's blood is free from impurity, the poisonous air
outside can have no effect on it. That is why, during an epidemic, some people
are attacked while others are not. Likewise, had we been incorruptible, the East
India Company could have done nothing and at the present time, too, officers
like Michael O'Dwyer would have lost their jobs" (CWG 20:428). This striking
rendering of his biomoral politics returns us to Gandhi's thought about blood purity, formulated here in relation to colonial rule. If the purpose of dietetics and
exercise was to purify blood, blood thus purified was itself transformed into a
powerful agent against poisons, snakebites, and epidemics. Properly circulating
pure blood stood in contrast to vaccines that were "poisons" introduced externally via a British public health system. Thus read, the real epidemic was not cholera or smallpox but colonial rule. What is striking here, however, is that the

purpose of drawing this analogy between epidemic and British colonialism was not to criticize colonial policies but rather to describe the impurity of the *antico-lonial* project. As impure blood succumbed to the outbreak of epidemics, so did the "corruptible" anticolonial response to colonial rule. And if the impurity of blood as bodily substance was a result of bad dietetics and exercise, the impurity of the anticolonial struggle was demonstrated in the inability of its supporters to sacrifice themselves readily for the cause of nonviolence. This criticism of the anticolonial project was all the more provocative since it was issued in response to the Jallianwala Bagh massacre in 1919 and was meant to characterize its victims.

The Jallianwala Bagh massacre occupies an important place in both popular and scholarly narratives of the Indian anticolonial movement. In 1919, Gandhi had issued a call for a one-day strike in the country against the Rowlatt Act—legislation that indefinitely extended wartime counterterrorism measures put in place in 1915. Strikes against the act were particularly powerful in Punjab, which then led the lieutenant governor of Punjab, Michael O'Dwyer, to expel two prominent nationalists from the province. In Amritsar, the anticolonial response to this expulsion had turned violent. This violence then became the pretext for Brigadier General Reginald Dyer to fire without warning into an unarmed crowd that had assembled in an enclosed public meeting place known as Jallianwala Bagh. While figures of the death toll vary considerably, reliable estimates suggest that over a thousand in the crowd were killed and several hundred were seriously injured. As Kim Wagner demonstrates, the massacre was not an isolated military action, but part of a long history of spectacular colonial violence intended as punishment (Wagner 2016). In his analysis, these demonstrations of mass violence were exemplary of the weakness rather than the strength of the colonial state and undermined colonial rule by turning its victims into martyrs for the national movement.

Popular accounts of Gandhi's life consistently stress the importance of the event in radicalizing his anticolonial commitment, inaugurating the so-called Gandhian phase of the Indian independence struggle. That the event roughly coincided with Gandhi's first mass mobilizations in India fuel such speculations. However, more careful historical accounting tells a less unilineal story. Six months transpired between the event and Gandhi's visit to the site, during which Gandhi had already started mass mobilizations that did not draw upon the Jallianwala Bagh massacre for inspiration. During this time, rather than martyrize those killed by the shooting, he issued several public declarations condemning the anticolonial violence that had ostensibly provoked General Dyer's retribution. "No penance will suffice for the evil that has been wrought by *our* hand in Amritsar," he wrote on 14 November 1919 (emphasis added). "It is true that a large number of our people were killed in Jallianwala Bagh. But we ought to have maintained peace even if everyone present had been killed. It is not right, in my opinion, to take blood for blood" (CWG 19:112).

This admonishment against taking blood for blood would recur in a formal report to the British government the following year: "We cannot too strongly condemn these excesses. Drunk with the blood of their innocent victims, these rioters proceeded to the revenue offices, and burnt them" (CWG 20:111). As became clear in Gandhi's writings, the opportunity to strike and the subsequent massacre had afforded Indians a perverse opportunity to demonstrate their strength and capacity to suffer without inflicting suffering. In such a calculus, strength was defined as the difficult act of fearlessness in the face of violence. In condemning the "drunken excesses" of the anticolonial protestors, Gandhi sought to demonstrate that General Dyer's retribution was an act of weakness and thus beneath the ethics of the warrior-*satyagrahi*. Following from this, Indians that were capable of exercising restraint in the face of violence were more powerful than the arms-bearing General Dyer, who was given to excess in that he could not perform the difficult act of withholding violence in the face of violence. The warriorlike gesture then was not the spilling of blood but rather the capacity to not spill blood. Further, the proper response of the *satyagrahi* to the massacre would be to forgive General Dyer unconditionally; only through forgiveness could the *satyagrahi* give up the sovereign demand and act of violent punishment. The thorny question that remained for Gandhi was whether Indians had developed the capacity and strength to forgive at that historical moment, since they lacked the power to punish in the first place. Much like the broader relation between nonviolence and violence, forgiveness could only be gifted by those that had the power to punish. Finally, and most importantly for our argument, demanding blood for blood was not just a contravention of the ethics of nonviolence in the calculus of Gandhi's anticolonial philosophy, but it also was a sign of weakness to be overcome in the practice of *satyagraha*. Later in this chapter, we will find contemporary Hindu nationalists returning to this invocation of mimetic bleeding in order to marginalize Gandhi from anticolonial historiography. Instead, we will find them proposing a counterhistory from which they are able to find precedence for their own calls for violence in historical actors they imagine as their proper ancestors: those engaged in acts of violent and masculine anticolonial bloodshed.

Yet, returning to Gandhi's thought—and his description of the potential of blood to demonstrate a quality of anticolonial immunity—how was the *satyagrahi* to cultivate a purity of the blood that could withstand the corruption and poison of colonial violence? In other words, beyond Gandhi's admonishments against taking or spilling blood, what constituted its positive biomoral variant? Eight months after the Jallianwala Bagh massacre, Gandhi began to sketch the rubrics of an answer to precisely that question: "There flowed in this Bagh a river of blood, the holy blood of innocent people. Because of this the spot has become sanctified. Efforts are being made to obtain this spot for the nation" (21 December 1919) (CWG 19:190). The relation between blood and violence appears here in a very different register than when the former was spilled in a gesture of "drunken" violence. The substance exceeds its status as a sign of violence (blood of innocents was spilled) and is transformed into an agent of sacral resignification (it flowed and touched the earth, turning the Bagh into holy ground). The sacral purity of the substance is derived from the "innocence" of those that were killed, where innocence within the rubrics of Gandhi's *satyagraha* is to be read as the warrior-like heroism of those who had sacrificed themselves in the face of violence. The sacral quality of those who were martyred certainly was a strong rhetorical gesture, but it also had practical consequences. In 1920, Gandhi led efforts to procure the site of the massacre and convert it into a pilgrimage ground. In his appeals to raise funds to purchase the land, he would repeatedly invoke the ritual function of sacral blood in turning the site from a "rubbish dump" to hallowed ground. Describing the gatherings of people at Jallianwala Bagh in the months after the massacre, Gandhi painted a ceremonial picture: "Many applied to their foreheads the dust of the place, as if it were sacred ash; many took away with them some earth made holy by the blood of innocent people" (CWG 19:301). The resignification of the Bagh from rubbish dump to a scene of pilgrimage successfully dissuaded Indian prospectors who had floated the idea of selling the Bagh land for money rather than placing it in a public trust. Gandhi's rebuke was understated but unmistakable: "There was not a corner of that garden which had not been stained by the blood of innocent men and it would be improper, therefore, to exploit it for financial gain" (CWG 19:393).

Through the long career of his writings, Gandhi's representation of the killings consistently foregrounded the material spillage of blood at the site while simultaneously invoking the substance's sacral purity. Indeed, his single-minded focus on the substance was remarkable in its omission of other available foci of symbolization. Postindependence artistic representations of the event memorialized at the site focus on the heaped piles of bodies left in the aftermath. The monument that stands at the site is a thirty-foot-high pylon with the words "In memory of martyrs, 13 April 1919" inscribed on all four sides. Memorialized physical reminders of the event include a wall riddled with bullet marks and a well into which many running from the bullets had jumped and died. The wall and the well were reminders of the helplessness and panicked flight of the victims of the shootings, fearful and without the capacity to return the violence as equals. For Gandhi, these could not serve as the proper objects of memorialization; they could only remind visitors of the incapability of the victims to offer *ahimsa* (nonviolence) to those that inflicted violence upon them: "If they had died knowingly and willingly, if, realizing their innocence they had stood their ground and faced the shots from the fifty rifles, they would have gone down in history as saints, heroes and patriots" (CWG 19:410). Thus, blocked from finding valor in the actions of those who were killed, Gandhi turned to their bodies and their spilled blood. While it could not symbolize fearless self-sacrifice, since the gathering was known to have drawn people across religious communities, the blood spilled at Jallianwala Bagh could index India's communal solidarity: "The most experienced doctor, even he could not have determined whether it belonged to a Hindu or a Sikh or a Muslim." Blood spilled at Jallianwala Bagh could sacralize the ground *because* it was mixed: "The blood of Hindus, Muslims and Sikhs mingled at the place. No one could tell how much blood of which community was spilt there. If a blood sample were to be sent to the most experienced doctor even he could not have determined whether it belonged to a Hindu or a Sikh or a Muslim. In other words, all the Indians became fellow-martyrs in Jallianwala Bagh" (CWG 94:292). He explained his insistence on memorializing the site thus: "The 13th of April saw not merely the terrific tragedy, but in that tragedy Hindu-Muslim blood flowed freely in a mingled stream and sealed the compact" (CWG 19:451). From 1919 onwards, the idea of an ever-expanding consanguinity would become ubiquitous in Gandhi's writing, centrifuging Indians of varied communities. Time and again, Gandhi returned to the idea that Hindus and Muslims were united by ancient ties of blood, instituting a term for this proximate other that would recur through the rest of his life: blood brother.[9]

Crucially, however, the ease with which blood dissolves difference in these formulations does not reflect Gandhi's deep ambivalence about interfaith and intercaste miscegenation. In chapter 1, we introduced the idea that many colonial and postcolonial projects of social reform advocate communal harmony between caste and religion through the mixing of blood. In later chapters, we will find such reformist claims proliferating biomedical discourse. At the same time, we described the limits of these projects, as they often reified rather than transcended inequality. For example, as we wrote in chapter 1, if the great Dalit leader and architect of India's constitution B. R. Ambedkar suggested that blood-mixing through marriage could be a radical step toward "dissolving" inequality, most reformist projects we describe in this book occur at a safe distance, requiring little or no contact between castes. Gandhi's imagination of reform falls somewhere between these two poles of political possibility. Gandhi's position on marriage rules and interdictions of marriage was that a "safe rule of conduct" would be to respect taboos (CWG 71:247). In the same year of the Bagh massacre, Gandhi wondered whether a piece of legislation introduced to permit intercaste marriages was worth the consternation it was causing caste Hindus (CWG 17:270). His position on the issue would evolve slowly through his lifetime. Even until 1932, he could only with great reluctance bring himself to support marriage within subcastes and remained wary of interreligious marriages (CWG 55:418). As late as 1937 he explicitly came out in favor of intercaste marriages as a route to social reform (CWG 71:393), and only in 1947 was he able to unequivocally support interfaith marriages (CWG 94:23).

Gandhi's conservative thinking about boundary-crossing marriages conjures the global spirit of eugenics contemporaneous with his lifetime. His writings demonstrate a deep familiarity with eugenic philosophy. For example, he expressed his preference for Malthus's original emphasis on continence, and his suspicion of neo-Malthusian use of artificial means to restrict reproduction (CWG 36:210). But as Sarah Hodges's work has shown, the trajectory of eugenic science in India was fundamentally different from that of its global counterparts (Hodges 2010). Indian eugenicists in the early twentieth century did not endorse adjudicating and sterilizing the racially unfit. Rather, their focus was on overpopulation, and their hope was to control that problem by promoting the use of contraception. Gandhi, however, was ambivalent about this nativization of eugenic theory; specifically, he consistently opposed contraception as a method because he feared it would promote moral licentiousness (Hodges 2017). Further, he understood birth control as evidence of a moral weakness to exert control over oneself (CWG 36:210–13). Taken together, then, Gandhi's ambivalence about interfaith and intercaste marriage and his inflexible emphasis on sexual abstinence represent blockages in his imagination of social reform through the mixing of blood. If the mixing of blood through intermarriage carried the potential of radical reform in Ambedkar's thought, Gandhi's conservative social imagination did not contain the erosion of communal boundaries as its telos; the transformation of the self and the flourishing of an anticolonial politics did not require radical caste reform.[10] Rather, the deployment of blood as politics performed only a demonstration of the truth of an anticolonial politics of *ahimsa* and *satyagraha*. It was as if blood could transcend the problems of religion and caste altogether, if not in life at least after death.

Violence as Nonviolence

We have begun to see how Gandhi's imagination of blood as a biomoral substance offers a glimpse into his biopolitical imagination and the relation between violence and nonviolence in the anticolonial struggle (the place of *ahimsa* in the conduct of *satyagraha*). Blood figures as a marker in his struggle to achieve equilibrium without desire and without attachment to any form of sovereignty—be it over another or over one's own self. Blood also offers the dream of transcending difference through a politics directed at the self, rather than toward radical social reform. Further, blood figures as a marker of strength, when its nonspillage is a demonstration of a warriorlike capacity to withhold violence. In these varied imaginations of blood, nonviolence begins to appear as something more than the negation of violence. Instead, as we continue to elaborate here, paying attention to blood helps clarify Gandhi's politics of nonviolence as not the negation of violence but of the possibility of violence *within* nonviolence, and even as the necessary precondition for nonviolence.[11]

Gandhi's first important political tract written, *Hind Swaraj* (1909), is typical of his early thinking about nonviolence as distinct and separable from violence. That is, if little acts of violence were an inescapable and unavoidable aspect of everyday life, the aim of the *satyagrahi* was to strive constantly for the impossible ideal of relinquishing such violence—in the end to "die without killing," as far as such a death was possible. Yet because one could never completely renounce the will to live, the *satyagrahi* participated in these inevitable acts of everyday violence, but always with the impossible horizon of absolute nonviolence in mind. The years immediately following the publication of *Hind Swaraj* marked a radical change in Gandhi's thinking about this relation between violence and nonviolence, such that violence no longer remained external to nonviolence. Concerned that *satyagraha* and *ahimsa* were being equated with weakness and an incapacity for violence—possibly a regrettable consequence of his own initial translation of *ahimsa* as "passive" resistance—Gandhi found it necessary to further refine and articulate his thinking about the relation between the two concepts. In his writings after *Hind Swaraj*, Gandhi emphasized that a truly nonviolent *satyagrahi* had to first possess the capability to inflict violence and thereafter relinquish this capability—that is, only those capable of killing could give up the desire to kill. In July 1918, in a letter to his closest disciple, Maganlal Gandhi, he goes as far as to parse his new realization as "Violence is in fact nonviolence" (CWG 17:150). Skaria's reading of Gandhi across Gujarati and English demonstrates that the fundamental constituent of *satyagraha* was not nonviolence in the sense of a passive antipathy to violence. Rather, *satyagraha* was a religious concept, one that involved a complete self-surrender that relinquished sovereignty, will, and autonomy over self and other (Skaria 2016). If such an abandonment of mastery enacted a form of *unwilled* violence, then so be it; such violence was in fact nonviolence. Thus, Gandhi was able to read as nonviolent the mythic act of Raja Harischandra raising his sword to kill his wife Taramati on the behest of a divine injunction. As Harischandra relinquished his desire and love for his wife, as well as his own wish not to enact violence, he became the paragon of the nonviolent *satyagrahi*: nothing but a cipher, without will and beyond all reach of sovereignty—be that of reason or faith. In Skaria's final reading, for Gandhi the true *satyagrahi* was the warrior that had relinquished arms and was able to live without desire or fear, completely surrendering the self while at the same time transcending the possibility of the self's subordination to another.

With this new shifting analysis of the relation between violence and nonviolence, Gandhi's imagination of blood as both a political and biological substance developed and coagulated. In the early years of his mobilizations against the British in South Africa, Gandhi often drew upon both Lord Salisbury and Dadabhai Naoroji's descriptions of colonialism as an act of extractive bleeding. Remarking on Lord Salisbury's death in 1903 in his newly founded newspaper *Indian Opinion*, Gandhi reprinted Lord Salisbury's description of colonialism as an act of bleeding in full, along with his own extensive commentary. In it, he invoked the bleeding metaphor not as a criticism of Salisbury's complicity in the colonial impoverishment of India, but rather as an example of Salisbury's honest and frank self-assessment of the failures of well-intentioned colonial policies (CWG 3:225). In other words, Gandhi's generous reading of Salisbury ignored the lord's injunction that the bleeding continue, only with more precision. Rather, Gandhi chose to emphasize the incisive power of the metaphor itself, the image of violence it conjured, and its enduring relevance for the colonial situation. Through his later years in South Africa, Gandhi would turn again and again to the bleeding metaphor. For example, the institution of the financially extractive poll tax was akin to squeezing blood out of stones, South African landlords were uncaring bloodsuckers that fed on labor, and British law was like a bloodthirsty monster with a special fondness for Indian blood. In 1908, he gave Salisbury's medical and surgical metaphor fuller treatment in an essay titled "Veins of Wealth": "Thus the circulation of wealth among a people resembles the circulation of blood in the body. When circulation of blood is rapid, it may indicate any of these things: robust health, [effects of] exercise, or a feeling of shame or fever. There is a flush of the body which is indicative of health, and another which is a sign of gangrene. Furthermore, the concentration of blood at one spot is harmful to the body and, similarly, concentration of wealth at one place proves to be the nation's undoing" (CWG 8:342).

The slippage here between the *colonial* circulation of wealth and the *biological* circulation of blood was not just cosmetic. It marked Gandhi's growing (and subsequently lifelong) attentiveness to blood as simultaneously a marker of political as well as biological well-being. In this regard, by 1930 the Salisbury metaphor would become far more incisive, as Gandhi invoked it to describe a brutal colonial rule that applied the lancet especially at sites that had been almost bled dry (CWG 49:62).

If Jallianwala Bagh stymied his desire to read spilled blood as evidence of the fearless *satyagrahi*, other opportunities presented themselves. In South Africa in 1908, the same year that he wrote "Veins of Wealth," Gandhi was attacked by a Muslim follower, after which he was physically incapacitated for several weeks. Writing soon after the attack, he felt that it had served a purpose in helping him overcome his persisting fear of death. The attack, he hoped, had brought him closer to an embrace of death, not as something to be desired, but as something to be accepted without fear. Soon after, he developed the idea that the shedding of blood was a necessary precondition for freedom: "It must be remembered that the British people won what they consider their freedom after they had let rivers of blood flow. . . . We, on the other hand, have shed no blood, endured nothing, for the sake of freedom, real or imaginary" (CWG 11:454). Just a week before the Bagh massacre, a crowd in Delhi had responded to Gandhi's call for *satyagraha* against the repressive Rowlatt Act that extended British wartime emergency powers. In response, the British police had opened fire on the gathering. There are conflicting accounts of the nature of the mobilizations and of the degrees of violence perpetrated by the crowd and the police (Kumar 1971). These conflicting accounts led to conflicting responses from Gandhi. But when convinced of the crowd's temperance, he was overjoyed at the violence: "I am now happy beyond measure over it. The blood spilt at Delhi was innocent" (CWG 17:378). The blood of innocents (later refigured to "treasures of blood") became a theme of joy and pride in Gandhi's writing about the Rowlatt Satyagraha in a way that the blood spilled at Jallianwala could not. Indeed, it rose to the status of aesthetic beauty. For example, after the 1930 Salt Satyagraha, he described the clothes of his companions Mahadev Desai and Jairamdas Daulatram as "beautifully splattered with fresh warm blood" (CWG 49:190). And while he condemned a lathi charge that left Gangabehn Vaidya (an elderly widow and a manager of his ashram) bloodied (CWG 51:84), in private letters to her, the same wound produced unbridled joy:

> How shall I compliment you? You have shown that you are what I had always thought you were. How I would have smiled with pleasure to see your sari made beautiful with stains of blood. I got excited when I knew about this atrocity, but was not pained in the least. On the contrary, I felt happy. (CWG 51:94)

> By the time you get this letter you will have been out of jail for many days. If it again becomes necessary to let your clothes be stained with blood, let them be. This colour is more pleasant than that of *kumkum* or *sindoor*. (CWG 51:194)

He would continue to invoke Gangabehn's defiance as a martial act worthier than the violent uprisings of those such as Bhagat Singh (CWG 51:306). For her part, Gangabehn had described the merciless blows to her head by the police, the blood that streamed from her wound, and how she peacefully sat in the police station when arrested, "allowing the sun's rays to fall on the bleeding part" (CWG 51:441).

This tripartite thinking would characterize Gandhi's political imagination of blood for years to come: first, a substance indexing the violence and extractive quality of British rule; second, a marker indicating the consanguinity of the *satyagrahi* with the other; and third, its spillage as the duty and precondition for true *satyagraha* and *ahimsa*. By 1918, he was clear that the idea of nonviolence—when conceptualized as the opposite of violence—enacted its own variant of violence: "We commit violence on a large scale in the name of nonviolence. Fearing to shed blood, we torment people every day and dry up their blood" (CWG 17:145). He was clear then that nonviolence was the true domain of the warrior (*Kshatriya*) and that only the one who could shed blood could take the decision not to spill blood. At a speech occasioned by the killing of the Arya Samaj reformist Swami Shraddhanand in 1926 by a Muslim, Gandhi refused to mourn his death and wished instead for such a death for himself if it came to him. In almost every reference to it in the years to come, Swami Shraddhanand's blood too was sacralized, as Gandhi asked for it to purify his heart (CWG 37:445) and for it to cleanse the division between Hindus and Muslims (CWG 37:457). Later in 1929, in an essay titled "Did Rama Shed Blood?," he returned to the idea that nonviolent cooperation was only for the strong, not for the weak. And when his optimism wavered in the face of continuing internecine violence—for example, when the Indian journalist Ganesh Shaknar Vidyarthi was killed in an attempt to intervene in such a riot—Gandhi wondered whether the poison of division had gone too deep for even the noblest of blood to purify (CWG 51:361).

This tripartite conceptualization of blood—as a measure of equilibrium and of fearlessness in the face of death, and as an index of communal solidarity— remained a dominant theme in Gandhi's writing. In a speech in Karachi in 1920, he asked the crowd, "What do you understand by giving blood?" The answer was simple: a martial readiness to sacrifice one's own life, a sacrifice proper to the "soldier" but not the "professor." In Gandhi's thought, we find exemplified the simultaneous biological and moral, material and figurative properties of blood. Let us track its biomoral iterations. It appears as material through an act of violence— the highest taboo and the product of the transgression of the *satyagrahi's* primary interdiction. Yet at the same time, once spilled, it is rendered pure and sacral as an index of communal solidarity and selfless sacrifice. Thus potentiated, blood sanctifies the land upon which it is spilled, transforming the site into a place of pedagogic pilgrimage whose lesson is that the sacrifice of blood becomes an anticolonial duty: "To fight these British, we shall have to make our blood as cheap as water" (CWG 33:343). Blood as substance holds the potential to both purify and contaminate; it is a reminder of violence to be abhorred as well as a sign of anticolonial martyrdom and an element of a new reformatory form that transgresses communal boundaries. At the same time, the telos of blood-mixing is not caste reform but rather a dream of the transcendence of hierarchy through an ascetic control and reform of the self and its desires.

Gandhi's imagination of blood is perhaps best captured in an image that recurs through his writing—that of rivers of blood. The image refers simultaneously to the unjust blood spilled by the colonizer *and* the joyful blood sacrificed by the *satyagrahi*. For example, "rivers of blood" were on the one hand convincing proof of the unparalleled barbarity of the Second World War (CWG 81:151). Gandhi was particularly struck by Churchill's speech at the end of the war, when the latter compared the war to a "blood-letting" that weakened and whitened Europe (CWG 90:431). Yet Gandhi redeployed the metaphor toward another end: such a "blood-letting" would not be in vain if it had taught Europe the power of joyful blood sacrifice, when the blood sacrificed was one's own and not another's (CWG 90:328). His commitment to this provocative idea was unflinching, even in the months before his death. It revealed the presence and viability of a certain kind of violence within his politics of nonviolence. In this instance, violence was an explicit formulation in Gandhi's thought. At the same time, his imagination of communal reform through blood spilled and mixed in the practice of nonviolence reveals another kind of implicit violence: the misrecognition of caste inequality as a problem of self-control rather than of social reform.

In April 1947, a few months before his death, Gandhi wrote, "Let them kill me. Will they drink my blood? Let them do so. That will save some food and I shall consider that I have been of service" (CWG 95:310). After his death in early 1948, the blood that flowed from his body at the time of his assassination was collected and preserved. It remains on display in Madurai—a material, biomoral reminder of a Gandhian hemo-politics suffused both with paradox and possibility.

Consanguine Martyrdom

Metaphors of blood sacrifice were famously central for another competing anticolonial figure—Subhash Chandra Bose. *"Tum mujhe khun do, main tumhen aazadi doonga"*—"Give me your blood, and I will give you freedom." These words, spoken at a political rally in Burma in 1944, are some of the most quoted in relation to the Indian anticolonial struggle. At the time of their utterance, their purpose was to stimulate a willingness on the part of the Indian masses to engage in armed struggle in order to bring to an end long-standing British colonial rule. To assert that it is an iconic phrase hardly does it justice. In fact, the very possibility of its forgetting became the matter of public interest litigation against the Indian iteration of *Who Wants to Be a Millionaire?* When the game show's promotional video featured a contestant unable to ascribe the quotation to its speaker, a Bombay resident brought forward a case to restrain its screening that was heard at the city's high court and attracted much media attention.[12] Our aim is not to rehearse this familiar narrative of Bose's invocation of blood as anticolonial metaphor. Rather, our interest is in what this invocation precipitates in a contemporary political world dominated by religious nationalism (Hindutva), in the long shadow of an anticolonial struggle associated with Gandhian *ahimsa*. Proponents of Hindu nationalism allied with India's ruling political party (the Bharatiya Janata Party, or BJP) have campaigned to appropriate Bose's armed insurgency within Hindutva history (Gupta 1996; Panigrahi 2017). For Hindutva ideologues, valorizing Bose's insurgency as armed, masculine, and violent allows for a counternarrative to an anticolonial struggle dominated by Gandhi—a figure with which the Hindu right has had a fraught relationship. The historian Sugata Bose argues that despite their differences, Subhash Bose and Gandhi both relied on a discourse of blood sacrifice and blood brotherhood to bridge ethnic differences and promote a common anticolonial nationalism (Bose 2011). In the present, however, as resurrected by Hindutva history, Bose is counterpoised to the effeminacy and weakness of Gandhian nonviolence, and is exhibited as a more proper exemplar for the Indian nation state in the present. In what follows, we describe why Bose's exhortation toward a nationalism coagulated by blood sacrifice makes him particularly appealing to contemporary Hindutva ideologues. Second, through the material and metaphor of blood, and building on our description thus far of a Gandhian hemo-politics, we counteract the Hindutva polarization of anticolonialism into its nonviolent and violent variants. Finally, paying attention again to the material politics of blood, we describe a fundamental difference between the Gandhian and Hindutva versions of sacrificial politics. We argue that the deep chasm that divides their politics becomes visible once we acknowledge the potent multivalence of blood as political substance and the contrasting political visions it reveals.

The Red Fort

A quotation, states Karin Barber, "is only a quotation when it is inserted into a new context"; it involves both detachment and recontextualization (2005, 274). Inserted into present-day political contexts, Bose's words "precipitate" (or constitute the rhetorical occasion for) various sorts of "shedding." Our focus here is on an example of blood portraiture that was directly inspired by Bose's utterance—an exhibition of blood portraits staged in Delhi in 2009. The subjects of the portraits, Bose among them, were "freedom fighter" martyrs—sacrificial heroes of the independence struggle. The following details concerning the exhibition derive from our visits to it, when we spoke at length with its organizer and visitors, but also from newspaper accounts and the visitors' book, with its thousands of entries, to which we were given access. In chapter 1, we placed blood within a complex matrix of interdictions and permissions regarding caste and personhood in South Asia. In that regard, the use of human blood for "art" and mass political communication may evoke some surprise. We suggest here that it is in part *because* of such sociocultural interdictions that the genre possesses expressive force. As with Gandhi's valorization of blood spilled and mixed, blood portraits that draw upon anxieties about the mixing of substances give such a form of political art a particularly powerful material force.

Artworks have long formed an integral feature of nationalist narratives. Idols and images from India's past "continue their lives resituated as art objects in Indian museums," playing a key part in "the colonial and postcolonial project of constructing an Indian national identity" (R. Davis 1993, 45). There is also a well-established tradition of explicitly patriotic art, insightfully documented by Pinney (2004) and Ramaswamy (2008). Such art often depicts nationalist heroes having spilled, or in the act of spilling, their blood. The patriotic art that we explore here likewise depicts martyrs revered for having shed their blood, but it differs in also being composed of human blood. If these literally bloody patriotic works differ from mainstream Indian patriotic art, they also differ from the use of blood in Western art. Discussions of the use of bodily substances (particularly blood) in Western art typically argue that it marks a return to primitive ritual (e.g., Siebers 2003) and/or that it results "naturally" from the trauma consequent on the cataclysmically bloody events of the twentieth century. The flow of the blood of performance artists such as Marina Abramović is often analyzed according to its "shock value" (Weiermair 2001), while more recently "bioart"—a field existing "at the intersection of the creative arts and the bio-medical sciences" (Palladino 2010, 96; see also Anker and Franklin 2011) that frequently employs as media human (and animal) substances, sometimes in biomolecular or diseased form—has been considered to offer the potential to reconfigure, even to subvert, the constraints of "bio-political governmentality" (Palladino 2010, 106). There are no doubt points of connection between these genres and Indian blood portraiture; all of them, for instance, raise questions concerning distinctions between presence and representation, while questions of loss, ritual, and shock value are certainly raised in the Indian case. We want to suggest, however, that unlike the forms of body art described above, the Indian case presents us with a direct political intervention (if bioart does provide radical political commentary, it does so only obliquely). The Indian case also speaks to a very specific political history and present-day situation and possesses its own unique set of representational and mnemonic complexities that we unpack.

A great seventeenth-century Mughal structure, the Red Fort possesses dense nationalist associations. On the day of Indian independence on 15 August 1947, Jawaharlal Nehru hoisted the national flag at the fort. Every year since, Indian Independence Day is commemorated with the Indian prime minister unfurling the flag at the site, followed by a nationally broadcast address from its ramparts. The Red Fort's iconic association with the anticolonial movement began at the end of India's first war of independence in 1857, when the British government tried the last Mughal emperor Bahadur Shah II at the site for his support of the war. But the fort's association with nationalism draws force not only from its association with precolonial Indian sovereignty but also from the prominence it derived from the 1945–1946 public trials of Indian National Army (INA) soldiers. Bose's call for an anticolonial uprising had led to the formation of the INA. The army comprised for the most part Indian prisoners of war who had served the British Army in Southeast Asia but had been captured by Japanese troops; these Indian prisoners of war had been released by the Japanese to aid the INA's war against Britain. After the end of the war, the government of British India hoped to make an example of three INA soldiers by publically trying them for treason at the Red Fort. In historical retrospect, the decision proved fatal to an already diminished British claim to legitimacy; the British government had decisively miscalculated the sentiments the trials would catalyze in postwar India (Bayly and Harper 2007). Moreover, the government's miscalculation was magnified by its choice of the three accused—Shah Nawaz Khan, Gurubaksh Singh Dhillon, and Prem Sahgal—a Muslim, a Sikh, and a Hindu. If the Gandhian call for interreligious and inter-sect unity had been challenged before and during the Second World War (Jalal 1985), the Red Fort trials offered an opportunity for a legal dramatization of nationalist unity. These trials stand as a final moment of solidarity between the Muslim League and the Indian National Congress before the two parties fractured to govern the divided nation-states of India and Pakistan.

The contemporary Red Fort bears many physical marks of its history, not least a museum commemorating Bose's Indian National Army. The exhibition of blood

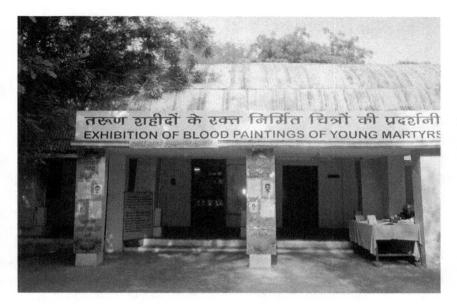

तरुण शहीदों के रक्त निर्मित चित्रों की प्रदर्शनी
EXHIBITION OF BLOOD PAINTINGS OF YOUNG MARTYRS

FIGURE 1. Outside the exhibition. (Photo by the authors.)

portraitures within the fort ran from October 2009 until the spring of the following year, drawing in visitors in the hundreds of thousands (three thousand to four thousand per day, according to official figures). The sign outside the tin-roofed exhibition hall, framed by an elongated Indian tricolor, stated in Hindi and in English, "Exhibition of Blood Paintings of Young Martyrs" (figures 1 and 2). Few of these visitors, however, entered the complex with the express intention of visiting the exhibition or in the knowledge that it even existed. The primary purpose of nearly all the visitors was to inspect the symbolic historical buildings of the Red Fort. The exhibition hall was set up just past the fort's famous Lahore Gate and a row of stalls selling tourist memorabilia but prior to the main set of buildings, convenient for many tourists to make the impromptu decision to pay it a visit (there was no additional cost). Most visitors were Indian; a good proportion of them had arrived on coach trips from the provinces, visiting the Red Fort as part of a nationalist itinerary that included other notable sights in the capital, such as Mohandas Gandhi's memorial.

It was Bose's famous utterance, "Give me your blood, and I will give you freedom," from which the organizer of the exhibition, Ravi Chander Gupta, took his original inspiration (*prerna*). Indeed, the very first portrait he gave his blood for—painted by his friend and colleague the artist Gurdarshan Singh Binkal—was of and for Bose, painted for Bose's birth centenary in 1997. Significantly, the painting

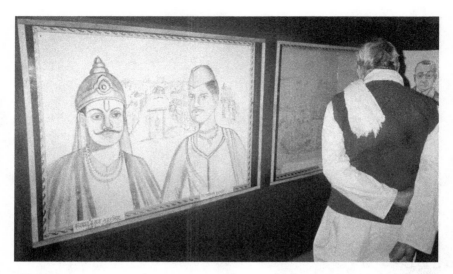

FIGURE 2. A visitor at the exhibition before a portrait depicting Raja Nahar Singh of Ballabhgargh and Seth Ramji Das Gur Wale, both of whom were involved in the Indian Uprising of 1857. (Photo by the authors.)

was made in the physical presence of Delhi schoolchildren. As Gupta, a retired schoolteacher, explained to us, the children's dispiriting ignorance of former patriotic sacrifices was one of the motivating factors behind the portraits: "The biographies of martyrs should be included in course curriculum. Paintings, posters and calendars of freedom fighters should be promoted so that more and more people know them and read about them." As one news report put it: "Gupta feels that very few people are aware about our freedom fighters and especially the youth."[13] Another reported that Gupta's organization hoped to take the 150-portrait "*shaheed*" exhibition across the country: "Those born in the post-Independence era cannot feel the struggle of freedom fighters."[14] A selection of the eighteen books Gupta has written on the martyrs, several of which were published by the Indian government, were on display at the entrance to the exhibition alongside the visitors' book (figure 3). Gupta has been particularly concerned to highlight the role played by child martyrs in the independence struggle, most of whom barely register in official accounts. He lives alone; as he put it to us, "The martyrs are my family."

At the entrance to the hall was positioned the very first blood portrait made: that depicting Bose in his classic military pose (figure 4). The exhibition's rationale was displayed at the side of the artwork:

> Why use blood as ink? (*Rakt ki syahi se hi kyun?*). Those martyrs could have supported their old parents. They could have led a life of luxury with their families, could have become high-level writers, industrialists,

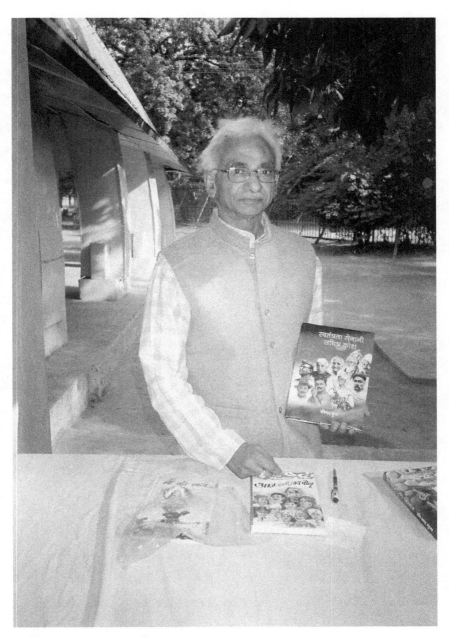

FIGURE 3. Ravi Chander Gupta with books he has written on the martyrs. (Photo by the authors.)

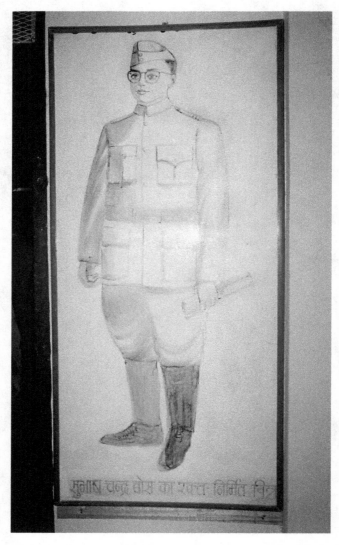

FIGURE 4. Subhash Chandra Bose (Gupta's first painting). (Photo by the authors.)

businessmen, or leaders and earned money and fame. But they chose something else . . . the path of sacrifice. They loved their country more than their families. They wanted to see the future generations as citizens of a free and prosperous nation. We heard that the history of the sacrifice made by the martyrs would be written in gold letters. But where has it been written? I thought, if not in gold letters, it can be written in blood letters . . . and the process started. This exhibition is a humble tribute to the martyrs.

The lament "But where has it been written?" takes us to the heart of Gupta's project—his fear that knowledge of the noble sacrifices of the many citizens who died fighting for freedom is fading away:

I am spreading awareness through this exhibition. This is to remind the people who are forgetting. The [sacrifices of the] *shaheed* (martyrs) are not taught on the curriculum. It is the need of the time to bring these stories onto [school] courses so that children may gain inspiration from them. The government is sleeping on this.

Another of Gupta's concerns is the impression he has of youthful martyrs as having been scripted out of the nationalist narrative. To right this wrong, he undertook twelve years of research on their histories, documenting more than five hundred children and young adults (from the ages of six to twenty) who died in the freedom struggle. Many, though not all, of the portraits in the exhibition depict these hitherto neglected child martyrs.

Speaking of the very first portrait for which he provided blood, that of Subhash Chandra Bose, Gupta told us, "I wanted to use my dearest thing (*sab se priya vastu*)—to offer it to Neta Ji. The dearest particle of my life—this is blood only. I can do this for him." Too young at the time of Bose's call, decades later Gupta is perhaps finally able to participate in a glorious cause. This is, then, a sacrificial portraiture: for the martyrs and for the nation. But the use of blood is also understood to be efficacious in respect of Gupta's larger concern to remember the martyrs:

The public is attracted to portraits of blood. I started this to attract the public and get their attention. People are more interested if the portraits are in blood; they are more motivated, more curious if blood is used rather than paint. Blood creates sentiments; sentiment (*bhavna*) is attached to blood. It acquires social value and importance if done in blood.

Of further note are the patriotic songs, mainly from Hindi films of the 1950s, that played continuously in the hall and that added to the multisensory nature of the exhibition. When we asked Gupta about his choice of music, he responded, "I am playing these songs to inculcate love for the country, to create an atmosphere. When you enter a *mandir* (temple) you light incense and transform the atmosphere. Like that, these songs create an atmosphere of patriotism." A song we heard numerous times during our visits is the classic "*Ai mere watan ke logo*" ("O! People of My Country!"), sung by Lata Mangeshkar, which commemorates Indian soldiers who died during the 1962 Sino-Indian War and was famously performed before India's first prime minister, Jawaharlal Nehru, on the country's 1963 Republic Day. Its themes correspond closely to those emphasized by Gupta, focusing as they do on blood and memory:

> O! People of my country! . . .
> Unfurl our beloved tricolor, but don't forget that at the borders brave
>   people have lost their lives. . . .
> When it was [the festival] of Holi they played [it] with their blood.
> When we were sitting in our homes they were being pierced by
>   bullets. . . .
> Some were Sikh, some were Jat [a cultivating caste] and some Maratha
>   [hailing from Maharashtra], some were Gurkha and some from
>   Madras.
> Whosoever died at the border, every such warrior was an Indian.
> The blood that fell on the hills of the Himalayas—that blood was
>   Indian. . . .
> Lest you forget them this story has been recounted. . . .
> Victory to India, victory to the Indian Armed Forces.
>
> —"Ai mere watan ke logo"

Holi is a spring festival celebrated in honor of the god Krishna in which playful reversals of gender, generation, class, and caste are enacted in a variety of ways (L. Cohen 1995a, 401). It usually involves the throwing of various brightly colored substances—vividly reimagined in "Ai mere watan ke logo" as bright red blood. Usually considered particularly pleasurable, or *masti*, the festival is here melded with the high seriousness of national sacrifice. Of further note is the song's integrative aesthetic, with its references to different religious, caste, and regional "types" of fallen hero—Sikh, Jat, and so on. The song thus introduces and enfolds themes of memory and integrated difference (by way of an idiom of blood) that are reminiscent of Gandhi's invocation described earlier in this chapter and are critical to our analysis below. In referring explicitly to the Sino-Indian War of 1962, it also underlines the important point that while Gupta is principally concerned to remember those who fought and died during the anticolonial movement, his portraits also memorialize Indians who died in subsequent conflicts. The most recent of his portraits depict martyrs of the 1999 Kargil conflict between India and Pakistan.

Martyrs and Memory

Anthropologist William Mazzarella describes how the achievement of Indian independence in 1947 was not only a moment of victory but also "in a very important sense a moment of loss"—a "loss of the loss," as he puts it (2010, 1–2). This is useful in helping us to understand the predicament of Gupta and other members of the organization he has formed to produce and look after the paintings. Scholars have been active in emphasizing various sorts of alienation and loss consequent upon colonial rule (e.g., Nandy 1983); at the same time, however, it can be argued that "colonization enabled a fullness of nationalist subjectivity. . . . In this paradoxical sense, British colonial rule was for India the loss that made possible the affective plenitude of mass nationalism" (Mazzarella 2010, 2). Gupta and his colleagues seek to revivify this affective plenitude in a kind of delayed challenge to, and contemporary variant of, the "loss of the loss." Of particular concern from Gupta's point of view is what he considers to be the popular and bureaucratic failure to remember past sacrifices—sacrifices that are the occluded condition of a present relentlessly future-oriented national situation. To paraphrase Engelke (2007), Gupta's blood portraits speak to a problem of nationalist presence.

Recall now the lines from Gupta's exhibition rubric: "We heard that the history of the sacrifice made by the martyrs would be written in gold letters. But where has it been written? I thought, if not in gold letters, it can be written in blood letters." The portraits are thus objects in the service of memorialization. The memorializing thrust of the portraits is necessary because existing memorialization processes are experienced as inadequate or tokenistic. Their purpose is to invoke a memory that is not passive but active, as the stimulus of a revivified sacrificial spirit. This is memorialization as a call to action.

Gupta recalled to us his days as a schoolteacher in a government school in east Delhi: "I felt the children knew nothing. They thought we achieved freedom without lifting a finger. They sang popular songs about Gandhi and *ahimsa*. They thought we got freedom without picking up a weapon! And so I said, well, I need to tell the children it's not true." This is, then, an explicitly anti-Gandhian project of reeducation and historical revision. Nationalist historiography—at least in terms of its manifestation in school curricula—thus hinges on what Gupta sees as a Gandhian perversion, to be corrected, in part, by the exhibitions he stages. It is not only Gupta and his organization who are alarmed by this apparent national forgetting. A blood donation camp in 2009 was staged in a spatiotemporal conjunction saturated with nationalist significance: the place was Jallianwala Bagh; the time was Mohandas Gandhi's birthday (Gandhi Jayanti). The camp's organizers stated that its aim was "to awake the government from deep slumber to grant the status of freedom fighter to the martyrs killed during the massacre of 13 April 1919."[15] If Gandhi began the resignification of the victims of the shootings as martyrs, the project continues until the present.

Yet this need to remember appears within a fraught contestation of memory in Indian historiography and gives it its particular religious nationalist force. As several historians of India have pointed out, memorials such as the Red Fort have been powerful sites of confrontation between Hindutva nationalists, secular elites, and subaltern subjects (Kavuri-Bauer 2011). Gupta's organization aims to intervene in the negotiation process of collective memory in order to revivify and stabilize a particular body of remembrances. His project is not only one of restoration but rather exists to counter transformation with transformation. Specifically, an ongoing complaint of Hindutva activists has been that "secular" Indian historians have offered a false narrative of Indian history that appeases minority groups such as Muslims while victimizing the Hindu majority that had been under Muslim domination in the precolonial period. Hindutva historiography thus strives to resuscitate an ancient, masculine, and proud Hindu identity, one that does not fit well with Gandhian calls to nonviolence. Thus, as we describe below, Gupta's desire to invigorate the history of martyrs and armed revolutionaries apparently is in sympathy with Hindutva historiography.

Coming Together to Bleed

By the mid-2000s more than a hundred portraits had been completed, with Gupta busying himself exhibiting them in schools and elsewhere. By this time, he had also formed an organization, the Shaheed Smriti Chetna Samiti (Society to Awaken Remembrance of the Martyrs; henceforth "the *samiti*"), in order that the paintings would be cared for after his passing. Until 2004, all the paintings were formed of Gupta's blood. However, after two bypass surgeries (Gupta is now eighty) doctors forbade him to provide any more of his own blood, so the artist Binkal now uses his own blood to paint the martyrs. But a problem arose—the paintings were fading, and the artist could hardly be expected to provide *all* the necessary blood for their retouching. There is a telling irony here: blood is the ink with which to redeem the promise of "gold letters" for the immortalization of the freedom fighters, but blood as artistic material is inconstant and ephemeral, partaking of the flux that is the hallmark of materials (Ingold 2007). Analogous with the faded memories the paintings are supposed to enliven, blood, too, fades. However, the potential danger of simply *re-presenting* the fragility of memories of the martyrs' timeless sacrifices in material form was turned into an opportunity. In 2008 in Ghaziabad, a district of Uttar Pradesh state adjacent to Delhi, a special "blood camp" was staged in order to collect blood for use in retouching the portraits. The blood of 125 people was collected. As Gupta noted to us: "There were a lot more people, but we didn't need more. It was organized for making national sentiments. We used bottles—only 20 ml each. We put an anticlotting chemical into it; there was just that, and the blood. We mixed the blood together and directly used it. First of all you sketch on the paper with a pencil, and then you paint over it with [regular] paint so that there is only a very faint outline, and then you paint over the faint outline with the blood."

Despite an effort to distinguish between blood collection and medically useful blood donation, this was, in a sense, a blood *donation* camp, but with recipients who were dead rather than living. More specifically, the donation was to their memories; the call was for donations that would keep the dead (rather than the precariously living) alive (in people's memories). The element of exchange is fairly explicit: the martyrs gave their blood for the nation; contemporary Indians are exhorted to give them their blood to keep their memory alive. Depicted on the banners adorning the event were the words "*Shahido ke liye rakt sangrah shivir*" ("Blood collection for the martyrs"). "People came running to contribute for the martyrs," says Gupta. Blood was donated, then, *for* the martyrs. Also of interest was the use of 20 ml collection bottles—far smaller than the medical limit. As Gupta explained to us, "We collected 20 ml only [from each person] so that many people could be involved—only one syringe each." Gupta was clear, then, that multiple sources of blood, though not strictly necessary, were nevertheless desired (and facilitated).

Importantly, Gupta was keen to stress that women, Muslims, and children all contributed. (The backgrounds of the contributors were *alag-alag*, "different-different," as he put it.) This was thus an example of the spatial concentration of difference that is characteristic of the Indian nationalist ideology of national integration more generally (Copeman 2009a, chap. 7). "Difference" (e.g., of caste, religion, or geographic provenance) among blood contributors was actively encouraged, with the portraits—now composed of multiple mingled bloods—becoming sanguinary microcosms of the national *unitas multiplex*. As we discussed in chapter 1, in many situations in the subcontinent, bodily mixing is anathema. However, partly because of this very negative power attributed to the mixing of substances, there inheres within the politics of substance a marked utopic potential (Alter 1992, 258; Mukharji 2014). It was this politics of substance that Gandhi had invoked in his call to memorialize the blood of those that had been martyred at Jallianwala Bagh. Mixing in the form of, say, an intercaste marriage or a transfusion sourced from different religious "types" (see L. Cohen 2001) can carry powerful messages about nationhood, reason, and civic-mindedness. The Nehruvian integrative nationalist or rationalist activist can gain great satisfaction from transgressing restrictions in flows of substance, but in "constructively" inverting the typical pattern of restrictions, the pattern can, paradoxically, be reproduced; it is simply the valuation of the transgression that is altered. Perhaps, therefore, what Gupta saw when he looked at the (retouched) paintings was an exemplary saturation, one that reasserts rather than contradicts Gandhi's sanguinary imagination. Thus, even if Gupta's explicit aim was to counter a narrative of Gandhian nonviolence, our examination of Gandhi's sanguinary politics allows us to identify ideological resonances between Gupta's project and Gandhian *ahimsa*.

Traces

For Gupta, the use of blood is important for gaining people's interest; it is, in this sense, a tactical usage. But it is also significant because in being formed through acts of bleeding, there is a key sense in which the portraits constitute themselves the emulation they call for—adding to their hoped-for precipitative force. There is a venerable tradition of patriotic Indian portraiture, a genre that gathered in intensity during the struggle for independence and that made similar demands on the contemporary viewer, who was encouraged to make sacrifices of a comparable nature to those depicted (particularly iconic are those depicting Bhagat Singh offering his own bloody head to Bharat Mata [India as mother goddess] [see Pinney 2004; Ramaswamy 2008]). While Gupta's paintings certainly connect to this lineage of didactic portraiture, they also obviously differ: first, in being of far more recent provenance from the perspective of historical nostalgia; and second, in being literally composed of the blood they seek to elicit from others. Moreover, these are metonymic extractions: a small part of one's blood is indicative of the larger deficits the giver is willing to offer in the future if necessary. This is a kind of memorialization that, as we have noted, is also a call to action.

Leafing through the visitors' book with Gupta—a favorite occupation of his during the long days of the exhibition, at which he was always present—we asked him which of the thousands of comments he found most gratifying. He guided us unhesitatingly to the words of an eight-year-old schoolboy from Delhi: "These paintings are from the heart, when the time comes to sacrifice my blood for the protection of my country I will sacrifice my whole life." As Gupta put it to us: "This exhibition is to inspire the people to make sacrifices. Sacrifices are not all over now. You can still do it; you *should* still do it. The sacrifices are not only in the past; even in the future there is a time for sacrifice for the country." In other words, Gupta is calling for the retemporalization of sacrifice. The paintings are thus a form of enactive remembering; they are depictions of blood sacrifice that perform the bleeding they represent and seek to inspire. We have referred to the hoped-for precipitative force of the portraits, so it is important to consider where such a force might come from. As we noted earlier, the portraits are (among other things) a retort to "weak" Gandhian nationalism. And the retort appears to "work," in part, through their being imitative of the bleeding they seek to inspire.[16] This then is a kind of mimetic bleeding art—"mimetic" insofar as "originary" blood sacrificers are paid homage to by bleeding in turn, but mimetic also in terms of the willingness to sacrifice one's blood that it is supposed to incite in the viewer. The paintings call for emulation as models of and models for sacrificial bleeding. Consider Alfred Gell's famous delineation of the aniconic symbol, which he compares to the foreign diplomat: "The Chinese ambassador in London . . . does not look like China, but in London, China looks like him" (1998, 98). Similar to the ambassador, who is a "spatio-temporally detached fragment of his nation," aniconic works of art, such as religious idols, make gods present in visual form. One can "represent" in the manner of a painting (iconically), but one can also "represent" in the manner of an ambassador (aniconically). Blood portraits are both iconic and aniconic: iconic because they visually depict fallen martyrs; aniconic because the artist is present in the painting not only in terms of conceptualization and technique but also as physical residue. That the corporeal self of the artist is mixed with the primary subject of the portrait, thereby "entering into" the subject of representation, suggests that what results, paradoxically, may be considered a kind of self-portrait.

We can discern here a quite familiar South Asian template. Hindu rituals contain identification between worshipper and deity as a central theme and objective (in *puja*), with identification reinforced subsequently through the offering of substances such as food and flowers (*prasad*). *Puja* (worship) aims to "create a unity between deity and worshipper that dissolves the difference between them" (Fuller 2004, 57). If Gandhi's imagination of blood sacrifices invoked its ritual power of sanctification, there is, we suggest, a *puja* element to the portraits, with the blood of which they are composed a kind of offering to the depictions it comprises. In this sense, the sign and the flesh are one, or one might say that the iconic and aniconic elements lose their separate identities in the space of the portrait-as-*puja*. Recall that the sense of an offering was explicit at the special re-touching event discussed above, with the public asked to give blood for the martyrs in return for the blood they sacrificed in the work of securing national independence. That the wider Indian genre of patriotic art, of which Gupta's works constitute a subspecies, incorporates nationalist heroes into the Hindu pantheon substantiates the argument that a *puja* element might inhere within the portraits. Ramaswamy refers to a portrait in blood depicting Mohandas Gandhi exhibited in the National Gandhi Museum in New Delhi. The "literally bloody painting shows Gandhi with not one but three heads (two of them painted in the colors of the national flag), signifying his apotheosis into the Hindu pantheon with its many multiheaded and multilimbed gods" (Ramaswamy 2008, 838). While it is rare for such patriotic portraiture to use blood as its representational medium, it is not unusual for the martyrs depicted to appear transfigured into Hindu gods. It is therefore reasonable to suggest that Gupta's blood portraiture, as offering, connotes a form of communion analogous with that of *puja* and its transfer of substances. Like the idols of gods discussed by Gell, the portraits are not only depictions. There is an aniconic element, too, for the portraits index, quite literally, the artist's spatiotemporal presence as substantive offerings to the icons they comprise. The painting itself is transactional in this sense; it enframes *puja*. Recall also Gupta's comparison, referred to above, between exhibition hall and temple space, with the music of *desh-bhakti* (patriotism) considered to be analogous to the way incense helps create a mood of devotional communion. The need for re-touching resulted in collection of blood from several hundred others. That there are multiple bloods mixed into the image collectivizes the *puja* that is enframed in the space of the portrait.

Were the portraits efficacious in the manner intended by Gupta and his *samiti*? The responses we obtained at the exhibition at the Red Fort do not provide a clear-cut answer. Some of the visitors we spoke with were not aware that human blood had been used for the portraits, despite the information displayed. However, to some degree this particular staging of the exhibition was not typical of the other occasions in which the paintings have been displayed (school classrooms, stand-alone exhibitions, etc.). Attendance here tended to be an epiphenomenon of the primary purpose of the tourist's visit (i.e., to see the main Red Fort buildings). Many attendees, then, could hardly be said to have been stimulated to attend by the novel prospect of a sanguinary mode of portraiture, though that is not to say that others have not been so at other perhaps less atypical display venues.

Responses gained from discussion but also in (mainly Hindi) written form in the visitors' book were mostly of a manner that Gupta would find gratifying— that is, they offered evidence that the "correct" nationalist interpretations and sentiments had duly been stimulated by the works on display. One visitor from Punjab stated, "Old memories are being refreshed." Another, from Bihar, stated similarly, "These people gave their lives to liberate the country—we should take inspiration (*prerna*)." Even more pleasing for Gupta was this: "I wish that my name was also included among these *shahids*. Then I could have called myself a true child of Mother India." Another comment, this time in English: "I am proud to be an Indian and also proud of those persons who forgot about themselves and gave the whole of their blood for our motherland. *Jai Hind* (Hail India)." A further observation, from a visitor from Faizabad, reflected similar sentiments to those of Gupta concerning memory and willingness to sacrifice: "This exhibition is in the blood of the artist! It is inspiring for the new generations. If any other country raises its evil eye (*buri nazar*) toward India, the entire young generation will be prepared to hang." Other visitors made similar comments concerning a present situation characterized by forgetfulness and consequent lessening of willingness to sacrifice: "These portraits in blood are inspiring. It is important that these ideas reach the new generation, as it is straying (*binak*) from its path." In respect of the precipitative aim of the exhibition, comments such as "I want to be like them and give my life for the country" are strongly indicative of the kind of positive response Gupta was looking for.

Beyond Violence and Nonviolence / Purity and Mixture

Blood extraction in mass political contexts (principally for purposes of medical donation, petitions, or paintings) is a key present-day form of political enunciation, for such extractions—speaking as and on behalf of a subject position (Bairy 2009, 112)—are intensely communicative. In the particular field of Indian party politics, Gupta's *samiti* is joined by Hindu nationalist organizations in their proclivity for blood as media for ideological communication. While it is important not to impute internal consistency to a highly differentiated set of groups and pragmatic alliances, Hindutva activists have, broadly speaking, been at the forefront of developing a political aesthetics of blood portraiture and speech. During political demonstrations in 1992 that led to the destruction of the Babri Masjid mosque in Ayodhya, Hindu nationalist youth group the Bajrang Dal welcomed Bharatiya Janata Party (BJP) leader L. K. Advani to the city by applying a ritual mark (*tilak*) of blood on his forehead (Fuller 2004, 272). On other occasions, they have offered him cups of blood. A protest rally against Islamic terrorism organized by the BJP and Rashtriya Swayamsevak Sangh (RSS) in 2001 featured the collecting [of] signatures in blood on huge banners proclaiming the "death of terrorism." . . . A three-wheeler equipped with loudspeaker and manned by a BJP worker did the rounds of colonies around [politician] Khurana's constituency, inviting people to sign their names in blood. "Campaigners first allowed blood to be drawn, saw it being put in a test tube and then dipped cotton padded needles to sign on the banner. And as they did so they were drowned in a chorus of nationalistic slogans," while the wasted blood was poured down the drain. . . . Even schoolchildren were included in the "sacrifice" of blood. All this in a city where the government has been repeatedly announcing a shortage of blood for accident victims.[17]

Consider also how in 2015 the BJP government in Rajasthan decided to organize a compulsory blood donation campaign in private and public colleges on the day of Baqr-Eid, barring Muslims from observing the holiday.[18] These are just a few of the many instances in which blood is invoked as a biomoral substance to assert the rights of a Hindu majority. Many activists of the Hindu right, then, see themselves as "people of blood" (Heuze 1992, 2261) and employ human blood for a wide variety of enunciative purposes. In several instances of political blood shedding such as this, extraction seems to communicate metonymic intentions, by which we mean that the portion extracted indicates the whole the agent is willing to give; it is a demonstration of intent (see the discussion of Bajrang Dal activists' blood portrait of Lord Rama in chapter 1). Blood as media may enact a premonitory bloodshed, a sanguinary forewarning.

The *samiti*'s use of blood is thus inescapably caught within the symbolic universe of right-wing political mediations of blood as biomoral substance. The transactional enframement of the blood painting, and its metonymic threat, are both also features of the wider Indian sanguinary politics and can be used in order to articulate far narrower political visions than that of the *samiti*'s apparently broad and inclusive "secular" nationalism. Further, perhaps such shared features should cause us to reconsider whether the *samiti* is in fact as broadly secular and inclusive as it is presented by its founders. While conducting fieldwork, Gupta informed us that he had recently received the promise of a permanent home for his portraits in Vrindavan at the ashram of Hindu ascetic Sadhvi Rithambara. The location she offered would place the portraits firmly under a Hindutva sign. Sadhvi Rithambara is a Vishwa Hindu Parishad activist of particular notoriety known for her anti-Muslim rhetoric. She was legally charged with and widely regarded to have been instrumental in fueling the anti-Muslim tensions that resulted in the destruction of the Babri Masjid. For Gupta, this was a welcome solution to a practical problem: "Very few people come forward with money. I have to spend Rs. 400 a day [roughly $7]. We found it very difficult to get land for [a dedicated] museum in Delhi. But we will go to Vrindavan. . . . Sadhvi Ritham-bara, who has an ashram there, has spent 30 lakhs [$45,000] [on housing the portraits and contributing to their upkeep]. She is protecting this heritage for the coming generations."

While generous, Sadhvi Rithambara's grant should be measured against her Vrindavan NGO's annual revenue of over $60 million from wealthy Hindu diasporic donors alone. In 2010, Gupta took the Sadhvi up on her offer, and the National Martyrs Museum was opened within her sprawling NGO complex in Vrindavan. The inauguration of the *samiti*'s exhibition was attended by the uppermost echelons of Hindu nationalist politicians, including current prime minister Narendra Modi, then–BJP president Nitin Gadkari, Vishwa Hindu Parishad president Ashok Singhal, RSS leader Mohan Bhagwat, and BJP general secretary Vijay Goel.[19] Further, Sadhvi Rithambara's recontextualization of the paintings is explicitly anti-Muslim: "It is a rare work; the atrocities of past rulers have been exposed through portraits prepared in blood and it is praiseworthy; it is a symbol of committed patriotism."[20] The vague term "past rulers" is a well-known Hindutva category that seeks to encompass not only colonial rule, but a putatively violent precolonial Muslim rule. Thus, despite Gupta's claims toward a nondiscriminatory politics, his close complicity with Hindutva figures poses questions about the *samiti*'s claims of a secular universality. What the *samiti* and the Hindu right share is a commitment to the principle of bloodshed (of one's own and of others) as a prerequisite for national integrity; in their rendering, this is a resolutely "anti-Gandhian" stance. Explicitly, both Hindutva activists and Gupta's *samiti* share a commitment to a revisionist historiography that aims to foreground armed insurgents over nonviolent Gandhian *satyagrahis*. This revisionist impulse ties nonviolence together with weakness, effeminacy, and passivity, foregrounding the masculine ethos of the insurgents and finding in such insurgents a nascent commitment to a Hindu nation to come. Thus revised, Hindutva historiography calls upon past bloodshed to legitimize bloodshed in the present and to threaten its possibility in the future.

Hemo-politics and Hemophobias

Janet Carsten (2011) calls attention to the unbounded properties of blood as a liquid form (both corporeally and conceptually). Employing this suggestive terminology, we might say that these portraits provide intimations of unboundedness. In Gupta's portraits, the part given is an indication of the whole that is not given but that one is nevertheless willing to give if called upon. While the portraits may be considered a contemporary analogue of the call made by Bose for the citizenry to shed its blood, they are more representationally complex than Bose's refrain: blood is the medium that exhorts further bloodshed. Such bleeding is thus mimetic in two senses: in imitating the bleeding of one's sacrificial forebears, but also in terms of the willingness to sacrifice one's blood that it is supposed to incite in the viewer. The explicit aim of such mimetic bleeding—both in Gupta's formulation and in its later amplification through Sadhvi Rithambara's project—is to counter the dominance of Gandhian nonviolence in representations of the anticolonial struggle. In its stead, such projects of mimetic bleeding seek to counteract weakness in the face of violence and to enact a bloody Hindutva revision of anticolonial historiography. This revisionist Hindutva history divides the leaders of the anticolonial movement into two opposing camps: those affiliated with Gandhi's "effeminate, passive nonviolence," contrasted against those committed to a "masculine and violent" nationalism. This division allows Hindutva nationalists to write a more active role for themselves in the Indian anticolonial struggle.

To elaborate, histories of the anticolonial struggle have been written along three axes: the first foregrounds the role of Indian elites as collaborators in colonial rule, the second lauds the anticolonial ideologies of Gandhi and the secular Indian National Congress, and the third (in response to the first two), emphasizes subaltern consciousness and practices that are not easily assimilable into the pan-Indian categories of nationalism, secularism, or religion (Chakrabarty 2000). The pre-independence founders and leaders of Hindutva nationalism do not have a privileged position in any of these narratives; they are either considered irrelevant at best, or more committed to securing Hindu interests than opposing colonial rule. Thus, Hindutva nationalists find it difficult to find a lineage for their own brand of nationalist politics in all three dominant accounts of India's anticolonial history. Thus, in claiming Bose as one of their own, contemporary Hindutva nationalists seek to appropriate a figure from the conventional anticolonial pantheon and refigure him as a Hindu nationalist ideologue. That Bose formed alliances with the Axis powers during the Second World War against the British helps the Hindutva case, as they metamorphose him into an ally for their exclusionary vision of religious nationalism. But as Benjamin Zachariah has shown, Bose's relationship to fascism was very ambivalent: while he admired the early success of the "strong leaders" in Germany and Italy in 1935, by 1938 he recognized that those experiments had embarked on their own imperial missions. He clarified then that he might have somewhat misunderstood fascist politics as only "an aggressive form of nationalism" and nothing more (Zachariah 2010). The contemporary Hindutva revival of Bose is not attentive to such historical nuance. As resurrected by them, Bose is transformed into a resolutely anti-Gandhian armed insurgent willing to shed blood in the name of an exclusionary nationalism, a better exemplar for India's present than the contemporary heirs to the Congress legacy. Contemporary critics of Hindutva religious nationalism have strongly resisted this revisionist Hindutva narrative, stressing Bose's robust nonsectarian and socialist credentials and discrediting Hindutva attempts to establish Hindu nationalist roots for his revolutionary insurgency (Daniyal 2016). Yet while such a defense resists Bose's "saffronization" as a Hindutva ideologue, it leaves unchallenged the primary Hindutva polarization of anticolonial politics into the categories of nonviolent and violent. Significantly, it is this foundational divide that allows for contemporary Hindutva ideologues to build claims about the weakness and strength of the two kinds of anticolonial politics. And since this bifurcation is a necessary foundation for Hindutva revisionist history, defending Bose against saffronization leaves the door open for further appropriations of other nationalist figures and movements and for the castigation of secular and nonviolent politics as passive and ineffectual.

Foregrounding the liquid form of blood offers a different way to think of the relation between anticolonial and Hindutva politics: it leaks and congeals a messier set of relations. It is rarely the case that a neatly demarcated Gandhian nationalism stands diametrically opposed to a neatly demarcated nationalism of the Hindu right (or any other variety of Indian nationalism); rather, nationalist sensibilities manifest in various dialectical combinations (L. Cohen 2008). At a surface level, and in contradiction to its explicit intent, Gupta's paintings really present a relation (rather than an opposition) between Gandhian and Hindutva hemo-politics. As we have shown, Gandhi's imagination of blood takes a tripartite form—it indexes violence to be abhorred, seeks a machinelike steadiness in its hydraulic circulation within the body, and rejoices in the spillage of blood when it indexes that same steadiness in the face of sovereign power. Our rendering of Gandhi's hemo-politics challenges the division set up by Hindutva nationalists and, indeed, Gupta's *samiti* as well. In the Hindutva imagination, the spillage of blood was the provenance of the armed martyr, in direct opposition to the weak Gandhian who was unable to face such a violent prospect. As we have shown, based on this historiographical revision, Hindutva activists in the present decry an emasculated nation and seek a renewed spillage of blood—donated, painted, and sacrificed—so that the nation might again be made in the image of a blood-soaked nationalism. Our description of a Gandhian hemo-politics fascinated with the proper spillage of blood challenges the Hindutva depiction of Gandhian politics as hemophobic.

However, such a surface resemblance, even as it works to undo the Hindutva caricature of Gandhian nonviolence, does not leak deeply enough to erase the ideological gulf that separates Gandhian and Hindutva nationalisms. To clarify, in challenging the division of nonviolence and violence in Indian politics, we do not seek to collapse the two very different nationalist visions. As Joseph Alter reminds us, somatic nationalisms can take many divergent forms, even in the same regional context (Alter 1994b). Specifically, and in consonance with our effort here, Alter undercuts the superficial similarity between the practices of somatic discipline of Hindu wrestlers and that of Hindu nationalists. Focusing on the Hindu wrestlers' fixation with another biomoral substance—semen—he finds a deeper, richer biomoral world in which semen is understood literally as a national resource, empowering and sustaining both the ordinary citizen and the wrestler. Crucially however, even as such a biomoral imagination rests on Hindu concepts of substance and balance, it is fundamentally different from that of the Hindutva nationalist obsession with the exclusion of those outside the Hindu regional, linguistic, or upper-caste community.

In the same spirit, our intention here is to nuance the biomorality of blood such that we shift the grounds of difference from the polarity of violence and nonviolence to something more fundamental: the telos toward which their hemopolitics are directed. In the Hindutva imagination, the sacrifice of blood is always an event that intends to inaugurate a mimetic sovereign form in the future. Through portraitures and donations, blood circulates in the Hindutva imaginary to clear the ground for a Hindu nation and community to come: one united by blood. In contrast, Gandhian hemo-politics establishes a biomoral model within which the proper circulation of blood rests on a detachment from sovereignty and an achievement of a machinelike state of equilibrium in which the self dissolves into *satyagraha*—the force and quest for truth. In other words, if Hindutva hemopolitics aims at the foundation of a new community defined around blood—a means to an end—means and ends are inseparable in Gandhian hemo-politics. As we have described, the act of spilling blood was a demonstration of reconciliation with one's own finitude and a willing subordination to one's own death. Skaria describes this orientation of the *satyagrahi* as "surrender without subordination," or as the "gift of death" to one's enemy (Skaria 2016). As we have seen, the Hindutva sacrifice is directed at another and for a mimetic outcome—boundary-marking against Muslims, revivifying a Hindu nation, and reenacting past putatively masculine strength in the present. Much in contrast, the Gandhian sacrifice of blood was a sign and index of the propensity and ability to sacrifice for the sake of sacrifice.

Thus, our reading of Gandhi's sanguinary politics dispels Gupta's characterization of Gandhian nonviolence as timidly averse to bloodshed. Further, when the polarizing binaries of violence and nonviolence collapse, new spaces open in their stead that reveal the potent biomorality that inheres in blood as a substance.

Its spillage might index not only a willingness to be martyred but also conflicting theories of sovereignty, violence, and community. The Hindutva martyr's sacrifice clears the space for territorial and ideological consolidations, whereas the Gandhian *satyagrahi* rejects the sovereign command over self, territory, and ideology. If the Hindutva blood sacrifice testifies to Hindu nationalism, the sacrifice of the *satyagrahi* is a critique of nationalist forms that congeal to establish centers of power and peripheries—both colonial and anticolonial. Blood in Gandhian hemo-politics is a biomoral fluid that flows best when unencumbered by the clotting of power and sovereignty that afflicts both colonialism and the anticolonial movement with "meningitic" outbreaks. The Gandhian imagination of the automaton powered by perfect hydraulic equilibrium portends a politics beyond nationalism, sovereignty, and territory, enlivened only by the subordination of sovereign will. In stark contrast, the Hindutva body does not self-regenerate or self-purify; it fades easily unless revivified through the continuous reenactment of sacrifice. Finally, through portraitures and donations, blood circulates in the Hindutva imaginary to clear the ground for a Hindu nation and community to come, one united by blood and that unites biology with territory. In contrast, Gandhian hemo-politics disengage the proximate relationship between blood, community, and territory; pure blood is that which is impure, and sacral territory is that which is purified by death and the relinquishment of the will to territory.

3

SUBSTANTIAL ACTIVISMS

Our focus in this chapter is on bodily transactions—particularly of blood—that illuminate gaps between the given and the withheld, gaps that become the basis of political critique. The critiques they stage are of absences and deficits—where blood donated by religious groups indicates a deficit in familial giving, where paper hearts gifted by survivors of the Bhopal gas disaster to the prime minister signal his lack of one, and where portraits of politicians employing the artist's own blood are gifted in expectation of previously denied political patronage. The gift that is given critiques that which is ungiven: family members unwilling to donate blood for their transfusion-requiring relative, the care not provided by the Indian state for Bhopal survivors, and the denial of patronage by politicians to their constituents. We draw here on the works of John Davis and Alberto Corsín Jiménez on the proportionality of transactions (Davis 1992; Corsín Jiménez 2008, 180–97). As we noted in chapter 1, Corsín Jiménez elaborates upon Davis's work on partonomies in and out of balance in material exchanges in observing that "the part that we give is an indication of the whole that is not given—that is, what you see (the gift) is what you do not get (the larger social whole). Gift-giving is thus an expression and effect of proportionality" (186). We extend this insight to illustrate how acts of bodily giving over may operate critically by way of partonomic relations between the given and not given, with that which is given underscoring that which is not (the deficits and absences we referred to earlier).

Such scenes of bodily giving over constitute a historically significant genre of political performance in relation to the ebbs and flows of other modes of activist signification. Jonathan Spencer describes an extreme negative valuation of the political in the subcontinent, describing people of diverse backgrounds as at once "appalled and fascinated" by political goings on, frequently commenting on the unsavoriness of politics ("dirty work") and on the moral failings of particular politicians (Spencer 2007, 22). Jonathan Parry, meanwhile, comments memorably on the moral pollution associated relentlessly and invariably with politics in the region, recounting Banaras funeral priests' description of the great difficulty in making a politician's body burn due to "the enormous burden of sin accumulated with his corrupt earnings" (1994, 127). If political sincerity is considered to be in such deficit, strategies such as the political fast have long aimed to redress this arrear. For Mohandas Gandhi, performed as a component of *satyagraha* (truth force), fasting was the mass political tool par excellence. Whereas if a politician now fasts, so the saying goes, he only does so between breakfast and lunch. If a political fast appears to be of a notable duration, the figure concerned has likely been "stealthily eating all night long" (Ramaswamy 1997, 230). Thus, one mode to evidence political sincerity becomes its own undoing. But if a political fast contains easy avenues for sleight of hand, the visual spectacle of politicians or party activists "bleeding for a cause" seems not to leave room for such speculation: the evidence is before your eyes—the bag is filled. Which is to say that the felicity of the presentation successfully supplements the constative substance of the statement or appeal. Extraction as enunciation could thus appear to move beyond the critique of political signs. Not unlike the promise that once attached to photographs as records of facts "about which there could be no doubt" (Pinney 2011, 54)—"every photograph . . . indisputably a document of an event, an event that could not be denied" (80)—political extractive events appeared to be "seared" with "reality" (Benjamin, cited in Pinney 2011, 86) in a way that the fast could never be. We suggest then that blood donation spectacles act as "rituals of verification."[1] It is because the blood extracted on political occasions holds an elusive promise of political transparency that we may term it *promissory matter*.[2]

Yet as we shall show in this chapter, blood—even while performing a ritual of sincerity and verification—exposes itself to accusations of dissembling and deception. When used as a substance of political communication, blood indexes conviction and an interior moral truth. But when used for the same effect by politicians perceived as corrupt, it drains the communicative medium of its material intimacy with sincerity. Further, in our discussion of explicitly activist actions, we track how the promise of truth and interiority in blood goes hand in hand with its ability to index violence. Specifically, in our discussion of activism in the aftermath of the Bhopal disaster, we show how blood comes to materialize the violence of the long unfolding event, at the same time as it evidences the political transparency of its consequent activist mobilization. And in our related discussion of activism around menstrual politics, we show how blood becomes a matter of celebration that verifies a feminist politics, at the same time as it stands in as an index of sexual violence. Through this chapter then, we trace this central tension in blood as political media: at the same time as the substance promises a performance of a sincere moral interiority, it simultaneously holds the potential to reveal the corruption and duplicity of political enunciations. And at the same time as it verifies the truth and transparency of activist claims, it exposes the violence that produces the need for an activist response.

Philanthropy

On 21 November 2004, at a Sant Nirankari *satsang* (devotional gathering) just off a busy arterial road in West Delhi, a group of young devotees visiting from Chandigarh performed a sketch on the theme of blood donation. The sketch dramatized the story of a young boy injured in a traffic accident. The boy's father declares that he is too busy to donate blood for the transfusion his son needs, but the two Nirankari devotees who brought the boy to hospital volunteer instead:

> DEVOTEES: We are willing. Take our blood. We are human beings. We are not related through blood, we don't even know him. But we have with him a relation of humanity.
>
> DOCTOR: That is strange. You are helping and his relatives are not. These days blood relations don't help, blood relations are finishing. You have come here and you are not his blood relations. A stranger is trying to help. Are you Nirankaris?
>
> DEVOTEES: Yes. How do you recognize us?
>
> DOCTOR: These days, Nirankaris are giving a lot of blood.
>
> *Later, after his transfusion and he is no longer critically ill, the boy begins to sob.*
>
> BOY: I'm crying because the persons related to me by blood didn't help me, but you strangers (*anjaan*) on the road who are not related to me by blood, you helped me. You gave blood. In my hour of sorrow all my relatives turned away. I will never forget your kindness.
>
> DEVOTEES: Do not be obliged. It is our guru's orders to help human beings with blood. He says humanity is the greatest relation. We have not done anything great; we have only done our duty. Perhaps God wanted to teach you a lesson: only humanity is the real relation. Now take rest.
>
> BOY: God is great. Now I realize the greatest relation is of humanity, not of blood.

The Sant Nirankari movement forms part of an inclusive reformist tradition that crosses formal "community" boundaries between Hindus and non-Hindus. Along with other likeminded reformist movements, the Sant Nirankaris relate to and draw inspiration from the *sant* tradition of North India: a loose family of nonsectarian saints, often from lower-caste backgrounds, who criticized elaborate upper-caste rituals and practices of idol worship. However, while rejecting idolatry in favor of a formless god (*nirankar*), Nirankari devotees coalesce around living *gurus* (*satgurus*) and attend his discourses in communal gatherings (*satsang*). And while gurus say that to donate blood is to participate in the service of humanity, devotees view it as much as a service or sacrifice to the guru (*guru-seva*), to his this-worldly glory, and for which, in turn, they will receive the guru's blessings and *gyan* (knowledge).[3] Blood donation as a philanthropic practice thus appears here at the conjunction of abstract altruism and concrete practices of self-interest.

Nirankari Colony, northwest Delhi, 24 April 2004—it is Human Unity Day (*Manav Ekta Divas*), a pivotal date in the Nirankari devotional calendar that commemorates the assassination of former guru Baba Gurbachan Singh on the same date in 1980.[4] The former leader's sacrifice is annually remembered through the staging of large-scale gatherings at which devotees are strongly encouraged to donate their blood. Many thousands of devotees give blood on this day in Nirankari Colony, where the guru will address gathered devotees, but also at scores of *satsang bhavans* around the world. The Nirankaris thus stage a positively revalued reenactment of the trauma of losing their former guru, converting his martyrdom from an experience of victimhood into one of self-initiated ennobling virtue. In doing this, they attribute to the successor guru an exhortatory aphorism about the transformation of violent bloodshed into spiritually meaningful donation: "Blood should flow into veins (*nari*), not drains (*nali*)." An announcement over the public address system declares, "When a brother, a sister, or a son in a family is in need of blood, everyone says take as much money as you want, but we cannot give [our own] blood. The relatives of some Nirankari donors say, 'Why are you giving blood?,' but it is great of them to give blood for humanity."

In both this loudspeaker announcement and the staged drama, Nirankaris imagine the possibility of constituting a social form through the act of giving blood. The relation between this constitution of a wider social form and bodily giving is partonomic: in our opening drama the gift of Nirankari blood gestures to, and is only required because of, a prior gift withheld by the family. The seemingly paradoxical final utterance of the boy only makes sense in the framework of this entanglement of the given and not given; the abstract social form of the *anjaan* is made sensible through the repersonalized figure of the errant family. "God is great. Now I realize the greatest relation is of humanity, not of blood."

But, of course, it *is* a relation of blood, if not a conventional blood relation. After all, this is a drama that seeks to performatively call into being future altruistic donations. The devotee-performers both mourn the passing of "true" blood relations (*khun ke rishte*) and celebrate the coming of the successor relation: the widened-out tie of humanity (*insaniyat ka rishta*). The bad family is vividly portrayed: too busy to care and donate for its own. The new abstract relations made possible by blood donation (*insaniyat*) rest upon a call to the passing of an older, more concrete relation of biological blood (*khun ke rishte*). If we call attention here to such a form of bodily giving as philanthropy, it is to suggest that the philanthropic imagination of anonymous giving is predicated on its particular repersonalizations. The *anjaan*, after all, is not the anonymous stranger presumed by modern philanthropy, but rather takes its meaning from the North Indian *sant* tradition. At the same time, the critique here of the familial order does not lead in a straightforward line to its rejection. In other words, the familial blood-relation (*khun ke rishte*) does not entirely eclipse the idea of a personal blood-relation but seeks to recuperate it as another kind of blood-relation (*insaniyat ka rishta*). The blood-gift critiques here by way of its partonomic form: the given indicates its entanglement with the not-given; the gift presupposes that it was previously withheld. Philanthropic critique—as we shall continue to argue in this chapter—is thus a partonomic relation between the concrete practice of giving and a prior failure of giving that threatens the constitution of a social whole.

The relation between the reform of blood donation and the social reformist agenda of the Sant Nirankari tradition here finds echoes in other alliances, or relations of reform, underpinned by practices of substance-exchange in contemporary India. Lawrence Cohen tracks precisely such a reformation of the body politic in postindependence cinema (2001). In his analysis of two films—*Sujata* and *Amar Akbar Anthony*—Cohen tracks at least two moments of a "nationalist recoding" of blood. In the dénouement of both films, an upper-caste mother figure lies in expectancy of a blood transfusion in a hospital bed. Until this point, the narrative burden of both films has been to relate how "traditional" forms of relation—caste and religion—lead to her malaise. Finally, in both films, the upper-caste mother figure is rescued by the donation of blood from the lower-caste daughter-in-law, on the one hand, and sons raised Muslim and Christian, on the other. In this postindependence imagination of India's political future, blood donation thus operates to dissolve the boundaries of caste and religion. Such an imagination is suffused with the Nehruvian imaginary of the times, where cinema played a pedagogic function to urge audiences to renounce dividing, subnational ties. In such cinematic gestures, the weakened and reconstituted mother figure often served as a powerful cipher for the nation and the future nation-making project at hand (Ramaswamy 2009).

But why do sanguinary politics serve as the privileged conduit for nationalist imaginations in India? Why is blood so particularly potent in conveying the weakening and strengthening of familial or national solidarity? As we discussed in chapter 1, McKim Marriott posited a "dividual," monistic (nondualist) nature of personhood in the region whereby people were understood as capable of both giving out and absorbing coded material substances—that is, substances imbued with personal character traits or particular moral qualities (Marriott 1976). In explicit contrast to Schneider's description of kinship practices in the United States, South Asianist ethnosociologists drew upon Marriott to distinguish "western" personhood from what they took to be a quite distinctive South Asian variety. For instance, it is well known that in many Hindu villages throughout India, caste boundaries continue to be maintained in part through restrictions on who eats and drinks with whom (Lambert 2000, 73–89). Scholars such as Inden and Nicholas declared code and substance to be inseparable in Bengali culture—for example, adoption, a "social" or "fictive" form of kinship, may take place only within and not between castes—and Marriott himself took to underscoring this inseparability through use of the term "substance-code" (Inden and Nicholas 2005). Brilliant as Marriott's Samkhya- and Ayurveda-inspired modeling of the implicit categories structuring South Asian life is, the sources drawn on can appear arbitrary and the categories and correspondences set in stone, while the possibility that South Asians might treat these reflexively and even dynamically deploy them in inventive ways seems entirely discounted.[5] In our description of practices of bodily giving over, we focus precisely on reflexive and inventive deployments that contravene the norms and correspondences modeled by Marriott. The licit and illicit flows of bodily substances that we describe carry the danger of contagious social contact—often contravening class and caste norms. For example, what we see in the case of Nirankari devotees' pedagogic performances is how a key category within Marriott's schema (substance-code) may persist precisely by way of an intervention that highlights a failure in the norm. The problem the performances address is that of the perceived disjuncture between substance and code—that is, between blood and its constitution of North Indian family relations. The performance of reform described above operationalizes an expansively redefined code—from the fallen modern Indian family (L. Cohen 1998)—to a widely conceived humanity, achievable through a more generalized diffusion of substance via voluntary blood donation. Similarly, in its official literature, the Sant Nirankari order is explicitly critical of the decoupling of duty and care (the order of law/code) from ties of blood (the order of nature/substance). It proposes a successor relation-form achievable through blood donation, with devotees' donated blood coded with knowledge, spirit, and intentions, enabling devotees "to establish blood relationship with other human beings" (Sant

Nirankari Mandal 2003, 20). And as we have seen, these will be "relations of humanity," a term that suggests a divorce between substance and code—with relational coding (duty, care) no longer dependent on substance (the blood tie)—but which, in fact, remain based upon substance (the blood tie). Thus, the reformation of the body politic through blood rests firmly upon an imagined form that already entangles substance and code.

In the Nirankari narrative, the contemporary family first divorces code from substance when relatives refuse to donate blood for one another (in replacement). It then rejoins substance and code in a perversely restricted manner when non-Nirankaris enjoin their Nirankari family members *not* to give blood "for humanity," suggesting that Nirankaris' care for unknown others would detract from their ability to care for their known dependents due to a damaging depletion of blood. The devotees reverse the archetypal demands of blood donation in the region—demands are not made on devotees for their blood; neither do they demand to receive it. Instead, they demand to give it. This, then, is a reflectively situated alignment of substance-code. Perceiving their contemporary detachment, the Nirankari response is to seek to restore their symbiosis via blood donation as a mechanism of promise and critique. The image is of donated Nirankari blood circulating outward, mixing with many other bloods to both restore and reformulate (for the scale is entirely different) the unity of substance-code—Marriott redux.

Performing Sincerity

While the scale of the nationalist imaginary is grander, the tension between the corrupt and the restorative functions of blood is equally at play in the political rallies that we first introduced in chapter 1. If the Nirankaris stake a future utopic humanity on the corruption of the contemporary family, political blood-donation rallies too are rife with the ambivalent entanglement of utopic futures and a dystopic present.

Political blood camp rallies, such as those conducted by the Congress and Samajwadi parties, suggest a reversal of the flow of forcible extraction that we described in the previous chapter, with vampirelike politicians (colonial and postcolonial) sucking the blood of the *janata* (people). If the *janata*'s blood/money is usually figured as flowing to the political class, part of what such rallies seek to communicate is a reversal of the flow. That is, the political class offers its own replenishing substance to the *janata*. The rise of the sanguinary political rally in the era of economic liberalization may thus be understood as far from coincidental. Critics responded to the Hindu far-right political party Shiv Sena's massive blood donation camp on Maharashtra Day in 2010 by stating that rather than taking people's blood, it should be providing them with water. As Nikhil Anand demonstrates, claims on matter form a vital part of Mumbai's city life, as its political ebbs and flows constitute a form of "hydraulic citizenship" that tie together material and semiotic urban infrastructures (Anand 2017). The blood donated at such rallies seemed to substitute for those substances of the civic and of development—water, electricity—that people really need. Rather than provide services, the political class instead provides blood via unpersuasive postures of commitment. A substance that had promised to demarcate a communicative sphere beyond symbolism, blood is relegated squarely back into the domain of the purely symbolic: political blood donation appears as a nostalgic attempt to reanimate the template of the "maa-baap" paternalistic-yet-benevolent state (Gould 2011, 182) in an era in which utilities are increasingly privatized. If marginalized groups in Mumbai exert pressure upon the civic state to provide water flows, the state in this instance responded with its own hydraulic imaginary—both desperate and strikingly out of place. The party's supremo (*pramukh*) Bal Thackeray responded to hydraulic citizenship claims by stating, "Blood donation is the real social work," while at the Bombay Municipal Corporation (BMC) "the leader of the house, Sunil Prabhu from the Shiv Sena, suggested that his party should get a pat on their back from the BMC for a successful blood-donation drive."[6] Indicative of its public-spiritedness and ethos of *seva*, the blood drive is the sovereign gift of the party. But a Congress corporator responded, "*Sena ko Mumbai aur Mumbaikaron ka khoon chusne ki aadat hai. Toh isme nayi baat kya hai?*" ("Sena is known for sucking the blood of the common Mumbaikar. There's nothing new or praiseworthy about this?"). We are back, then, with the more familiar practice and metaphor of illicit extraction. The accusation is that the party sucks the blood of city dwellers, which it then passes off as a gift from itself; the donated blood is framed as a gift to the very janata, or Mumbaikar, it is extracted from. But that was not all. Another Congress corporator "alleged that the blood donation drive was conducted by luring union workers in the Shiv Sena with the promise of a permanent job."[7] Whether or not there is weight to the accusation, it contains more than a faint echo of the forcible deals of Emergency-era India, in which the granting or regularization of plots of land might be dependent on undergoing sterilization (Tarlo 2003). The very means by which the party seeks to show it does constructive *seva*—providing for, not extracting from, the people—is reduced back down to the level of (literal) *khuun choosna* (sucking blood). In such scenes of fake and extractive giving, the partonomic logic of bodily philanthropy becomes dangerously transparent. The gift presented as a remedy is reframed itself as poisonous due to its prior illicit extraction. In the political camp, it is no longer easy to distinguish between the remedy and the poison, or the gift that is given from that which is extracted, or the reformist part from the suspended whole.

This prompts further reflections on witnessed bleeding. In 2002 a controversy arose when Hindi film icon Amitabh Bachchan inaugurated a series of blood donation camps for the Uttar Pradesh–based political outfit the Samajwadi Party (SP). They were staged during a state assembly election campaign, a time when the election commission's model code comes into force, which is meant to prohibit "vote buying" by candidates eager to hand out "electoral freebies" (frequently saris, cooking vessels, alcohol, and cash). The SP's rival, the Congress Party, lodged a complaint with the commission, alleging that "Mr. Bachchan and the SP leaders were using the blood donation camps to gain political mileage. . . . These camps are being synchronized with the election campaign and they amount to an offer of allurement to the voters."[8] The complaint was that blood donation was being deployed to legitimate otherwise forbidden political bribes. One implication was that since the event was associated with the SP, the blood collected might be viewed as a "gift" to the public from whom it seeks votes. More significant, however, is how the "token of regard," which by law is quite acceptable for blood camp organizers to offer to blood donors on completion of their donations, can be used to set up an exchange that otherwise would be obstructed. At a time when gifts to voters are explicitly forbidden, and this indeed being the only time that political functionaries would want to make them, the exchange is performed obliquely in the guise of another exchange (which legitimately inheres within the setup of blood camps). That is, taking the donor-voter's blood allows the party in turn to offer back what they would not be allowed to give (e.g., saris, cooking vessels) if there wasn't a blood donation event acting as an "exchange cover," whilst at the same time also making visible an electorally useful association between the party and social service.

The intimacy between blood donation and corruption reappears in the following news story, which made headlines in December 2013:

> Plumbing new depths of sycophancy, dozens of Mahila (women) Congress activists happily posed for photographs claiming that they had donated blood to mark the birthday of party president Sonia Gandhi, at Gandhi Bhavan in Hyderabad on Monday. The problem, however, was that very few of them—three by our count—had actually donated blood. The rest merrily posed for pictures on the stretcher. State Mahila Congress president Akula Lalitha said that 15 activists had donated blood. She said it was common for publicity hounds to pose for pictures with fake claims. Doctors from Red Cross Society, Barkatpura, who collected the blood, said that they had faced such situations many a times.[9]

As we noted earlier, party-organized blood donation camps are liable to be canceled if a leader is unable to attend, and if the leader does attend, they often break up immediately upon the leader's departure. The above example is of the same genus as such (abortive) camps, but its cynicism was more glaringly ripe for media exposé. The *actually* posed blood donation camp seemed to underscore its logical extension—the posed nature of the rest of the sanguinary politics. What was in any case a thoroughly gestural politics, here we finally locate its "purest" fake form. We quote now a selection of the reader comments below the main text of the online version of the article:

> by Indian_anna on Tue, 2013-12-10 12:52
>
> we should thank them for not giving the genuine blood, as we do not need a corrupt blood from these liars . . .

> by nsrivastava2 on Wed, 2013-12-11 09:24
>
> You are so true. Those 3 who donated shall take back their's.

> by a k shetty on Tue, 2013-12-10 16:12
>
> these ladies are behind all these scam . . .

> by TS on Tue, 2013-12-10 16:38
>
> What else can you expect from them when they are working under the leadership of "Amma" Fake people. . . . Shame on you all . . .

> by WP on Tue, 2013-12-10 17:52
>
> Seriously? Blood donation is one of the easiest things you can do to help a fellow human being. It hurts as much as a mosquito bite, does not leave scars and best of all, you can start your normal work right after you donate. If these ladies feel the need to fake even that, I am at a loss for words.

> by Shah minhaj on Wed, 2013-12-11 19:35
>
> . . . its funny and shameful how desperate they are to get in the picture!!

> by BG on Wed, 2013-12-11 22:17
>
> These might be the same people who say "we need a change" without any contribution . . .

by VKV.Ravichandran on Thu, 2013-12-12 04:55

Nauseating. Shame on the part of Congress. When will people reject out right this kind of shameless politicians. What gives them confidence that people can be fooled and cheated by enacting such cheap drama. These hypocrites suck your blood out.

by SoniaGoBackToItaly on Thu, 2013-12-12 05:52

With that fake smile and intention they look like "those types" waiting in the bed, pathetic!! I hope no one would need to receive their blood, it is all dirty with politics.[10]

Clearly, different axes were being ground in the forum. The avatar names of the commentators themselves provide interest: "SoniaGoBackToItaly" is suggestive of the Hindu right's interest in the story, from which it unsurprisingly sought to draw political capital. Likewise, "a k shetty" employs the language of the scam. This and the headline itself ("Fake blood donation shames Congress in Andhra Pradesh") draws this event into the sort of national conversation that issues of fakery and duplication (L. Cohen 2012; 2017) enjoy in the country. These are conversations that take in, among other things, fake gurus, fake milk products, and most notoriously "fake encounters," which refers to the staging of extrajudicial executions in Kashmir and elsewhere *as if* they had been enacted in combat situations. If those army and police personnel who enact fake encounters are said to do so in order to gain professional advancement ("to collect bounties and add stars to their epaulets" [Duschinski 2010, 124]), a similar logic inhabits the staged blood donation camp through which party workers seek advancement in the party.

Visible here is a kind of degenerative symmetry: in chapter 1 we noted that on Sonia Gandhi's birthday in 2003, Youth Congress activists organized blood donation events at which they signed anticorruption pledges. In that instance, the enactment of blood donation helped register a message of committed anticorruption. However, the same leader's birthday ten years later generated comments declaring that the "corrupt blood of these liars" must remain uncollected: "I hope no one would need to receive their blood, it is all dirty with politics." "Those 3 who donated shall take back their's [sic]." Their body parts, dirtied by their bad characters, must not be allowed to circulate and infect others. Corruption means that politicians' bodies don't burn in Banaras (Parry 1994); it also means that their blood must not be transfused into the body politic. We noted above the currency of the phrase that politicians suck blood (*khuun choosna*), an image featured in cartoons in which corruption is figured as transfusion into the politicians' body. Here the commentator VKV.Ravichandran reiterates the sentiment in English

("These hypocrites suck your blood out") as a means of explaining: Well *of course* their blood donation was fake—political parties only *take* people's blood.

Finally, WP asks why the activists were in any case reluctant given that "blood donation is one of the easiest things you can do to help a fellow human being." And here we can gain a sense of why the sanguinary politics, despite the public circulation of such discreditable stories, retains at least some vigor: verifiable extractions enact political commitment and truth because of one's own reluctance to do likewise. If the Congress members *had* donated, it would have been a sacrifice, a "giving over" (Cohen 2013) to the leader and to the *janata*. As it happens, their alarm at the prospect of donation overcame their willingness to enact it, and the media was willing and able to register this. What we mean to say here is that *the scandal was to do with the extraction not happening, not with the "truth" of it if it had.* To assert that the sanguinary politics has been recast wholesale as a dissembling political form would be going too far; its continued enactment in a large variety of mass political settings suggests it continues to possess some degree of communicative efficacy. Consider, for instance, the case of the high-profile Maharashtra Committee for the Eradication of Superstitious Practices (*Maharashtra Andhashraddha Nirmulan Samiti*, or MANS), which campaigns across the state to expose the spuriousness of what it sees as irrational and dangerous religious practices that exploit the credulous and vulnerable. The major aim of the organization is to pass legislation in the state parliament that will make illegal precisely these forms of religious practice. In 2005, MANS succeeded in persuading the Maharashtra State Legislature to approve the "Eradication of Black Magic and Evil Aghori Practices Bill." However, due to a concerted and sometimes violent campaign on the part of right-wing Hindu organizations who claim that the bill was specifically targeted at Hindu forms of religious worship, which it would effectively criminalize, the bill has not yet—to MANS's dismay—been signed into law.

MANS sought an appointment with the chief minister to press its case. Finally, it resorted to a letter-writing campaign using activists' own blood. The movement's then-leader, Narendra Dabholkar, recalled to us a particular campaign:[11]

> We decided to write letters to the chief minister [CM], [Congress leader] Sonia Gandhi, and [local "big man" politician and then-central government minister] Sharad Pawar with our own blood, from MANS workers. We took out just 3 ml of blood from the vein in a special syringe— enough for three to four sentences only. Then, using small brushes, we wrote letters to the CM. More than a thousand letters were sent to the CM. Nobody objected or ridiculed the idea, but everyone was now sure of the integrity of the organization, so ultimately the result was that the CM was compelled to discuss with us.

This is to say that, finally, MANS had found the right elicitory form and obtained the appointment. To cite one report, "Dr. Dabholkar informed that about 300 such letters would be written to the Government, where the 'number' is not an issue but the issue is about the 'pain.'" Physical self-subjection thus also formed a component of the correct manifestation. However, number and endurance were insufficient in themselves. Rather, it seemed that activists' use of their own blood was critical for demonstrating an "integrity"—a "congruence between avowal and actual feeling" (Trilling 1971, 2) made tangible and discernible via externalization of moral interiors ("actual feeling") as bloody text ("avowal") that "compelled" the chief minister to pay attention. MANS had finally located the correct performative supplement to the constative. In what follows, we take a closer ethnographic look at another such "successful" performative linkage of moral interiority with blood. In doing this, we trace how certain actors are able to continually deploy blood as a material ritual of verification, despite the accusations of dissembling that have come to be leveled against its deployment by politicians perceived as corrupt.

Persuasive Portraiture

Shihan Hussaini of Chennai, Tamil Nadu state, is a karate and archery teacher, but he also runs a fine arts academy offering instruction in sculpture, dance, and painting. We waited for him in his office, which displayed swords, guns, arrows, daggers, and a huge Buddha head. Through a window we watched an attendant arrange fifty-seven paintings of the former chief minister (state-level head of government) of Tamil Nadu, Jayalalitha—all painted using the artist's blood. There were mirrors on each wall, which multiplied the bloody images (figures 5 and 6). Why did he engage in such an exercise? The reason, he explains, was simple: he needed land for a karate school. For this he required an appointment with the chief minister.

> After I had 101 cars run over my hand [Hussaini is known for such spectacular feats] I did a portrait of Jayalalitha. Had I just done a painting and no blood, it would have achieved nothing. She brought me to her residence and promised me 1 million dollars. . . . She asked why did I do it. I said I knocked on your door several times, but there was no reply. I had to run trucks over my hand and paint your portrait in my blood! [However,] once [the promise] was announced, some bureaucrats changed the decision and the land was taken [from me]. The next year she turned fifty-seven, so I did fifty-seven portraits. But she was

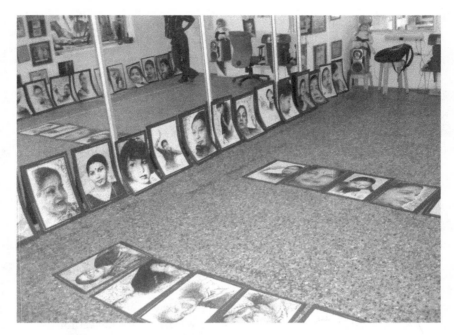

FIGURE 5. Hussaini's paintings. (Photo by the authors.)

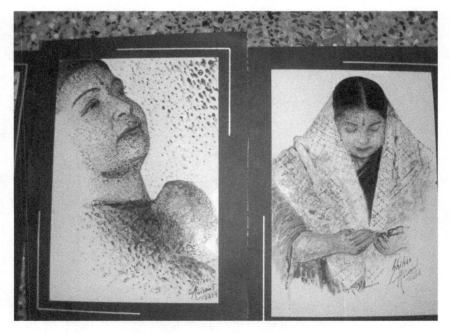

FIGURE 6. Portraits of Jayalalitha in blood. (Photo by the authors.)

subjected to sixty [legal] cases, so couldn't give me the land. When she comes back I will influence her to get the land. This is to influence decision-making.

Hussaini is explicit concerning his theory of art:

Blood art is a tool of propaganda, communication, and influencing decision-making. . . . I go and ask for a favor, and I give them a painting in my blood. I have influenced several people with my own blood portraits of them. For me, it is not aesthetic—it is to influence thought, decision-making, people, an entire idea to be implanted in people.

In other words, this is interventionist art, created in order to compel particular outcomes. Hussaini's portraits thus attempt, with some success, to compel or oblige via aspects of their form. First, there is the sheer number of them:

[Jayalalitha] was fifty-seven years old, so I did fifty-seven blood portraits. . . . I'm adding them up every year. My very first portrait was for land, and I got it, but subsequently I had an exhibition in 2001 and the Karunanidhi [Jayalalitha's successor and fierce rival] government was so offended by the blood painting they raided my place and took this painting. . . . I said, you take—I will make fifty-seven more. Till now I have never got it back. The original one is lost forever. So in defiance of this daylight robbery by the state machinery, I did fifty-seven more paintings [in blood of Jayalalitha]. . . . With an election coming, [Karunanidhi] thought it was only for propaganda. The paintings were taken. I fasted [to protest]. I was forced [to stop] by friends because the police were arranging and putting false [legal] cases on me. My riposte was to do fifty-seven more paintings of Jayalalitha and another every year on February 24—Jayalalitha's birthday.

With one portrait for every year of the chief minister's life, an acutely personal formula is set up between quantities of lifetime and offering. Its enumerative form seems to help make the gift compelling (in the sense of the adjective but also the verb—force or oblige). Yet each image forms only a small part of a larger concern, for another is added every year. There is, in this sense, only one (ongoing) collective portrait. But enumerative form is also a site of vulnerability for Hussaini. The critical mass of "sixty legal cases" against Jayalalitha meant that she couldn't make good her promise to him, while the very need to create more portraits was a result of their initial theft by Jayalalitha's political opponents, an action seeming to demonstrate the superior efficacy of his competitors over his own artistic efforts at political influence. It is not surprising that media reportage found in Hussaini's literally bloody art an excess that reconfirmed the perversity of Tamil Nadu's modes of political expression. For instance, the paintings were bracketed by both the BBC and local newspapers with a case from 2003 in which a man from Vellore was reported to have cut off his tongue as a birthday offering to the chief minister.[12] Initiating a user-led discussion with the title "Why Do Tamils Burn Themselves?," an Indian news website has enlisted Hussaini's paintings as further compelling evidence of Tamil Nadu's status as politically pathological.[13] It is worth pointing out that it was also in Chennai (the capital of Tamil Nadu) that Lawrence Cohen conducted an interview with a female slum dweller who, already having sold one kidney to settle a debt, invoked Jayalalitha's predecessor as leader of the All India Anna Dravida Munnetra Kazhagam Party, the former chief minister M. G. Ramachandran (MGR), and his need for a kidney transplant, in making the following startling admission: "He was dying, and received one from his niece; they did the operation in America. At that time, I did not know about kidneys. If I had, I would have given him both of mine" (1999). Elsewhere Lawrence Cohen (2004, 167) has analyzed such ideational-corporeal political relations in terms of a citizen's operative form, where one's body is always potentially a countergift to the state, "in some cases as a sacrifice resurrecting a failing or absent sovereign." Hussaini's portraits point toward the variety of media employed in enacting such a corporeal exchange relationship.

We use "enact" advisedly. Hussaini enacted his devotion in compelling fashion. He attained an audience with the chief minister—no small feat. He provided media-friendly quotes: "'There were times when I passed out [when having blood drawn]. But I persisted.' Mr Hussaini says that he worships the Chief Minister as 'Ma Shakti,' or the goddess of power. . . . 'It shows my admiration for Ms Jayalalitha, who is a woman of great courage.'" Moreover, the BBC article on Hussaini treats his portraits as a quintessential example of the way in which in South India, "the dividing line between politics and cinema is blurred [with] fans often going to extreme lengths to display their affection." Yet in conversation with us, Hussaini was explicit about the performative nature of his "fandom": "The reports were wrong. I am not a fan! [i.e., he did it not out of devotion but because he wanted land]. All poets play praise for rulers. Unless you eulogize and iconize your kings and CMs, you're not going to get your commission. I did not draw her portrait because I am a fan—but because it is a tool." While such a utilitarian analysis surely accounts for the ends the artist sought to accomplish, it hardly does justice to the means. The material presence of the artist in Hussaini's portraits was necessary for achieving something very particular: a relation to the subject of representation in the "space" of—which is to say enframed within—the portrait. In a consideration of John Berger's (2007) writings on drawing, Michael Taussig (2009) highlights the intimacy between drawer and thing drawn: "Each confirmation or denial brings you closer to the object, until finally you are, as it were, inside it: the contours you have drawn no longer marking the edge of what you have seen, but the edge of what you have become. . . . A drawing is an auto-biographical record of one's discovery of an event, seen, remembered, or imagined" (Berger, cited in Taussig 2009, 269). In drawing, one gets close to an object. The drawing forms an intimate material relation. In the case of Hussaini's portraits, the act of representation no doubt brings the artist closer to the represented in the manner suggested by Berger. But there is an intensification of the relation achieved by way of the artist's indexical physical presence within the portrait—substance delineating subject. The aniconic element—the sanguinary medium as literal index of the artist—is present as substantive delineation of the icon it comprises, the relation both formed and displayed in the space of the portrait itself. The image objectifies a relation and is that relation; as Marilyn Strathern puts it, one can "not only perceive relations between things but also perceive things as relations" (2005, 63). This relation—made and displayed in the image itself—is integral to its ability to affectively persuade. Hussaini ultimately might not have obtained the land he sought, but the mere granting of an audience with the chief minister attests to the success of what might be called the propaganda of the image. As Michael Carrithers points out, direct access to Indian political leaders—ordinarily extremely difficult to secure—may be "vital for life chances, in politics, in business, or in education" (2010, 255). The fusing of subject and object in the medium of the portrait forces a relation upon the anticipated viewing subject/recipient. Hussaini's portraits compel not by invoking the wider relationships out of which the presenter/giver is made up, but by materializing (and inflicting) a relationship between the corporeal self and the recipient onto the recipient. A priori encoding of the form of the relation in the image was thus, in Hussaini's own words, a tool. Strathern, too, explicitly defines the relation as the anthropologist's tool, for anthropologists "use relations to explore relations" (2005, 7). Specifically, anthropologists "operate two kinds of relations at the same time" (2005, 7)—the conceptual and the interpersonal. The relational portrait, toollike, caused an invisible (conceptual) relation between ruler and unknown subject to become a visible (interpersonal) relation between ruler and known subject—the portrait a kind of relational intervention.

We have stated that the portraits objectify a relation; let us now consider more carefully the properties of the "blood tie" created in the images. First of all, Hussaini's portraits form a part not only of the wider sanguinary politics but also of a tradition of political praise offering in South India that is characterized by relations of "hierarchical intimacy" (Bate 2002). Preminda Jacob describes the particularly intimate association of visual culture and political power in Tamil Nadu, pointing out, for instance, that all five politicians that have headed the state's government since 1967 have been products of the film industry (Jacob 2009). Poems and images printed in local newspapers by local political functionaries or low-level community leaders in honor of these film-stars-turned-political-leaders (in particular, Jayalalitha) "aestheticize power as an intimate being, such as a family deity or mother, who will grant us the benefits of her presence and respond to our appeals" (Bate 2002, 309). Locating its roots in the medieval bhakti tradition of devotional love, Bate describes how images of Jayalalitha are framed in ways that underscore her royal-and-divine identity. Yet such "hierarchical distancing" of the leader is fused with tropes of intimacy: Bate offers the example of a central print of Jayalalitha surrounded by sixty smaller images of exactly the same image, with their warm gazes seemingly directed downward toward the advertiser himself—the head of the Tamil Nadu Sales Board—whose image is located at the bottom right of the advertisement (318). If, once again, quantity is a key quality of an image that is both many and one at the same time, in tying the advertiser's name to that of great political leaders, what such images and their attendant poetry achieve is, of course, a relation. In other words, these "portraits" are not simply of the leader; neither are they simply self-portraits. They are portraits of the advertiser in relation to the political leader that also create this relation.

Hussaini's portraits, indeed, partake of this genre—the relation both made and made visible in the space of the portrait. But the use of blood heightens the intimacy of the relation discussed by Bate. The portraits adhere to—but critically exceed—the regional convention of political praise offering. This brings us back to Berger's account of drawing. As was noted earlier, the material qualities of Hussaini's portraits embody an intensification or literalization of the process described by Berger: Hussaini "adds substance" to the already intimate process of physical portrayal. Indeed, Hussaini repeatedly emphasized to us the provenance of his artistic material in the heart: "This is an amazing and personal medium; when you draw people it is said it should come from your heart, and this literally comes from the heart." He has faced criticism from several quarters; in particular, for "wasting" a medically valuable substance and for proliferating new icons—not an uncontroversial practice for a Muslim who claims direct descent from the Prophet Muhammad: "People have said it's sacrilegious. But I say it is the most special substance because it comes literally from the heart." And again: "They say that you can see the artist in the art, and when I do my art it is literally true." That the substance of his paintings derives from his heart is a key aspect of his self-presentation in media interviews as much as in interviews with us, and the connection, far from being only his own, is a recurrent motif of the Indian sanguinary politics. For instance, the attention paid by the public to the provenance of artistic material in the heart was a notable feature of its response to the exhibition of freedom fighter portraits in blood that we described in chapter 2. To paraphrase

Hussaini, then, what we witness in his blood portraits is substance literally from the heart commingled with—and intimately delineating—the features of its subject. Of course, even works considered by critics to dismantle long-standing aesthetic conventions are assessed according to an authenticity criterion—they must be "from the heart." For Richard Handler, "modern art is required, not to please, as in earlier aesthetic theories, but to provide its audience with examples of authenticity" (1986, 4)—hence recent controversies concerning Damien Hirst's spot paintings, famously made by a team of assistants. Defending himself against accusations that he was making millions of pounds from artworks he had little to do with, he is reported to have stated, "Assistants make my spot paintings but my heart is in them all."[14]

Well, not literally. In Hussaini's case, because the medium of the portraits has literally passed through his heart, the sentiments of the works are considered to be more forcefully conveyed and faithful. Indeed, there is the suggestion that the blood medium does not merely connote the sentiment that gave rise to its extraction but that it is, quite literally, that sentiment as unmediated affect. We have discussed elsewhere understandings in South Asia that see the heart as the literal repository of genuine sentiment.[15] From love and pride to shame and fear, feelings "belong to the body and they flow [literally] from the heart" (Krause 1989, 568). The de-metaphorized portrait's material composition from a substance delivered literally from the heart, and partaking of the sentiment it embodies and produces, lends force to its affective efficacy. Certainly, it was central to the propaganda of the image in Hussaini's own terms. Such running together of the contiguous and the representational is, of course, not unique to Hussaini in India's wider sanguinary politics. The example offered earlier of the Bajrang Dal's collective portrait of the god Ram in activists' pooled blood suggests a similar underscoring of a demonstrable relation and aesthetics of commitment via the blood medium: a portrait of neither Ram nor the activists but of the activists in relation to Ram—a blood tie made literal.

Portraits of what, then? Strathern's approach to images is one that pays great attention to the instability of figure and ground (Strathern 1990; Wagner 1986). Hussaini actively builds in, or encodes, a figure-ground reversal; we are directed to concentrate at least as much on the substance of composition as on the "figure." To employ Kath Weston's (2013a) formulation, the extracted blood that is used in portraits and petitions is metamaterial because it forces reflection upon the material properties of the artifacts it forms. If in the classic understanding of portraiture "the portrayer makes visible the inner essence of the sitter" (Van Alphen 1997, 241), in Hussaini's case the portrayer makes his own "inner essence" visible in relation to the portrayed. That the word for heart, *dil*, is frequently used for "I" in parts of South Asia (Krause 1989, 568) might further support a figure-ground reversed understanding of Hussaini's paintings as nonrepresentational self-portraits (forming part of an epidemiology of nonrepresentations, so to speak). There is an echo here, then, of those artworks that contain "a miniature replica of [themselves or their authors], as in Velazquez's Las Meninas" (Ssorin-Chaikov 2013, 8), even if in Hussaini's case the artist's appearance in the work makes no reference to the artist's own likeness. Hussaini's paintings, indeed, are not self-portraits in any simplistic sense but "self-in-relation-to-another" portraits. The key point here is that the instability of figure and ground is an important facet of Hussaini's relational industry. The easy switches from figure to ground, and vice versa, remind the viewer of the relation the image comprises— that is, the portraits make evident not only the one who is represented. Matter here is a kind of relational reminder.

Of course, one might object that the toollike nature of the relation does not square with Hussaini's insistence that the portraits are composed via "the most personal medium" and our own insistence, with reference to Berger and local understandings of the human heart, upon the achievement of relational intimacy. But it is not simply a question of either relation as tool or relation issuing pristinely "from the heart." The relation works so well as a tool precisely because it elaborates an aesthetics of presentation and commitment and is undergirded by an artistic sensibility fully cognizant and reflexive of the persuasiveness of form. Issuing "from the heart" via "the most personal medium"—this is precisely how the tool works. The portraits—as emotive instantiation of a relation between icon and iconizer—thus possess affective power; the chief minister was emotively compelled to respond. To conclude this section, then, we briefly consider the nature of the image-maker's sway. Van Alphen explains how the portrait conventionally bestows power on the portrayed: "It is because we see a portrait of somebody that we presume that the portrayed person was important and the portrayed becomes the embodiment of authority. Thus, authority is not so much the object of portrayal, but its effect" (1997, 240). It is possible that Hussaini's portraits did augment the chief minister's authority and that her prestigious invitation to the artist and promise of property were merely acts of noblesse oblige. Such a view, however, discounts the capacity of the affective image to influence or compel its viewer to action. Rather than augment her authority, the portraits demonstrate her essential vulnerability when subjected to the relational industry of another. This was not a relation she chose; Hussaini acted according to the principle that "one cannot point to a relation without bringing about its effect" (Strathern 2005, 64). The image was the occasion for a kind of relational binding—a blood *tie*.

One can thus gain a sense of the continued potency of extracted blood as promissory political matter, despite our prior description of its association with political dissembling in "fake" camps. The extraction of blood as enunciative act continues to promise to provide material access to the truth of the donor's moral interiority and convictions. This argument is congruent with Van de Port's observation about the critical role of the body in seeming to "precede" all argument and therefore in "upgrading the reality caliber of social and cultural classificatory systems" (2011, 86). In the following section, we explore how this logic of the material intensification of moral interiors suffuses the activist work of the survivors of the Bhopal gas disaster.

Activist Faux-Philanthropy

In 1984, a poisonous cloud of methyl isocyanate leaked out of a negligently maintained Union Carbide plant in Bhopal. Over the course of the night the gas cloud quickly engulfed the slum settlements that surrounded the factory, leading to the immediate death of over two thousand people. Since then, more than twenty thousand have succumbed to the slower effects of the poison, and about 100,000 more have been left with varying degrees of disability and impairment. The corporations responsible have continued to evade responsibility for the tragedy; the U.S.-based corporation Dow Chemicals bought Union Carbide in 1999, claiming responsibility over only Carbide's assets and not its liabilities. The site, upon which the survivors have no choice but to continue to live, remains toxic and the groundwater poisoned. The corporations involved have cited "trade secret" clauses in refusing to divulge the results of their investigations into the nature of the toxic gas. Very little of the settlement negotiated between the corporation and the Indian government has trickled down to the survivors. For its part, the Indian government has failed to provide adequate health care to the survivors. The funds reserved for that purpose from the settlement have gone toward creating a hospital from which the survivors are excluded. Further, the government refuses to recognize obvious signs of second-generation effects and has also failed to deliver upon promises of public medical research into the chronic effects of this poisoning (Hanna, Morehouse, and Sarangi 2005).

Faced with these circumstances, the survivors have organized a highly charged and widely networked international "campaign for justice" over the last thirty years. Within the affected slums, they have set up a health clinic that warns against excessive pharmaceutical use and dispenses free multimodal treatment to all those who live in the area. This is consonant with the broader tenor of the activist movement; its ongoing effort has been to link the original disaster of 1984 to the abuses of multinational pharmaceutical companies in the present. The Bhopal activist network is comprised of several subgroups that come under a broader conglomerate organization known as the International Campaign for

Justice in Bhopal (ICJB). The prominent subgroups of the ICJB are Bhopal Gas Peedit Mahila Stationary Karmachari Sangh (Bhopal Women's Gas Victim's Stationary Labor Organization), Bhopal Gas Peedit Mahila Purush Sangharsh Morcha (Bhopal Men and Women's Gas Victim's Struggle Forum), and the Bhopal Group for Information and Action (BGIA). The BGIA, which takes center stage at moments of heightened activism, is led by charismatic leaders Satinath Sarangi (Sathyu) and Rachna Dhingra; they determine the broader direction as well as the practical daily life of the movement. While the ICJB has conducted protests and actions with remarkable regularity over the last three decades, we focus here on a set of actions that we were able to follow ethnographically in 2008.

In February that year, the ICJB gathered about fifty survivors and activists and set out on foot from Bhopal. The destination was New Delhi, the capital city, which lies about five hundred miles north. The street in the capital on which they converged (and do so almost every year) lies not far from the administrative center of Rajpath and India Gate. Called *Jantar Mantar*, it is named after a historic eighteenth-century astronomical observatory that it circles. In recent decades, Jantar Mantar has been administratively marked, cordoned off, and policed for a very different purpose; it has been designated by the city administration as the space within which groups of civil dissenters can make public displays of protest. The Bhopalis were not alone there; among many other organizations, they were flanked by a group of Tibetan protesters on one side, trade union organizers on the other, and a group of disgruntled civil servants farther down the road. We focus here on two strategic actions led by the second-generation victims of the disaster, children in their early teens that organize under the suborganizational umbrella of Children Against Dow-Carbide (CADC). The broader activist collective formed CADC earlier that year, well aware of the persuasive moral figuration of the child activist. Further, the institutionalization of the group was also motivated by the Indian government's ongoing refusal to recognize second-generational effects, thereby delegitimizing an entire constituency of survivors. In later years, CADC would go on to the United Kingdom and the United States, talking at events and canvassing congressional representatives, urging them to put pressure on Dow Chemical. In the first action of their Delhi campaign, CADC reached out to their peers in elite schools in New Delhi. Sareeta, Rafat, Yasmin, and Safreen, some of the leaders of the suborganization, painstakingly detailed the effects of the disaster to their Delhi peers. Questions and conversations followed their presentation, after which both the Bhopali children and the schoolchildren from Delhi wrote letters to the Indian prime minister (the de facto addressee of most Bhopali public interventions). However, while the Delhi children wrote letters in conventional pencil and ink, CADC used blood collected from young Bhopali adults at the protest site. The moment of the taking of blood was dramatized by the young adults by red headbands, photographed and captioned later with aggressive messages such as "Look into our eyes, Prime Minister." With this blood-ink, Sareeta and other children from CADC wrote a letter to the prime minister asking in the most courteous of tones for a long-denied appointment. The text of the letter read as follows: "Dear PM, We are people poisoned by Union Carbide. We have walked more than 800 km just to meet you. For the last 19 days, we have been sitting at Jantar Mantar. Would you please take one hour out of your busy schedule to meet us at Jantar Mantar? That is all I wanted to say. On behalf of the Bhopal victims—Yasmin Khan, on behalf of Bhopal Survivors." In this strategic action, the violence of the disaster was routed first through the contaminated bodies of those directly affected and then through the pen of eleven-year-old Yasmin, who knew its effect since birth. In a public event, it was then inscribed as a public letter addressed to the prime minister. Along with the letter, the medium of the writing (blood) was prominently displayed in medical container vials. The children then carried this letter-in-blood to the residence of the prime minister and had it sent in via emissaries, after much wrangling with security.

The medical instruments in the moment of writing—the syringe, the vial, and so on—point to one valence of blood that the activists are well acquainted with: its evidentiary quality. In addition to serving as a ritual of verification in political theater, the medical testing of blood is well known as a standard evidence-gathering trope, as it plays a part as evidence of contamination and suffering, allowing for claims to be made for compensation and future medical care. Here, this evidence was imaginatively redeployed as a medium of expression, rather than as an object for scientific examination. Thus deployed, blood-as-writing rejected the supposed transparency of medical evidence; instead, writing with blood established an alternative technique for making suffering visible. Crucial to this alternative technique was the sarcastic content of the address: "Would you please take out one hour from your busy schedule?" Roland Barthes has suggested that a fundamental condition of modernity is that sarcasm became a possible condition of truth (1972). In other words, Barthes describes sarcasm as a critical deconstructive tool from *within* language that denaturalizes how languages often naturalize dominant ideologies. Resonantly, Yasmin's sarcastic utterance served as a mode of critique: as a linguistic technique, it revealed the absurdity of the polite address from her to the prime minister. In the face of the history of neglect that various prime ministers have practiced toward the children of Bhopal, sarcasm in the letter pointed to a failed possibility of an ideal relationship between the writer and the addressee.

By itself, this might be a commonplace observation. What makes this striking, however, is that the letter takes its force not only from the sarcasm inherent in the linguistic address (in the disjunction between apparent content and intent) but also from the disjunction between the apparent politeness of the message and the violent materiality of its writing: blood. To underscore the particular stakes of using blood for communicating political content, we find it crucial to further unpack this disjunction between message and medium. The Bhopali deployment of blood as material and medium is a distant cry from the substance's association with Nehruvian nationalist integration, as described by Lawrence Cohen in the context of early postcolonial India (2001). With the Bhopal disaster, and the subsequent collusion between the Indian government and multinational corporations to evade responsibility, the integrative imagination of blood gives way to one that is suffused with violence. The closest and most immediate referents for this new sanguinary imagination is the blood spilled on the night of the disaster and the subsequent blood that indexes ongoing contamination in the bodies of the Bhopal survivors. The fiery red bands that the activists wore while donating their blood for this campaign evidence an anger at odds with the polite address of the letter. Thus, while writing with blood here attempted a mode of biosocial relationality between the poor and their government, the mode in which this was attempted was not through the invocation of an inherent biological commonality but rather through calling attention to the violence of contamination and the insistent possibility of death.[16] In other words, in taking recourse to blood, Bhopali activists animated its potential to *both* remedy (asking for political representation) and critique (describing the prior failure of political representation). If the government had pushed the poor into zones of "thanatopolitical" neglect, writing-through-blood sought to counter such a practice of invisibility by intensifying the substances of the body, demonstrating an activist biomoral interiority, and revealing a history of violent deficits in the proper functioning of the body politic. The gift of Bhopali blood exemplified the potential and power of the partonomic gift in its most pointed form—where the gift given not only highlights that which is not given but also demonstrates the vast biomoral chasm between the part and the whole.

CADC's strategy of a critical bodily giving over was exemplified again in a following activist action—the "Have a Heart" campaign (figure 7). This action once more involved the activist-children canvassing at city schools for support. After explaining the complexity of the issue and the seriousness of their concerns to fellow teenagers, they asked for volunteers to cut out large paper hearts of various colors. Once several such hearts were carved out, the children from Delhi reflected on what they had just heard and penned a letter on the cut-out heart to the prime minister. The name of the campaign gave away its affective ploy. The

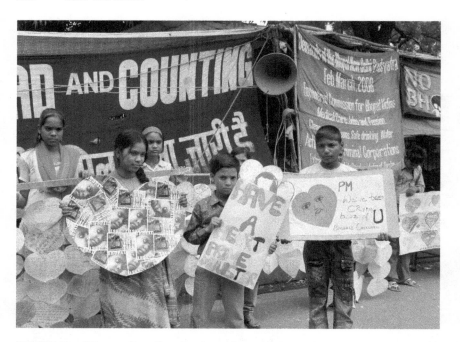

FIGURE 7. "Have a Heart" campaign. (Photo by the authors.)

"Have a Heart, Prime Minister" campaign played with the idea that these carved hearts were a donation to the prime minister, to make up for the lack of his obviously missing organ. If his heart were indeed in its place, it would not allow him to turn a deaf ear to the suffering of the activist children. Gifting in this activist mobilization stalled at the heavily guarded gates of the prime minister's residence, just a few miles from the site of the protest. The survivors could only look on as an aide finally took the hearts into the guarded compound and disappeared down the long pathway toward the residence bungalow.

Resembling the blood-writing campaign, the "Have a Heart" campaign was sarcastic: it entailed medical philanthropy (altruistic organ donation) from Bhopali children; those that had been denied care from the government, to the highest functionary of the government—the Indian prime minister. The paper hearts offered a metacommentary on the indissociable relation between the gift of blood as a ritual of sincerity on the one hand, and of graft and dissimulation on the other. In other words, if we saw how the heart vis-à-vis Hussaini might carry the weight of an "inner essence" of a person, in the Bhopali action we see how its absence can index a most crippling biomoral deficit. It is no accident that the heart is not a replaceable organ; in a biological sense, its "donation" implies death for the donor. In a biomoral sense, the absence of a heart indicates a moral death. In a faux-philanthropic gesture that was both playful and sobering, the poorest and most medically deprived donated a pseudo-organ to the person they saw as responsible for their deprivation. The "philanthropists" here were those without the resources to gift in the first place.

While Cohen points out the symbolic valence of blood donation as a marker of solidarity in early postcolonial India, he goes on to argue that such an integrative imagination is succeeded by one that is extractive and exclusionary (Cohen 2011a; 2011b; 2013). That is, if blood was linked to an ethics of secular citizenship in the heady first decades of decolonization, as the promises of caste and class solidarity failed to materialize, the imaginary of a forcibly extracted organ took center stage in the country's disillusioned later years. Cohen's ethnographic engagements in contemporary India detail the illegal organ trade economy, as the poor sacrifice bodily material for temporary relief from debt. The gift from a child to the prime minister—from the politically "naive" to the highest functionary of the state—refigures this practice of bodily deprivation to powerful effect. The faux donation of the hearts revealed the intimacy of donation and extraction under duress and identified a biomoral pathology in the recipient of the gift—a corrupt government unwilling to relate to its citizens.

Rethinking Bodily Evidence

While so far we have detailed blood writing as an unstable and shifting art of moral persuasion, the most successful of the activist strategies was an indefinite hunger strike. In beginning this chapter, we gestured to the particular capability of the fast as an activist form to index a conviction unto death; while bloodletting promises transparency, it very rarely evidences the same principled intimacy with death. Yet we indicated the breakdown of the fast as a medium of communicating political sincerity. The Bhopali activists at Jantar Mantar were well aware of the deficit of public trust in this activist mode. Since they shared the bathrooms at Jantar Mantar with other protesting groups, they were privy to a common practice among politicians ostensibly on hunger strike: privately devouring glucose biscuits in the enclosed stalls. How then were they able to rescue the fast from accusations of corruption and dissemblance?

The 2009 strike was led by nine of the more experienced activists at Jantar Mantar; several were experienced in the form, having conducted similar fasts in preceding years (figure 8). The only nourishment they allowed themselves was water mixed with hydration salts—a concession to the scorching heat of the Delhi summer. The veteran hunger strikers among them told me how the first few days were the most trying. If one could tide over the first five days, the body stopped

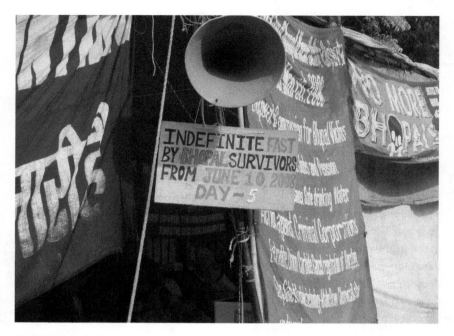

FIGURE 8.   Relay hunger strike carried out by Bhopali protestors. (Photo by the authors.)

producing the sensation of hunger. By the second week, the bodies of the hunger strikers had begun to produce ketones. Ketones are compounds produced by the body when carbohydrate intake drops dangerously. They assist in the metabolic breaking down of fatty acids for energy in states of fasting and starvation. While ketones are not known to be harmful by themselves, prolonged production might lead to ketosis or ketoacidosis—conditions in which ketone production has reached dangerous and unregulated levels.[17] After three weeks, these conditions could lead to a variety of possibly fatal complications, including the disastrous consequences of protein metabolism. A report from the thirteenth day of the hunger strike showed already dangerous levels of ketone production among two of the hunger strikers at the Bhopal site. Thus, over these weeks, the hunger strikers allowed their bodies to produce a substance that simultaneously kept them alive and could have led to their death. The levels of this toxic product—ketones—were recorded meticulously every day by a roster of doctors who had agreed to come to the site to monitor biomedical measures (figure 9). It was precisely through this quantification and medicalization of the hunger strike that the Bhopali activists could validate its authenticity and fatal possibility, as opposed to those that undercut it with private eating. At the same time, ketones—like blood—became a scientific mode through which a previous history of biomedical triage was con-

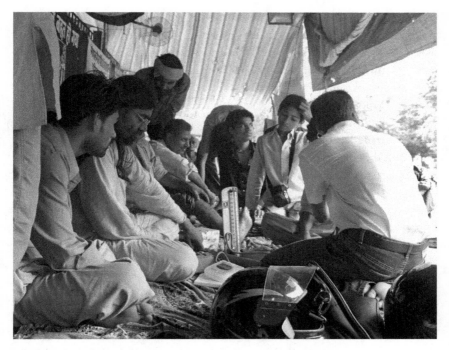

FIGURE 9.   Ketone-measuring and health checkup of Bhopali protestors during the hunger strike. (Photo by the authors.)

tested. One might read this practice as both guided by and critical of the increasing metric-driven orientation of public health, where the bare facts of bodily vulnerability must speak in numbers to evidence the quality or lack of care. Regardless, during the strike, the body became a medium of communication, authenticated and disseminated through the medical document. The deployment of ketones through fasting is crucial to understanding the substantial politics of the fast. It shows an innovative resignification of fasting as itself a verifiable ritual. If the verifiability of blood extractions helped the practice accrue the moral weight of authenticity and sincerity, the hunger strike indicated a fascinating response. Like blood, ketones were demonstrable and verifiable enactments of the fast. In much the same way as blood, ketones were a gift that produced an insistent and urgent demand of intimacy, reciprocity, and obligation from its addressee. In the same way as blood, ketones addressed a deficit in public trust about activist mobilization (a trust eroded in part by the participation of corrupt politicians), promising a new economy of transparency and sincerity.

After twenty-two days and close to the imminent possibility of long-term medical damage to their bodies, the activists began a relay, with a fresh set of strikers taking over from the previous ones. Finally, after 172 days of relayed hunger strikes, the Indian minister for chemicals and fertilizers arrived at the site, with sweets for the hunger strikers and an announcement of an empowered government commission that would look into Bhopal—a key demand of the campaign. Previous government commissions had lacked the ability to take immediate action; the introduction of the term "empowered" encoded the promise of swift redress. Among this and other victories, the negotiated truce also put in place a plan to pursue legal and criminal liabilities against Union Carbide and Dow Chemical (the current owner of the subsidiary), as well as a plan of action for the rehabilitation of the gas victims. In the years since, many of these negotiated declarations fell far short of their promise. This has led to repeated hunger strikes, actions, and campaigns in recent years, both in Jantar Mantar and in Bhopal; the story of governmental neglect and partial legal recognitions continues to unfold in the present.

Blood, Period

In 2015, the controversial Indian-Canadian artist and poet Rupi Kaur posted a self-portrait on Instagram that pictured her seemingly asleep, face turned away toward a wall, wearing pajamas stained by a spot of menstrual blood. This self-portrait was part of Kaur's final year university project that she had developed in collaboration with her sister Prabh. Their intention was to provoke a response from the social media site and its users—which it did. Instagram deleted the post within twenty-four hours, but not before Kaur had received a barrage of abusive threats in the post's thread. She then posted the photo once again, checking to see if the site's deletion had been an error. This time, Instagram removed the post almost immediately. In response, Kaur turned to other social media platforms to express her outrage. She posted the following statement about this short-lived social media visual experiment on her website:

> i bleed each month to help make humankind a possibility. my womb is home to the divine. a source of life for our species. whether i choose to create or not. but very few times it is seen that way. in older civilizations this blood was considered holy. in some it still is. but a majority of people. societies. and communities shun this natural process. some are more comfortable with the pornification of women. the sexualization of women. the violence and degradation of women than this. they cannot be bothered to express their disgust about all that. but will be angered

and bothered by this. we menstruate and they see it as dirty. attention seeking. sick. a burden. as if this process is less natural than breathing. as if it is not a bridge between this universe and the last. as if this process is not love. labour. life. selfless and strikingly beautiful.[18]

Kaur's controversial self-portrait was one of a series. Other photographs included images of her sitting on a toilet and dropping a sanitary pad into a bin, of blood in a pristine white toilet bowl, of a white washing machine with blood-stained clothes ready to be washed, and of drops of blood entering a shower drain flanked by her feet.

Responding in part to the widespread public controversy around Kaur's project, anthropologist Chris Bobel suggests that 2015 was "The Year the Period Went Public" (Bobel 2015). Bobel borrowed the title of her short piece from an article in *Cosmopolitan*, the popular global magazine marketed to women. In playing with *Cosmopolitan*'s title, Bobel signaled how a long history of feminist activism around menstruation—a central theme of her ethnographic work—had suddenly become mainstream. In other words, Kaur's project was not unprecedented. Menstrual blood has been a key bodily substance in feminist activism since at least the mid-to-late twentieth century (Bobel 2010). Kaur's aesthetic protest echoed the stance of two generations of feminists who have fought to destigmatize the bodily process and contest its pathologization. In this, Kaur's work aligns itself with particular groups of menstrual activists that Bobel studies who seek to establish that menstruation is not only normal but also evidence of women's intimacy with a deeper, natural world—in Kaur's description, "a bridge between this universe and the last."

At the same time, what was different about Kaur's entry into this longer history of menstrual activism was that she was a woman of color reaching out to a diverse global audience. As Bobel's work has shown, menstrual activists in the United States have been and are predominantly white (Bobel 2010, 10). Bobel conjectures that the absence of women of color from the movement has much to do with a historically derived politics of respectability. Drawing on the work of Evelyn Higginbotham, Bobel suggests that one response of women of color to racism has been to mask and mute their sexuality, rejecting historical constructions of their bodies as promiscuous, overly fertile, and sexually available. Such a politics of respectability, Bobel contends, has made it difficult for women of color to enter into the activist modalities of exposure and celebration that characterize menstrual activism. Further, Bobel shows how feeder feminist movements that comprise menstrual activism have traditionally been dominated by white women, adding another barrier to the entry of racially diverse activists. In this context, one might think of Kaur's work as an effort to bring a new demographic with whom she is especially popular—a global cohort of women of color—into an activist fold from which they might have previously felt alienated.

Over the last decade, Kaur's project has become more the norm than the exception; a significant number of women of color have joined the project of menstrual activism and similarly captured media attention. For example, Daniela Manica and Clarice Rios write about the performances of Spanish artist Isa Sanz and Brazilian artists Maria Matricardi and Carol Azvedo, among others, who use menstrual blood as an aesthetic medium of protest (Manica and Rios 2017). And the Indian diaspora has been a big part of this diversification of menstrual activism. In 2011, Indian-Canadian Miki Agrawal (who had started an underwear company to replace tampons) drew intense public controversy when she claimed that the New York transportation authority had tried to censor her menstruation-positive advertisements (Bellafante 2016). In 2015, Indian-American musician Kiran Gandhi ran the London Marathon without pads, to bring attention to the global taboo and shame that accrues to menstruation. And in 2017, Indian-American Amika George founded the #freeperiods movement in Britain, bringing attention to "period poverty" and the unaffordability of sanitary pads and even drawing a pledge from the Labour Party to commit £10 million to the issue (Ram 2018). In her ethnographic work, Bobel found a range of politics in mobilizations around menstruation in the United States: from feminist-spiritualist celebrations of blood as a source of female power, to consumer-rights and environmental-justice advocates, and radical third-wave queer and anticorporate activists. Mobilizations around menstruation across the Indian diaspora similarly occupy a diverse range of political positions. Kaur's project draws most apparently from the feminist-spiritualist celebration of womanhood that Bobel describes as a significant constituency of menstrual activism in the United States. Miki Agrawal's politics aligns more closely with a global discourse of socially minded business entrepreneurs. Amika George comes closest to the more radically minded activists that Bobel describes, as she frames access to menstrual hygiene as an issue of social welfare and class politics.

While many of menstrual activism's celebrity figures are in the Indian diaspora, our particular interest here is in how the movement has taken shape in the mainland. In 2015, the poet and writer Nabina Das began a piece in the *Economic and Political Weekly* titled "Blood, Period" with the claim: "Suddenly, blood is in the news" (Das 2015, 95). In part, Das was responding to Kaur's Instagram post. The photograph reminded Das of a widely publicized sexual assault on a Delhi public bus in 2012. The incident set off a series of national and international activist campaigns that ultimately resulted in some limited legal reforms (Roychowdhury 2015). Das, however, was drawn to a very particular aspect of the attack:

the spillage of blood on the bus that the perpetrators claimed that they had been shocked by and had even attempted to clean. This spilling of blood during an incident of sexual violence led Das to suggest that the misogyny responsible for rape was a product of the same patriarchal structures that lashed out against Kaur's aesthetic display. Through blood, Das linked two separate aspects of the relation between gender and blood: the substance could serve as an object and medium of feminist celebration while at the same time evidence and dramatize the violence of sexual assault.

Das was not alone in recognizing this political polyvalence of blood as an aesthetic substance. In early 2015, the same year as Kaur's project, German teenager Elona Kastrati hung sanitary pads all around Karlsruhe with messages such as "Imagine if men were as disgusted with rape as they are with periods." Her campaign—Pads against Sexism—caught the imagination of university students in Delhi. In March of the same year, a group of students from the city's Jamia Millia Islamia University reproduced the strategy, hanging sanitary pads on trees, walls, and campus buildings. When university officials took the pads down, the students took the campaign outside campus and around the city. Over the next weeks, the campaign spread to other universities across the country. The messages written on the pads contained variations on Kastrati's original theme. They included "Period blood is not impure, your thoughts are," "Menstruation is natural, rape is not," "Streets of Delhi belong to women too," "Rapists rape people, not outfits," "*Kanya kumari, gandi soch tumhari*—You talk about virginity, when your thoughts are dirty," and "Red here is just paint. But rape draws real blood."

For the activists Bobel follows in the United States and in the Indian diaspora, the targets of intervention include the pathologization of female bodies, heteronormative discourses around menstruation, and environmental and anticorporate justice. The Pads against Sexism campaigners in India share the aesthetic deployment of blood as a political strategy with their global and diasporic counterparts. And like their diasporic counterparts, their public display of menstrual symbols—red paint, sanitary pads—makes public a bodily domain usually understood as shameful and private. At the same time, this campaign identified as its target a controversy that has dominated mainstream media attention and public feminist mobilizations in India in recent years—namely, sexual assault. That is, while sexual violence is one of many concerns for the global and diasporic menstrual activists, it has emerged as the overwhelmingly central focus of attention for campaigns within India. Specifically, Pads against Sexism emerged in the aftermath of many other recent student mobilizations around sexual assault. In 2014, the "Let There Be Noise" protests after allegations of an on-campus sexual assault had led to the resignation of the vice chancellor of Jadavpur University in West Bengal. After the Pads against Sexism action in Delhi, students at Jadavpur University quickly mobilized around the same strategy. The same year also saw the "Kiss of Love" protests against the policing of public intimacy. The campaign began on the campus of Ernakulam Law College in Kerala and then spread to universities all across the country. Nabina Das and the Pads against Sexism campaigners in Delhi drew upon these prior mobilizations and adopted their framing of sexual violence as an immediate and urgent problem.

While Pads against Sexism attracted some short-term public visibility, another menstrual activist campaign in India has had a much more sustained public and political impact. In 2006, the Indian Young Lawyers Association filed a public interest litigation seeking the entry of women in the Sabarimala temple in Kerala. As anthropologists Filippo and Caroline Osella have described, Sabarimala is a South Indian all-male pilgrimage site, whose deity Ayyappan is hypermale, since he is the offspring of two male gods (Osella and Osella 2003). The temple has traditionally denied entry to women of menstruating age, citing the god Ayyappan's perennial celibacy, which leads to his disinterest in women devotees. The long convention was legally authorized in 1965 in the Kerala Hindu Places of Public Worship Act. The issue had come before the Kerala High Court in 1991. A canny move at the time by the head priest reinforced the practice of gender discrimination in temple entry. The priest had reasoned that "custom" dictated that only devotees who had practiced penance for forty-one days were allowed in the temple, and that menstruating women were temporally and biologically incapable of maintaining such a period of purity (T. Singh 2016). As is often the case with litigations in the slow-moving Indian legal system, the 2006 petition was heard and debated several times. And over the next eight years, it seemed as if the issue had lost momentum. However, a set of incidents in 2015 catapulted the issue to international visibility. In 2014, a woman traveling in a state transport bus was forced out as it headed toward the temple. When she sought to file a police complaint, the local police refused to recognize her claim. A few days later, five female protestors rode the same bus but were detained by the local police before they could complete their journey. As Chitra Prasanna describes, the incident laid bare the inextricability of religious, patriarchal, and police authority in the region (Prasanna 2016).

These protests might well have remained a brief, localized reaction if the temple's board president—Prayar Gopalakrishnan—had not offered a novel solution to the problem: "These days there are machines that can scan bodies and check for weapons. There will be a day when a machine is invented to scan if it is the 'right time' (not menstruating) for a woman to enter the temple. When that machine is invented, we will talk about letting women inside."[19] This tone-deaf response was widely reported by the media and catalyzed a national backlash. In late 2015, a twenty-year-old student from Punjab—Nikita Azad—posted an open letter online to Gopalakrishnan protesting his remarks. Her letter was accompanied by a picture of her holding the words "Happy to Bleed" written in red across two sanitary pads (Azad 2015). Her letter was remarkable in how it expressed devout traditional values, along with her list of a range of pilgrimage sites that she had already visited with her family. She also sought to make clear that she had always carried her sanitary pads in a discrete black bag so as to "protect her honor" and never let her male relatives know when she was menstruating. In other words, she had "tried my best to uphold the sacred culture of our society." Why then, she asked, was she made to bear the responsibility of a curse—the murder of a Brahmin by Indra—in which she had not participated? (Azad was referring to a common origin myth of the ban on menstruation.) All she knew, she added, was that "blood flows out." Azad then turned a corner and, in consonance with the Pads against Sexism campaign, connected the issue directly to sexual violence:

> We live in a nation, "a democratic nation," where a woman is raped every twenty minutes, and every second woman is subject to domestic violence. According to you, perhaps the reason behind these is also blood. As you have given the solution to protect the sanctity of temple by not allowing bleeding women inside, do you propose that bleeding women should be caged in homes to prevent such incidents?

In a follow-up letter in 2016, Azad further clarified the importance of linking menstrual activism with the ubiquity of sexual violence:

> A man with equally active reproductive organs is allowed inside the temple while a woman is not. Is semen purer than menstrual blood? However, for us, it is not a question of pure v/s impure or men v/s women. Our fight begins from our homes and workplaces. Relatives who beat our mothers to abort us, to in-laws who burn us, to those who rape us, to temples that denigrate us, it is a struggle inherent to the struggle against patriarchy.

With the 2015 letter, Azad began an online campaign with the hashtag #HappytoBleed. The campaign gathered force and enlisted India's foremost feminist lawyer, Indira Jaising. They then filed a petition to the Supreme Court of India to be made party to the legal dispute over the temple (Rajagopal 2016). Partly in response to the public media attention that the campaign received, the Supreme Court brought the case of temple entry out of its long stasis in early 2016. The campaign has continued to receive sustained media attention since that time. Late in 2016, the *Washington Post* reported that an estimated five hundred women inspired by the campaign traveled by bus to Sabarimala to "storm" its sacred altar (Gowen 2016). That year also saw the return of the Marxist Left Democratic Front government to Kerala that reversed the prior government's opposition to women's entry to the temple. At the time of writing, the matter of temple entry remains under the adjudication at the apex court.

While the resonances between Kaur's art campaign and the Pads against Sexism and Happy to Bleed campaigns are clear, there remains one key difference. The first two campaigns took inspiration from a long history of menstruation-related activism whose vocabularies were explicitly secular and global. They framed the issue as one of the right of women everywhere in the world to menstruate without shame or stigma. The Happy to Bleed campaign adopted a different citational register. It approached the question of menstrual freedom from within the vocabularies of constraint that are operative in the experience of many groups of women in India. The anthropologist Sarah Lamb writes about meeting a woman on a bus pilgrimage to the holy city of Puri in Orissa (Lamb 2005). Controversy erupted at the pilgrimage one morning when menstrual rags were found near the guesthouse in which they all stayed for a night. The matter was dropped after a while. Lamb talked to the woman who was menstruating and found that she knew that she might begin her period on the journey but had really wanted to go on pilgrimage for a long time and took the chance that she might be able to conceal its onset. The woman added that she believed no sin or harm would accrue (*dos*) because her devotion was pure, even if the substance was not. This conversation led Lamb to reflect on her ethnographic work in Bengal, where menstruation played a key role in demarcating gender and caste boundaries. Lamb also looked back to the canonical work of Mary Douglas on purity and pollution and found that examples from India were crucial in developing the anthropological argument that impurity and pollution had often to do with violations of bodily boundaries and were therefore often tied to the bodies of menstruating and reproductive women (Douglas 1966 [2002]). Douglas's understanding has been refracted through the anthropological scholarship on India that demonstrates the close linkage between menstrual blood and the policing of caste and gender boundaries (Leslie 1989; Marglin 1977; Thompson 1985). At the same time, Lamb developed the work of Marriott and Inden we referred to earlier in this chapter to move beyond Douglas's insistence on the seemingly static correlation between substances and social order. In her discussion of the socialization of menstruation, Veena Das too argues for a dialectical relationship between the control of bodily boundaries and the possibilities of flux and transformation, as she traces it in a life course. Thus, both Lamb and Das emphasize the ethnosociological insight that substances are continuously transacted and constantly transform persons and their place in social hierarchies (V. Das 1988). And both document the small and furtive acts—transacted through veiled utterances and glances—through which women inhabit and subtly resist kinship and ritual gender norms around menstruation.

Unlike the practices of resistance, concealment, and negotiation at the everyday level that interest Das and Lamb, the campaigns we have examined here are mediatized political projects directed at disruptive and systemic change. They take place not in the give and take of everyday life but rather are performative and aesthetic strategies at a heightened and explicit register of a confrontation with norms. At the same time, this activist project is reflective of the ethnosociological insistence on flux, contestation, and transformation in the transaction of bodily substances. As we suggested in the beginning of this chapter, reformist and political projects that deploy blood imagine a rupture in the relation between substance and code and seek their realignment. While the projects of most diasporic activists and the Pads against Sexism campaign adopt a global, secular vocabulary in an outright rejection of "tradition," the Happy to Bleed campaign frames its intervention as reform. In her letter, Azad emphasizes that the "pollution" of menstruation and the "purity" of sacral space are not fundamentally contradictory but have been put in opposition by patriarchal conventions. In other words, much like the Nirankari activists we discussed earlier in this chapter, Azad suggests that substance and code are in misalignment. But differently from the Nirankari reformists who believe that substance and code have fallen out of alignment in contemporary times, Azad does not participate in a narrative of decline. Rather, she suggests that "traditional" norms around menstruation are incorrect from the point of view of a pious, feminist politics, even as they have been historically durable. In other words, even as menstrual blood is a substance out of place in the temple and its potential understood as polluting, the fact of convention does not in itself mean that the substance-code relation is in proper alignment. Further, her project then is not to throw out tradition entirely and reject religious conventions but rather more subtly to realign the substance-code relation in a way that menstrual blood no longer enacts temple pollution. Finally, the strategy through which she seeks to achieve this realignment is through the mediatization of menstrual blood as writing. By circulating a representation of menstrual blood in the domain of a visual public, Azad aims to achieve its authorization in the public space of the temple.

Further, we argue that the transformative alignment of substance and code in the Happy to Bleed campaign has had a persuasive impact also because it has deep roots in the region's political style. As Robin Jeffrey has shown, the lower-caste strategy of demanding temple entry as a cipher for equality and inclusion had proved extremely successful during the colonial period in the same region as the Sabarimala temple. From the 1860s to the 1940s, politically mobilized lower-caste college-educated men deployed the strategy of temple entry to widen the popularity of the anticaste movement. The strategy of inclusivity proved radically successful, rallying low-caste peasants and workers and finally leading to the Temple Entry Proclamation of 1936 (Jeffrey 1976). Azad's campaign for the entry of menstruating women to the Sabarimala temple astutely drew upon the long and successful history of political styles in the region that had previously sought in their own way to reorient the relationship between substantial purity and pollution in public spaces. The ethnosociological insight about the potentiality of flux and transformation thus plays out powerfully in two arenas that are explicitly about the control of boundaries—bodily and spatial.

While we have focused in this section on the activist association of menstruation with sexual violence and segregation, we would be remiss not to point out another mythic-religious imagination of menstruation in the region that understands bleeding as a source of divine, female power. Just as anthropologists have described the violence inflicted upon menstruating women across a range of contexts, they have also argued against interpreting cultural imaginations of menstruation as always repressive of female agency (Buckley and Gottlieb 1988). Scholars working in India have been keenly aware of the double-edged power and pollution that accrues around the substance. For instance, Nikita Azad's reference to the relation between menstrual blood and Hinduism's original sin of the god Indra's killing of a Brahmin is more complicated than it first appears. Wendy Doniger traces a Vedic iteration of the myth that describes menstrual blood as a route through which Indira's sin is expiated: women accept a portion of Indra's guilt upon his request as menstrual blood and receive in return the gift of reproduction and sexual pleasure (Doniger 1976). Thus, the substance bears both the sin of an original impurity as well as the powerful and generative capacity of its expiation. Contemporary anthropologists too have documented examples of this intimacy of power and pollution in menstrual blood. For example, Jeanne Openshaw documents the practice of the ingestion of menstrual blood among the *bauls* of Bengal, as the substance is understood as a vital gift and a marker of great abundance (Openshaw 2002). But perhaps the most well-known example of the potentially generative power of menstrual blood in India is through its association with the Kamakhya temple in the state of Assam. As Hugh Urban writes (2008), the goddess Kamakhya is an embodiment of divine female power (*sakti*). According to several mythic sources, the temple is sited on the goddess's sexual organ, which fell from the heavens when the overwhelming power of her body threatened to destroy the universe. As Urban explains, the contemporary goddess and temple represent a mixture of various religious traditions and their historical unfoldings—indigenous, tribal, and brahmanic. When she menstruates for three days each year, the temple is closed for her blood's impurity. At the same time, however, the same dangerous blood is understood as the source of life and creative energy; when the temple is reopened on the fourth day, red cloths representing the bloody flow are distributed to assembled devotees. Urban's broader project argues that the kind of power embodied in the goddess's blood erodes "modern Western distinctions between the religious and the political, and between the spiritual and the sensual." Instead, he finds, categories of religion, politics, and sexuality have come to be historically interlinked around the temple in Assam, as the authority of male priests and kings depends vitally upon the female power of the temple (531).

The activist projects around menstrual blood we describe here do not explicitly evoke the mythic sources of its divine power. Of the projects we have described, only Rupi Kaur's invokes the divine, cosmic power of menstrual blood. And even then, it does not do so through explicit reference to Indic traditions. And even as Azad evokes tradition, she writes of it as a "curse" that needs to be reevaluated and reformed. But we argue that in deploying the substance as a material and medium of protest, they implicitly express the double valence of blood identified by Urban in relation to the accrual of political power in Kamakhya. In a register they self-identify as Indian-feminist, the Happy to Bleed activists seek to reform through a reformulation of blood as substance-code. In this, their intervention resonates with those of the other activists in this chapter: they recognize the polyvalence of blood to connote violence and enforce segregation, while at the same time they deploy the substance as a medium of truth and a mechanism of exposure.

Blood as Critique

We have described a wide range of substantial activism in this chapter; the actors that have deployed blood as a material for critique have included the Sant Nirankaris, party politicians, Shihan Hussaini, activists from Bhopal, and menstrual activists. All of the practices we describe employ a partonomic script. That is, they address a prior deficit—in familial and national relations, or in political patronage and care. In the case of faux philanthropy—the Bhopali gifts of blood and hearts—the real and metaphorical bodily gifts seek to redress a prior failure in the extension of a biosocial relation of care. In the Bhopali case of faux philanthropy, the sarcastic undertone is in sharp contrast with the sincere intent of the Nirankaris. In the case of Hussaini and the Congress's "fake" camp, we encounter differential performances of transparency. Among these latter forms, the Bhopali faux philanthropic gift comes closest to resembling Shihan Hussaini's gift of portraits to Jayalalitha. Both share the hope that the excess of the gesture might compel a response. While such a compelled response might not promise a fundamental biomoral change in the recipient of the gift (an aspiration the Ni-rankaris cannot shed), it serves at least as a critique of the denial of prior patron-age and care. In other words, while the Nirankaris' partonomic script rests on a sincere faith in the ability of the partonomic gift to enact biomoral change, Hus-saini's gift and the Bhopali actions rely on the duress that blood ties imposed upon the recipients of the gifts.

Philanthropy and faux philanthropy blur at the edges, but the distinctions be-tween them are important. While both Hussaini and the Bhopali activists hope to put pressure on political figures, the substance-techniques of the Bhopali ac-tivists enact a further subversion: they undercut the association between blood and nationalism, between shedding and sacrificial devotion. In the broader san-guinary politics of contemporary India, many kinds of nationalist gestures of giv-ing, spilling, and sharing blood contribute to both broad and narrow visions of a secular nation-state. Hussaini's portraiture shares more in common with the na-tionalist portraits of Gupta discussed in chapter 2, since both seek to enlarge rather than curtail the power of those that they portray. While Hussaini might seek to compel and direct this power toward his own end, his intention is not to demonstrate the corruption of Jayalalitha but rather to become part of and ben-efit from it. The Bhopali faux-philanthropic gestures enact a far deeper criticism of political relations by seeking to reveal its biomoral pathology. In this, the Bho-pali actions form the perfect conjuncture of the "fake" and "true" blood dona-tion camp. They are inherently and intentionally paradoxical: they draw power from the indexical quality of blood to evidence sincerity, but they do so to com-municate sarcasm and cynicism about the addressee. As a partonomic form, the gift of a heart is best described not as a part given that indicates a whole not given, but rather a part given that indicates a deep corruption in the part-whole relation—a corruption not easily remedied through either exemplary or compulsive philan-thropy. It is as much a ritual of defamation as it is a ritual of verification; it aims as much to reveal the biomoral pathology of its addressee as it does to authenticate the addresser.

In focusing on the *how* of activism as much as the *why*, we have showed how donated and received bodily substances in different iterations are both reformist and remedial, extractive and poisonous. Disease is indexed by a disjunction be-tween the substance-code relation, magnified upon the body of the putative In-dian family, the divided postcolonial nation, and the corrupt postliberalization state. Its cure relies on an invocation of malaise, followed by the philanthropic donation that realigns cause, character, and the materiality of the substance at hand. We have called this form of exchange partonomic to characterize how that which is given indicates the whole that is withheld, thereby instantiating a mode of philanthropic critique.

Yet at every instance, substance-exchanges reveal the fragility of such scenes of critique. Thus, Nirankari blood donations sought to recuperate the family to the end of a common future humanity at the same time as they glorified a this-worldly *satguru*. The blood camps of political rallies too walk a fine line between sincerity and self-interest, between the camp organizers' desire for a universal philanthropic good and the messy extractive modes of realpolitik. The blood writing of Bhopali children made this relation between instruction and corruption starkly explicit, where activists deployed the material index of sincerity to communicate sarcastic critique. Finally, the hunger strike deployed another bodily material—ketones— to return an index of sincerity that the blood as an activist medium was perceived to have lost. The material giving of blood and the metaphoric donation of organs allow us to point to ambivalence and fragility within philanthropic practices. The bodily gift is both a marker of conviction and the bearer of its own undoing.

In other words, hemo-political critique carries with it a circular threat; the utopic and the corrupt are joined in a dangerous, substantial proximity. The promise of a future through the gift is fraught with the danger of invoking vio- lent pasts and revealing a divided present. The blood gift particularly points to a breakdown of the substance-code relation, a malaise at once material, biological, and political. But in the practices of its giving, its pedagogic and reformist aims never escape its messy origins. To understand the work of critique, then, is to un- derstand its conjunctive tense—a fragile state between embodied critique and bodily extraction in which the scene of critique is never cleanly detached from the scene of corruption.

In the reformed (i.e., voluntary, non-remunerated) mode of blood collection, one does not know but may imagine one's recipients. This widening aligns blood donation with the idea of service and sacrifice to broader imagined communities—the nation, the abstract entity of "society," and of a "family" larger than immediate kin. We showed how the bodily philanthropy of reformed blood donation is made congruent with both reformist agendas as well as with political party activists and other dubious characters seeking access to the ethical surpluses generated by voluntary blood donation, grafting the aura and status of such practices. This trajectory of the sanguinary politics is thus in tune with Jonathan Spencer's observation that one aspect of the opposition between "dirty politics" and imaginary antipolitics "is its constant productivity—new leaders constantly seek new ways to take the politics out of politics, yet each attempt ends in a different kind of failure as the amoral world of the political inexorably tarnishes the shiny new possibilities" (2008, 626). In the Bhopali case, writing with blood performs an interior, biomoral truth that enfolds a further threat; it aims to compel a response that promises not just political patronage but an acknowledgment of toxicity within the body politic. In each deployment of practices of bodily giving over, that which is given threatens to spin "out of place," causing witnesses to reflect on gifts not given and relations not established. These substances "out of place" gesture to an economy of recognition and misrecognition of substance ties and the unevenly distributed possibilities of political intimacy. As anthropologists know well, practices of gifting are hardly ever innocent. In the gesture of forming and reforming human communities, gifts reveal the vulnerability of social forms and stake the possibility of their deformation. As blood circulates in the social body in North India, we suggest, it acts both as remedy and poison; practices of blood donation hope to perform reformations of a national imaginary, while in the same gesture, counter-practices steeped in irony reveal the fragility of sanguinary visions.

4

HEMO ECONOMICUS

From Blood Sacrifice to Blood Science?

This chapter examines pedagogical projects that seek to encourage Indians to donate their blood voluntarily. Such projects strive to produce a perceptual shift away from an association between blood donation with "sacrifice," articulating instead its relationship with "blood science." The chapter locates what we call the antisacrificial redescription of blood donation as a productively compromised pedagogical project seeking to produce and convey new bodily understandings designed to persuade Indians of the safety of blood donation, so encouraging more people to donate. The campaign has achieved some success, particularly in Bengal. Yet close examination reveals something more complex than a simple linear shift from "sacrifice" to "science." Rather than being eliminated, sacrifice is sublated, finding new and subtle forms in the understandings and practices meant to replace it. Sacrifice as a mode of bodily practice, we suggest, is not absented but redimensioned in newer, "scientific" pedagogies of blood donation.

Our ethnographic focus is on a campaign featuring the descriptive reconfiguration of blood from being something like an organ (irreplaceable, its giving irreversible) to something that is economically productive and replenishable. The body is thereby reconfigured as something that is able to give, *and to give again*. As a blood-donor recruitment volunteer put it to us, "We have excess blood. If a person can survive from our excess blood, then this is not a sacrifice. It is just a donation." This chapter thus gives an account of a form of pedagogy concerned with shifting the public's proportional imagination of bodily blood quantum (from finite to infinite, from lacking blood to holding a surfeit of it) that simultaneously redimensions the gift of blood: a perceptual downsizing from a gift too big to the point of being ungiveable, to a gift so small to now barely register as such, but which, in a seeming paradox, still enacts a sacrifice.

We draw on ethnographic research in Kolkata and Delhi, where we followed voluntary blood donor organizations seeking to educate schoolchildren and others about the quantities of blood that can be safely donated. The key point they seek to convey is that the body produces more blood than it needs, and so a portion of this excess blood can be given without the body losing anything. This is an insight at odds with conventional understandings of blood excorporation in the region as involving irrecuperable loss, understandings that inform continuing perceptions of blood donation as a sacrificial gesture. To give blood without risking irrecuperable loss would seem to fundamentally undercut the gesture of blood donation as sacrifice. An imagination of blood as excess and surplus thus involves the antisacrificial redescription of blood donation. Employing Georges Bataille's notion of "excess" energy in *The Accursed Share* (1988), we seek to show how, for such campaigners, the body comes to be perceived as positively made for giving—that is, the body contains a (completely safe to give) gift-share of blood.

An enigma in the Indian experience of blood donation has been that while most medics are keen to dispel the popular local conception that blood is nonreplenishable (i.e., once donated, blood is gone forever), they also understand that they have depended on those very ideas; many who have given have done so *because* of its sacrificial connotations. It is worth underscoring this key paradox: the idea that it is safe to donate the substance can thus, counterintuitively, be a hindrance to collection. This has meant that donor recruitment agencies have not always spoken with one voice about the safety of blood donation. Some recruiters see its association with sacrifice as a means of increasing voluntary donation—for instance, drawing an equation between the god Shiva's drinking of poison and donors' giving of blood.[1] Such recruiters actively employ existing understandings of the perils of blood donation precisely as a means of recruitment, judging that comparing donors to a nobly self-sacrificing god is more likely to be efficacious than emphasizing that it is safe to donate blood. It is not a senseless strategy: sacrifice not only repels but attracts donors. Once again, part of this is religious, for the more the sacrifice the bigger the merit (Mayer 1981, 162). The shift away from sacrifice and toward "science" might thus also be construed as without religious merit, which is dangerous given that so many of the gains the voluntary movement has made come precisely from religious movements' involvement.

Yet for all the dangerous attraction of sacrifice, if one asks nondonors (in Delhi and Kolkata at least, our principal field sites) why they do not donate, they will almost always refer to the "obvious" dangers of the practice. For example, students frequently state that their parents have forbidden them—which though a convenient displacement of responsibility, is also likely in many cases to be true.[2] There is thus general agreement among blood banks and medical authorities that the perception that blood donation is an activity of irreversible depletion (that is, of very real personal sacrifice) is the principal factor hindering an increase in voluntary donation.[3] Making voluntary blood donation attractive to would-be donors, then, necessitates the antisacrificial redescription of blood donation—a specifically tailored pedagogy that involves the imaginative reproportioning of the body and its hemo-economic processes.

It is significant that our work here goes against the grain of most existing literature on divergent modes of biological exchange in the subcontinent, which tends to depict bodies as being made abject by giving/donation practices (e.g., L. Cohen 1999 and 2001 on organ donation and selling; and Sunder Rajan 2006 on clinical trials). In developing his work on organ transfers in India, Lawrence Cohen (2001) has highlighted, with characteristic acuity, the several ways in which such transfers intertwine with sacrificial registers. Cohen dwells in particular on prevalent public representations of the selling, or "sacrifice," of kidneys by family members anxious to raise dowry funds: the gift of an organ (*ang-dan*) to facilitate the gift of a daughter (*kanya-dan*) (or the traffic in women, as Cohen puts it). He describes how in the Hindi film *Saaheb* (1985), the hero sells a kidney in order to finance his sister's wedding: "The film cuts from wedding to operation and back again, repeatedly linking the sacrificial oblations of the marriage ceremony making husband and wife into a new body with the transfusion of Saaheb's anesthetized body" (26). Meanwhile, in their study of stem cell research in North India, Bharadwaj and Glasner (2008) argue that the concept of "biosociality" is analytically unsuited to describing the social relations that appear in Indian stem cell clinics if (as they suggest it generally is) it is understood to indicate the informed, consenting, and willed formation of biologically driven identities (D. Banerjee 2011, 489). For instance, in the New Delhi clinical sites of which Bharadwaj and Glasner write, it is frequently economically disadvantaged infertile couples who act as stem cell donors in return for gratis future in vitro fertilization cycles. (This arrangement does not quite accord with conventional informed consent or global protocols of voluntarism.) Thus, for good reasons, the picture of the body presented in this literature (from kidney and stem cell donors and vendors to clinical test subjects) leans toward an object of repressive body politics; donors are depicted as figures of abjection made to give by an asymmetrical ethics in a world divided into those that sacrifice and those that can choose not to sacrifice. This chapter pushes in a different direction in describing a project in which (Indian) bodies are depicted as precisely not needing to sacrifice. No longer abject sites of extraction in situations of constrained ethics, they are to be reconfigured into subjects of reproducible generosity.

The Association of Voluntary Blood Donors, West Bengal

The Kolkata-based Association of Voluntary Blood Donors, West Bengal (AVBDWB) is a special organization in the history of blood donation in India. Innovative and successful, it is not only a vanguard voluntary movement for the promotion of non-remunerated blood donation in Bengal, but it has spawned imitator organizations in other states such as Kerala and Tamil Nadu.[4] It also regularly stages workshops and conferences to share recruitment techniques it has honed at its Bengal "laboratory" with other state blood banks and donor organizations. To be sure, it is not only a story of success; as an amateur (albeit highly skilled) voluntary organization, it cannot account for inefficiencies and corruption elsewhere in the "vein to vein chain." But where, for instance, in Uttar Pradesh in 2014–2015 only 62,961 voluntary units were collected out of a total number of 900,142 (6.99 percent), in Bengal 498,224 voluntary units contributed to the overall total of 926,158 (54.8 percent). Only the Andaman and Nicobar Islands, Goa, Himachal Pradesh, Jharkhand, Mizoram, and Mumbai have comparable figures out of thirty-five states in total (DAC, Government of India 2015, cited in AVBDWB 2015). Bengal's comparatively high percentage is almost completely due to the campaigning and educational efforts of the AVBDWB. We have outlined some of its recruitment techniques elsewhere.[5] Here we will outline the techniques of other organizations as well but retain a focus on the AVBDWB's pedagogical efforts as emblematic of a process that involves changing the bodily meanings of blood donation, a process that may be thought of as, to paraphrase Spinosa, Flores, and Dreyfus (1997), disclosing new bodily worlds.

Simply put, while the AVBDWB's techniques overlap with those employed elsewhere in the country and beyond, it is this organization that is the most systematic and rigorous in applying them. It mobilizes the "new" knowledge of what it calls "blood science"—first, as a disabler of the notion of donation as involving irrecoverable depletion (i.e., as a sacrificial act), and second, in the academic institutionalization of blood donor motivation: schoolchildren and teachers are encouraged to study for and take exams in blood science and record the qualification on their CVs. Specifically with respect to its school programs, one of the organization's founders told us, "Our aim is to make them blood donors when they reach 18." Given their age, the emphasis is more on blood science than on blood donation, with the latter approached only allegorically. For instance, in tell-ing the story of how in 1912 a large boat ignored the *Titanic*'s SOS calls, resulting in the avoidable death of hundreds, the audience comes to understand through the allegory that if they are healthy but do not donate their blood, they will be indirectly responsible for avoidable death and suffering. The AVBDWB's mission is as much a moral one as it is about science communication.

Blood Science

We encountered in chapter 3 the view that Indians lack civic-mindedness and "don't give," or if they do give, it is only in order to help their "own" (family, caste, co-religionists, etc.).[6] When we met AVBDWB activist Ranjit at a blood dona-tion camp in Kolkata, he explained his organization's very different approach: "We ask, why don't people donate? (1) Is it because they are selfish? (2) Is it because they don't know blood science? Number 1 can be ruled out because when we ex-plain to them, many come forward. People are not genuinely selfish. They are just ignorant of the science of blood." This point of view is important because it is so markedly different from the defeatism and vicious circularity that charac-terizes the attitudes of many professional recruiters. For many recruiters, low vol-untary blood donor numbers substantiate their view that their fellow Indians are not philanthropically or civic minded and hence their own efforts are often un-reciprocated, and donation numbers remain low. Such a view is common among societies partly shaped by Orientalist discourses, where many have internalized a bifurcation of "civic" and "religious" sociality (Hirschkind 2001).[7] In postcolo-nial India, a chief political aspiration for many political organizations (including the Hindu right) has been to innovatively braid the two together as part of a new vision of an Indian nationalism that is strengthened by the overlapping of civic and religious vocabularies (Hansen 1999). The AVBDWB approaches the same problem, albeit with a contrasting aspiration for secular pan-Indian community.

Let us describe the central obstacle that promoters of blood science face in their aspirational quest. One of the very first blood donation camps we attended was at a Lord Ayyappa temple in Delhi, which largely catered to migrants from the south of the country. There we met a man in his late thirties, a bus driver origi-nally from Kerala. Busy diving into the donor refreshments, despite not having himself donated blood, he was the subject of some comment. He told us that if he were to give his blood to the doctor, then the doctor would have to give it back to him (i.e., he would need a transfusion), so it was better to not donate and so avoid what would be a pointless transaction. Another—legitimate—partaker of the refreshments interjected: "It's [the feeling of] taking something away from the body. They [nondonors] think they'll run out of it." The bus driver responded, "I have less blood (*khuun ki kami*). I actually need to take blood." "You see?" said the other. Proponents of blood science, then, must seek to counter, first, the notion that there is only a finite store of blood in the body (making blood donation akin to, say, the donation of a kidney), and second, the sense that many people have—especially those who are lower middle class and below—of themselves requiring more blood, never mind donating their own. They must go further still and explain that not only do such persons not have a deficit, but they have a surplus that is safely donatable. The pedagogy of blood science thus seeks to inculcate the perceptual reproportioning of blood quantum and generation.

On not requiring a transfusion: At a Catholic girls' school in Kolkata, an AVB-DWB member speaks (mainly in English) on blood science: "We need a scientific perspective. We all have a heart, whether it is in the right place or not. It pumps blood day in and day out. Our blood travels 12,000 miles in twenty-four hours, and 8,000 gallons gets pumped. People say, 'I should receive blood!' But if you were given an extra unit of blood, the 8,000 gallons that gets pumped would become 9,000 gallons per twenty-four hours, and if you got two more units, your heart would then fail." On another occasion, before a group of local schoolteachers (in a mixture of Bengali and English), a different recruiter from the same organization developed the theme: "Men have 76ml of blood per kilogram of body weight, and women 66ml. If you multiply your weight by 66ml, you can work out how much blood you've got. Everybody's blood is proportionate to his or her height. If you put a bucket of water under a tap for eternity, once it's full, you won't get more in it. You don't need more blood. Just as if you put a bucket under a tap and keep the tap on for all eternity and it won't ever fill two buckets, similarly blood cannot ever be more than 76ml per kilogram of body weight." In other words, do not ask for a transfusion unless you've suffered blood loss. We suspect that the recruiter himself would acknowledge that this is a simplification—it confuses quality and quantity, for an anemic girl from Himachal Pradesh might have a normal quantum of blood but still require a transfusion to raise her hemoglobin level—but this is nevertheless the method of explanation. Note the comparison with water. In chapter 3 we encountered the view that politicians should concern themselves less with blood and more with water as a substance of the civic. Here water and blood are in a different relationship. The comparison is not to show degeneracy; rather, it is pedagogical.

On the recuperative power of blood: Water imagery is also used in order to explain how blood, after donation, re-forms and returns. A recruitment professional at a government blood bank in Delhi shared with us the following poetic lines she had composed: "What difference does it make / If from the well one pot goes away? / You only benefit from this. / You lose the old and obtain the new. / The process brings benefit to the body / And happiness to the heart." Echoing Paul Ricoeur's (1966, 418) remarks on how life functions "in me without me"—"It is a wisdom of movement: the circulation of my blood and the beating of my heart do not depend on me"—AVBDWB's publicity materials state, "[Blood] is like a spring. What you use from within comes back automatically. You don't have to do anything." A member of the same organization expressed his frustration to us that "people don't give blood because they don't know that it is replaced automatically. They do not know that it is similar to the well and water. If I take water from the well, nobody puts water in the well. God puts it back. It is a system of the universe; earth-connecting channels put water [back] into the well. If water is not at a particular level, it gets balanced. They are not able to understand this." Blood donation is thus figured as an intervention in an already ongoing process of re-formation. Removing a portion stimulates new growth, like fresh water in a spring. Antisacrificial redescription of blood donation as a process for expelling the old and gaining the new can seem to portray it as a branch of therapeutics, almost akin to bloodletting, with donation a kind of blood-cleansing mechanism with connotations of *dan* in the classic Indic mode in which a giver gives partly as a means of self-purification. We will return to this question below.

The bus driver at the Lord Ayyappa temple camp who declined to donate did so in the belief that were he to do so, he would require a transfusion. In the AVBDWB way of thinking, the donor in fact does receive a kind of transfusion, but *from within*. The donor is infused with his or her own fresh blood consequent on the originating activity of giving itself. If blood, in such depictions, is like water in returning to find the right balance, one thing it is not like is money. As one AVBDWB member told an audience of students, "Money leaves us and is forever gone. Blood is not like this; there is re-formation very quickly." We can build here on Strathern's insights on "vernacular comparison" (2009). The AVBDWB compares different sorts of substance along an axis of their ability to return once parted with as a form of rhetoric. The dexterous recruiter deploys associations and separations in order "to move the social situation from one state to another" (Carrithers 2005, 581).

Supplementing the strategy of vernacular comparison, the tactic of demonstration has also formed a key force of rhetoric in the AVBDWB's attempts to persuade and convince nondonors to donate their blood. In the early days, AVBDWB members would appear before students in Jadavpur University lecture theaters to inform them about blood science, but not only to speak; blood science was demonstrated, with another AVBDWB member (accompanied by a medic) donating his or her blood on the stage beside the speaker. The very survival of the donor, witnessed by the audience, implied a proof of the blood science enunciated by the speaker. Donating itself was a force of rhetoric.[8] In a less dramatic mode, many AVBDWB members have themselves donated blood scores of times, some a hundred times or more, and this fact itself possesses demonstrative rhetorical value when invoked in blood science talks, for how could the speaker, having donated many times, be present before the audience if it were not for the recuperative power of blood? Further, if the very purpose of blood donation is the saving of life, why would its advocates seek to promote it (ask its advocates) if in fact it endangered the giver's life? A Delhi government blood bank recruiter addressed the matter in a self-penned Hindi poem used in promotional Video CDs shown in schools and colleges:

> We have to give life to the other.
> This does not mean we want to lose life.
> I don't want to wipe the vermilion off one woman
> To make life for the other (*dusra*).

Married Hindu women wear auspicious red vermilion in the parting of their hair. If they are widowed, the mark is removed. In stark terms, then, the message of the poem is *We are not trying to kill you*. The poem seeks to explain that blood donor and recipient lifetimes are not in a zero-sum relationship and to distinguish blood donation and blood banks from narratives that seem to posit a universal practice of extracting the vitality of underprivileged donors to extend the lives of privileged recipients. Similarly seeking to deterrorize blood donation, the umbrella website for state-run blood banks in Delhi contains an aphorism said to have been spoken by the Buddha: "Thousands of candles can be lighted from a single candle, and the life of the candle will not be shortened."[9]

The foregoing attempts at rhetorical persuasion are usually accompanied by a set of facts and figures. At a Youth Congress camp on Sonia Gandhi's birthday came a loudspeaker announcement: "It is believed by many that if you give blood then your own blood gets less—it's not so; this is a wrong conception. In forty-eight hours, scientists say, new blood gets formed. So there should be no worry or fear in giving blood." The figures vary a little; some medics say that the volume of the donation is replaced within seventy-two hours. Some donors we spoke with found this confusing: "If it comes back in seventy-two hours, then why do they want us to donate next time in three months?" In response, the AVBDWB attempts to make clear in its leaflets and lectures that when a person donates, half a gram of hemoglobin leaves the body, and it takes six to eight weeks to replenish this. In other words, quantity is restored within seventy-two hours, quality in six to eight weeks. But still, six to eight weeks is not three months—the required interval between donations. When asked about this discrepancy, medics and recruiters often made two points: First, Indians tend to have a lower body weight compared with Westerners and therefore have less of both blood and hemoglobin, so extra caution concerning recovery time is required. Second, since voluntary blood donors are a "minority community"—less than 1 percent of the Indian population—their interests must be protected in the form of extra precautionary measures.[10] The use of language most frequently heard in reference to the rights of cultural and ethnic minorities and their access to redistributive justice to describe the status of voluntary blood donors shows the reach and plasticity of rights language and claims in India. It also shows the way in which—perhaps partly due to the insistent slogans that exhort the fostering of a *culture* of voluntary blood donation—blood donors may be bracketed off in familiar terms of cultural difference as a distinct community.[11]

On the body's surplus of blood: If the recuperative power of the body complicates narratives of a blood donation that is sacrificial, the idea that the body holds a surplus of the substance might seem to kill off such narratives entirely. For according to the AVBDWB and other recruiters, it is not even a loss that is recuperated, but merely a portion of the excess all human bodies hold. "Excess" is thus redistributed from the excessive loss of sacrifice to excessive blood quantum, enabling a conception of blood donation as involving absolutely no loss at all. Recall the words of the AVBDWB officer quoted earlier: "We have excess blood. If a person can survive from our excess blood, then this is not a sacrifice."

A lecturer in engineering from Jadavpur University, also a member of the AVBDWB, described to us how most forms of bloodshed, particularly in West Bengal with its popular traditions of bloodthirsty Kali worship, carry connotations of sacrifice and how this is a double-edged sword. Such connotations can serve to ennoble the act, but they also underscore perceptions of it as harmful. Overall the extractive resemblance between them has proven to be extremely unhelpful, in the lecturer's view, for they are fundamentally different activities: "In blood donation you cause no harm to yourself. In sacrifice you harm yourself. We impress upon [people] that [blood donation] is nothing like a sacrifice, that in blood donation you are giving only part of a surplus." So how is this surplus figured to nondonors or future donors such as schoolchildren? And if blood donation is not a sacrifice, then what is it?

"'My God, we have no extra blood to give!' People used to think I was mad when I asked them to donate some of their extra blood, and it is still hard to explain this to them," a Delhi-based recruiter told us. At a blood science education event at a municipal building in Kolkata, an AVBDWB leader sought to explain to a slightly surprised public (for they had turned up believing that the event concerned science education more broadly): "For each kilogram of body weight, a male has 76ml of blood; while for females it is 66ml per kilogram of body weight. So if we multiply our weight by 66/76, that is our blood volume. But we only need

50ml of blood per kilogram of body weight. There is thus a surplus. In engineering terms, it is the *factor of safety*. If we slowly part with 8ml of blood per kilogram of body weight of this surplus, there is no harm." One middle-aged woman stood up to respond, "I currently have the correct amount of blood in my body," the implication being that she could not herself give for this reason. The speaker responded, "Blood cells have a life span of 120 days. Even if you do not donate blood, 1/120 of your blood is dying per day. On the 120th day we would have nothing left if we didn't have replenishment. Donating blood does no harm to us, and through blood donation we can save a precious life."

Part of what is being communicated here is that our blood *in any case* leaves the body, so why not put that process to use for the benefit of those who are in need of it? Other recruiters are more explicit about what is only suggested here in terms of avoiding waste. A medic at an NGO-run blood bank in Delhi put it like this: "Whether you donate or not, red cells have a life of 120 days, and after this they expire, break down; there is a burden and lots of work required to excrete these old cells. After three months you can donate for others—so you give, and 90 days after your red cells will be mature. Let it be useful for someone, let's not waste it." Or in the words of a poem read at a poetry competition on the subject of blood donor motivation at the government All India Institute of Medical Sciences (AIIMS) hospital in Delhi: "We don't even know that after some time / Our blood cells swell up and are destroyed by themselves. / They are extra (*zyada*), and if that excess (*bahut zyada khun*) is given away in donation, / It can save somebody's life." Apoptosis—programed cell death—thus enables blood donation. "Death and the regeneration of life" is here writ both small and large—on a cellular level, the "swelling up" and "destruction" that stimulate new growth, and in a hospital bed, the regenerative transfusion that piggybacks on a process of cellular death and rebirth.

Surplus, Waste, and the Gift-Share

The revaluation, or reclamation, of biological waste as a new source of therapeutic and commercial value has formed a focus of works on biological exchange (Konrad 2005; Waldby and Mitchell 2006; Hodges 2013). For instance, ova donors in the United Kingdom are told that they have "spare embryos" (Konrad 2005, 51). The treatment process is "predicated on the value of excess and the desirability of cultivating a surplus of eggs through superovulation" (58); women state that "if [they] didn't donate them they would go down the pan" (198). Konrad thus speaks of "remaindered form" and an "aesthetics of excess" (201). Influenced by Waldby and Mitchell's argument about the "commercial and epistemological value" of designating bodily tissues "waste," scholars have shown how such designations are often the first step in establishing their exchange value (2006, 115). Waste products, as "abjects," do not carry the donor's personality and so are alienable; their designation as "waste" justifies the creation of biovalue from them (Kent 2008, 1751).

It might appear as though we have been describing in this chapter a process akin to this: an attempt to redesignate understandings of blood donation away from intimate self-sacrifice to simple excretion of a waste product—a move from intimacy to alienability. Dixon-Woods et al. (2008, 61) have questioned such narratives for fostering an understanding of the sources of biological materials "as 'disempowered' and 'often-unwitting' individuals, disengaged from the scientific and commercial potential of tissue by its designation as 'waste' on removal from their bodies." Our view is that the focus on waste and biovalue can be both useful and misleading—misleading because it is useful: its easy generalizability may make us overlook the specific features of particular networks of biological exchange. The nuanced approach we seek is found in Klaus Hoeyer's (2009) work on bone donation in which he recognizes the importance of the designation "waste" in creating exchange value but holds that "waste" does not exhaust the meanings of the donated substance as such. Instead, "donors and doctors use the categorization to establish a shared understanding of the implications of a donation: the donor does not stand to lose anything by letting go of the bone" (244).

In concert with Hoeyer's approach, what we find in our case is the mobilization of a conception of excess blood—the very opposite of *khuun ki kami*—as a means of promoting the understanding among would-be blood donors that they do not stand to lose anything by letting go of some of their blood. We have already seen why this, alongside an emphasis on hematapoietic recurrence, is important for countering the perception that blood donation involves irrecuperable loss. What focusing on the body's surplus of blood also allows recruiters to do is to conceive and communicate the notion of a body and substance that is designed for giving—the excess is neither "mere" waste nor abjectly alienable. Rather, it forms a gift-share. To be sure, if that share remains ungiven, it is a loss and to be lamented; it would be a "waste" even. But it still must *be* given—shared.

Another oft-heard Indian recruitment slogan is that blood donation is like a mother's love moving from the healthy to the ailing—that is, the donor is like a nurturing mother. In more tangible terms, whereas a mother gives milk that has, so to speak, been made in order to be given, the donor's blood comes to possess similar connotations. This gendered motherly metaphor takes us well away from alienability and abjection, serving an indicative purpose in allowing us to consider what work the designations "extra" and "surplus" are doing in our specific case.

It is not only the rescaling (aggrandizement) of kin relationships, then, that is at stake here, with donor-mothers figured as substantial nurturers of recipient-children. Rather, just as a human mother's milk is made to image altruism and is a substance made to be given away, so the designation "surplus" performs a similar naturalizing function with respect to bodies "made to give." Significantly, many AVBDWB members understand this as a kind of *countermetaphor* to that of Richard Dawkins's *The Selfish Gene* (1976), a book with which numerous members are familiar.[12] Dawkins himself regrets the title of his book and the misleading impression it gives of a biogenetic justification for egoistic behavior. In his introduction to the thirtieth anniversary edition of the book, Dawkins (2006, vii–ix) lamented such reductive readings.[13] Nevertheless, such understandings dominate popular conceptions of the work. Again and again the text was mentioned with disapproval by AVBDWB members at lectures, seminars, and in interviews with us, who see its philosophy—at least, the one implied in its title—as antithetical to their mission of fostering the voluntary blood donation movement. For instance, at a public lecture given by one AVBDWB member (in Bengali), *The Selfish Gene* was invoked as a text communicating the idea that "we are slaves of our genes, but human beings have the power to rebel against the so-called selfish design of the gene. Human beings can be unselfish. . . . Blood donation is unselfishness. We know the surplus is there. It should be called 'the unselfish gene!'"

Bataille dealt with issues of excess and surplus in a very different and yet related way in *The Accursed Share* (1988). For Bataille, the "accursed share" refers to the "excess energy" an economy must disburse through wasteful consumption (e.g., expenditure on luxury goods). Such surplus energy is that which "cannot be deployed for a system's growth but which nevertheless has to be used up, rather like the heat that has to be used up thermodynamically in so-called dissipative structures" (Urry 2010, 207). We borrow Bataille's turn of phrase in suggesting the notion of the gift-share to describe the AVBDWB's countermetaphor to that of the selfish gene. It allows us to demonstrate the work that the designation "surplus" does in addition to allowing donors and medics to reach the shared understanding that blood donors do not stand to lose anything by letting go of some of their blood. The body's surplus, replenished after each donation, shows its purpose in being made to share. It is not selfishness that is predetermined, but sharing as revealed by the availability of the gift-share. As in Bataille's conception, there is a portion of excess, though here the excess is routed differently to a therapeutic end (in Bataille's terms, the "restrictive" and "general" economies are mixed together).[14] For Bataille, such excess energy "must be spent, willingly or not, gloriously or catastrophically" (1988, 21)—or, we might say, redistributively.

Many understandably view natural symbols and metaphors with skepticism—especially those in which blood figure (e.g., Haraway 1995). Natural symbols, suggests Douglas (1970), in conveying associations deriving from their organic roots can naturalize particular social processes; for instance, Weston (2013a) demonstrates how a pronounced discourse of blood in discussion of financial markets (e.g., the use of phrases such as "flow," "circulation," "liquidity," "the economy's lifeblood," and even "cash transfusion") is a factor in foreclosing debate about how things might be otherwise. The notion of blood's natural surplus, which we gloss here as its gift-share, partakes of these problematic logics, to be sure, though in the form of countermetaphor (or counteressentialism) as a rebuttal of conceptions of humans' innate selfishness. The "extra" blood designation is not (only) productive in terms of deactivating views of blood donation as physically harmful and for facilitating the alienability of blood and therefore its disentanglement from donor bodies, but also in promoting a view of bodies as designed or made to be unselfish. As a contestatory metaphor, it forms a part of the AVBDWB's own political hematology.

While the body's extra blood is foregrounded across the Indian blood-donor recruitment world, preoccupation with *The Selfish Gene* seems to be AVBDWB-specific. But one can certainly find echoes of it in other places. At the above-mentioned poetry competition in Delhi, for instance, these lines were spoken: "The extra blood says 'Use me / Give life to the other / And remove this land's pain.'" The biological-conceptual complex of surplus and recurrence is suggestive of a certain intentionality. The blood itself speaks—it *wants* to be used.

As we noted earlier, antisacrificial redescription of blood donation as a process for expelling the old and stimulating fresh growth might seem to make it into a branch of donor-oriented therapeutics. But in the case of the AVBDWB at least, we can see that, though a conception of donation as purgation apparently is hinted at through designations of surplus blood, this neither exhausts the meanings of the action nor de-gifts it as such. The AVBDWB message—which dominates understandings in Bengal—defines the surplus in terms of care for the other: one is not giving one's waste; rather, it is a waste not to give, since the portion of excess will in any case be lost. Moreover, it is not that donating blood is purifying for donors, but that they do not imperil themselves in giving it (because there is a portion that is safe to give). Indeed, as we have seen, for the AVBDWB the presence in the donor's body of an excess that can be safely removed, far from canceling the gift, proves that the body is made for giving.

We can compare this with Emilia Sanabria's (2009) work, which explores linkages between blood donation, class, menstruation, bloodletting, and ideas of well-being in Bahia, Brazil. Medics see the ascetic form of uncompensated blood donation, which they advocate, as continually under threat from conceptions of donation as generating some kind of benefit—in this case, the health benefit of purified blood. Sanabria reveals an acute gendering of blood donation in the region, which centers on the fact that, although menstruation acts as a bar to female participation (men donate almost twice as much blood as women), those women who are not menstruating may seek to donate their blood as a kind of substitute for that which they forego. Since menstruation is held to alleviate a physical and emotional condition caused by a build-up of blood, some nonmenstruating women see blood donation as a special means of achieving a similar effect. As is the case in India, so too in Bahia: blood donation comes to look like a mode of socialized bloodletting.

Particularly important to Sanabria's analysis is the practice of hormonal menstrual suppression, a medical intervention that is utilized by many Bahian women but that is also thought to cause a problematic build-up of blood in the body. While this latter understanding is not limited to Brazil, the association in Bahia between menstruation and blood purification heightens the concern about accumulation consequent on menstrual suppression. In this situation, as one of Sanabria's informants puts it, "giving blood gives relief." But the logic is not simply one of somatic introversion, the donor "cutting" the "transfusion relation" (L. Cohen 2001, 27) into a transaction with and within oneself (i.e., "giving" thick blood and "getting back" clean blood). For while evacuative perceptions of blood donation undoubtedly possess conceptual affinities with seemingly nonrelational bloodletting, giving blood in order to secure "relief" is also considered by Sanabria's informants to give "the otherwise useless menstrual blood a positive and altruistic function." Indeed, the availability of blood donation as a means to expel accumulated blood has made blood shed through menstruation appear wasteful to some. Once more, it is not that one is giving one's waste, but rather that not giving is wasteful. Similarly, so far as purgation and donor-oriented therapeutics are hinted at in both India and Bahia, it is not that blood donation has been made nonrelational in being rendered a form of bloodletting, but rather that bloodletting has been made relational in being turned into a form of blood donation.

Spillover Hematology, or a Return to Sacrifice?

Alberto Corsín Jiménez (2013, 130) explains how, according to economists, public goods "have a tendency to flow over their market circumscriptions, delivering their 'goodness' beyond their original catchment area." An example of such a spillover might be the skilled musician whose nightly practice of his or her instrument provides enjoyment to a music-loving neighbor (130). Such spillovers are "uncompensated benefits that one person's activity provides to another" (Lemley and Frischmann 2006, 2). Taking inspiration from this literature, Corsín Jiménez proposes a "spillover sociology," the better for taking account of the non-contained nature of social life. From such a perspective, the body's productive activity in creating "more blood than it itself needs," so allowing that excess to form a benefit for others, might be framed in terms of a spillover hematology: the AVBDWB characterizes the body's "extra" blood as a kind of public good, capable through donation of flowing over its originating biological province and helping others as well.

But now we must ask: Can the blood the body produces really safely spill over to form an infinitely extensible benefit for others? Consider the slogan that can be found on stickers attached to the rear windows of cars in Scotland: "Please drive carefully—I've already donated blood." The way of thinking embodied in the catchphrase is precisely contrary to AVBDWB's pivotal message—namely, that blood donation is a perfectly safe activity. The catchphrase implies that blood donation makes donors more vulnerable in temporarily removing a portion of their buffer stock: should they suffer a hemorrhage, they will more quickly bleed to death. The slogan constitutes a small act of donor care on the part of the Scottish blood service; it says to drivers, "Be extra careful—this person's surplus is depleted; their vulnerability to further bleeding is heightened." So can buffer stock qualify as surplus if that share is protective? The body's surplus of blood comes into view as both fact and fiction. If it is a fiction, it is perhaps a necessary one. The surplus might be described as a species of hyperbole in Quintilian's sense of it as lies told without mendacity (Johnson 2010, 346). To reiterate: it is easy to see why the AVBDWB would wish to eschew such a message as contained in the car sticker as being incongruent with its antisacrificial redescription of blood donation. This is because it seems to smuggle sacrifice back in, in the way it refers, however obliquely, to loss.

We want to suggest now that if the AVBDWB seeks to undercut the association between blood donation and blood sacrifice, its attempts to do so are themselves undercut by messages emanating from elsewhere in the Indian blood donation and transfusion field. In this way, sacrifice comes to retain a dangerous presence in the imagining of blood donation—but a rescaled, transfigured presence. This brings us back to questions concerning *dan*. As we shall see, blood banks' characterization of blood donation as a mode of *dan* (that is, as *rakt-dan*) is useful to them, but it reintroduces sacrificial connotations. So we see competing messages run together—one antisacrificial, the other insinuating sacrifice—that seemingly undercut one another. We want to suggest, however, that the different messages resolve one another.

Indic *dan* is very frequently characterized as a gift for which no return can be countenanced. Since blood donation was first practiced in North India, however, *rakt-dan* has been the euphemistic administrative label for all the varieties of blood donation: paid, replacement, and voluntary. For many voluntary donors and blood bank staff, the use of "*dan*" to denote paid and replacement donation was and is a disgraceful misapplication of a revered term and concept. However, the recent emphasis in India on the promotion of voluntary blood donation, necessitated by a 1998 legal ruling that forbade payment, has made the use of the term "*rakt-dan*" seem less reprehensible to these donors and staff. This is because in the emergent voluntary system, donors should receive no payment and should be unaware of the recipients of their donations. Voluntary donation thus promises to provide both the asymmetry and anonymity held to characterize many classical notions of *dan*. Indeed, the anonymity and asymmetry of voluntary blood donation, on a conceptual level at least, present striking points of convergence between *rakt-dan* and key features of classical modes of *dan*.

Blood bank staff actively seek to translate this conceptual convergence into a practical one. Voluntary blood donation, they say, must conform precisely to the highest ideal of disinterested *dan*, since it is seen to ensure the safety of donated blood. This is because of the medical policy axiom that offering donors incentives increases the likelihood that they will conceal risk factors which, if revealed, would disqualify them from donating. The characterization of blood donation as a *dan* thus becomes an imperative for reasons of the safety of the transfusion. We thus already see a point of difference between the strategies of the AVBDWB and other agencies: the AVBDWB's antisacrificial redescription of blood donation emphasizes the safety of the act of donation for donors; emphasis on *dan*, on the other hand, is a means of trying to enhance the safety of recipients.[15] What are seemingly pitted against each other are the competing imperatives of getting people to donate in the right way (the emphasis on *dan*) versus getting people to donate at all (the antisacrificial strategy).

Placing emphasis on blood donation as a mode of *dan* not only serves as a template for the ascetic form of uncompensated giving that medics desire, but it also becomes a point of vulnerability where the suppressed element (sacrifice) can creep back in. "New" forms of flesh-and-blood *dan* have accumulated rapidly in recent years. This, of course, reflects the increase in forms of donatable corporeal material now utilizable by biomedicine: in addition to *rakt-dan*, there exist *netr-dan* (eye donation), *ang-dan* (organ donation), *deh-dan* (body donation), *bhrun-dan* (embryo donation), and other categories. While these new variants attest to the extensibility of *dan*, existing precedents for these sorts of gifts in theory and in practice suggest that, in addition to defining a "new" terrain of *dan*, they reconnect with or revivify foundational corporeal features of *dan* that might have been downplayed (or at least metaphorized) in more recent times. *Deh-dan*, which in its present-day usage refers to postmortem gifts of the body for extraction of organs and/or dissection by trainee medics, is a particularly elaborated category of giving in literature such as the Dharmashastras. There are, in addition, literal offerings of body parts, as in the cases of Karna in the *Mahabharata*, the sage Dadhichi, and the king Jagdev Singh Panwar, who gave "even his own head in *dan*" (Raheja 1989, 97). There are also metaphorical gifts of the body, where in complex ceremonies the ritual patron divests himself of his impure self through the giving of "gifts (*daksina*) which represent parts of the body" (Heesterman 1985, 27).[16]

If, as numerous theories suggest, *dan*—as an unreciprocated gift—is "officially" a surrogate for both sacrifice and asceticism in the age of Kali, then the unreciprocated giving of corporeal substance, when it is defined and understood as *dan*, simultaneously refutes and implies the asceticism and sacrifice it replaces. Indeed, theories of *dan* lay emphasis on the substitutive function of the gift, for, in the words of Heesterman, "the men of our era are no longer deemed strong enough to cope with the heady excitement and terror of sacrifice. In the *dvapara* era, sacrifice was the foremost meritorious work, but in our age it has been replaced by the gift" (86). But blood donation as *rakt-dan* can appear to collapse into complex simultaneities the developmental sequence, whereby *dan* is said to stand in for asceticism, which in turn, stands in for sacrifice. Or in Corsín Jiménez's (2013, 20) terms, the developmental sequence is "reversible." In contexts of Hindu ritual, as noted by van der Veer (1989, 72), fire sacrifice and gift-giving are equal insofar as the Brahmin-as-receiver-of-gifts is considered to be one of Brahma's mouths, the other being Agni (the sacrificial fire). Further, Agni is present in Brahmins as the digestive fire through which they "process" the gifts they receive. If it is in the domain of Brahmin-directed gifts that sacrifice has retained more than a latent presence, the *rakt-dan* conceptualization similarly places sacrifice back within the orbit of the blood gift's signification.

We may recall here the enigma of the relationship between blood donation and sacrifice referred to at the beginning of this chapter—namely, that the dangerous appeal of sacrifice means that, for some, antisacrificial redescription can act as a hindrance to blood donation. At the same time, the AVBDWB is perfectly aware that the connotation of blood donation as an irreversible loss is deleterious to collection. Our argument is that if the AVBDWB's message were to be fully successful, it would no longer be successful; its success *must remain* only partial. Were the antisacrificial definition of blood donation to be fully accepted, the result would be an overwhelming "loss of the loss" (Mazzarella 2010, 2), which would itself be damaging to collection figures. The danger of downsizing blood donation from being a gift too big to the point of being ungiveable, to a gift inconsequentially small, can be seen in the counterproductive effect of a recruiter's lecture at a

Mumbai school. In an effort to encourage donation, this recruiter argued, "Every human being has five to six liters of blood, and there is a buffer stock, and donating 350ml makes no difference to you." He then displayed a poster depicting a young woman happily reading a book while donating blood. The accompanying Marathi text read, "It is very easy to donate blood—all you need to do is lie flat! And this blood is regenerated by itself." Later, after the lecture, he explained to us that "the poster has an impact because of the novelty—'Oh, I have an excess! I don't lose anything. I give from the buffer stock and it's only a small fraction of the excess stock!'" However, when we spoke with the audience, they seemed less impressed. "If we lose nothing," said one seventeen-year-old student, "then can the transfusion really help someone?" "I thought I was sacrificing for the other, but now I see it [blood donation] is nothing," said another student. In the light of such comments from donors and would-be donors, we argue that sacrifice, smuggled back into the frame through *dan*, and the countermessage of antisacrificial redescription, do not simply cancel each other out but rather modify one another in a kind of productive mutual undercutting. If the antisacrificial redescription of blood donation makes it possible to give, the reactivation of sacrifice through *dan* makes it attractive to give.

To return to the Scottish car sticker mentioned earlier: what it teaches us is that it is perfectly possible for loss and safety to run together. But sacrifice must be understood in an adjusted sense—as loss, to be sure, but only from an already existing excess, and only temporary; the dangerous appeal of sacrifice is redimensioned but not eliminated entirely. After all, Indic sacrifice is certainly a scalable phenomenon: animals may stand in for humans (Samanta 1994), and vegetables for animals (F. Osella and C. Osella 2003); in the *kuthiyottam* sacrifice of southern Kerala, performed in honor of the goddess Bhadrakali, the portion of human blood that is spilled metonymically stands in for the whole of a person's lifeblood that was spilled in pre-reform times (110). Meanwhile, in the same ritual, the blood of two young low-caste boys substitutes for the blood of the sons of the sponsor, which were it to have been shed, would also have been substitutions— for that of the sacrifier (119). Blood sacrifice is always being redimensioned.

Michael Lambek (2008, 150) suggests that blood sacrifice is a measure of absolute, as opposed to negotiable, value. In India, its value might well remain unqualified (for those who conduct it; cf. Babb 2004), though the conditions of its enactment seem more negotiable. Blood sacrifice gains such value, Lambek argues, because it is "something that, once conducted, is not retractable." He is not referring, of course, to blood donation, but even so, and to the extent that it is associated with blood sacrifice, we have perhaps found a retractable variant: one suffers a loss until one no longer does so, and then, ideally, one suffers it again. If one gives one's life, then that is that. But if one sacrifices that which recurs, one can perpetually sacrifice. Lambek (2008, 150) further notes that "in the post-Puritan world it is assumed that value is something to be gained at no cost to the self—as interest, dividends, or other forms of exchange value." If the antisacrificial strategy of the AVBDWB conveys the "new" truth that blood donation is something to be performed at no cost to the donor, then the language of *dan*, and its history of substitutions, modifies that truth even as that truth rescales and redraws the nature of the sacrifice.

The AVBDWB project depicts bodies as precisely not needing to sacrifice. Rather than abject sites of extraction, donor bodies are reconfigured into subjects of reproducible generosity. The problem here was that the AVBDWB's antisacrificial approach, in spite of its continued employment of gift rhetoric, overflowed, going further in seeming to de-gifting blood donation entirely: blood donors lose nothing but the time it takes to donate; the gift simply vanishes. Under the sign of sacrifice, it reappears. At the same time, however, the AVBDWB approach ensures that the sacrifice is no longer an abject one.

Variations and Fault Lines

Based on the statewide collection figures that we quoted, we note that the AVBDWB's attempts to educate Bengali schoolchildren and others about blood science have been quite successful. We explained how the AVBDWB's antisacrificial redescription of blood donation has focused on conveying three linked tenets of blood science: that bodies which have not suffered blood loss do not require transfusions; that bodies hold a reserve of blood from which a portion may be safely donated; and that once removed that portion is replenished. Of particular importance, for association members is explaining the recuperation of blood. In so doing, they undercut sacrificial understandings and so facilitate donations. Importantly, however, while they emphasize the fact of recuperation, they leave open to speculation the *how* of recuperation—the mechanism through which blood is replenished. In this section, we consider speculation about the origin of the replenished blood, speculation that diverges from officially sanctioned biological narratives, and also examine the nature of the AVBDWB's investment in the human origins of the substance.

1. Return

We have previously written about replenishment being attributed to divine largesse in specifically devotional North Indian contexts.[17] Part of the interest there lay in devotees' understanding that the blood returned because of their devotional relationship with a guru. Without that devotion, the donated portion would not necessarily be replenished. What we find in the recruitment contexts we have been discussing in this chapter is related but different. That replenishment happens is presented as a scientific fact, regardless of the donor's religious devotion. At the same time, replenishment is sometimes attributed to God. As a donor recruiter from Delhi put it to us, "Technically speaking there is always a reserve. Donation is my resolve. I donate, and the Almighty again provides me with the reserve."

So far as the AVBDWB is concerned, such understandings are uncontroversial. Though the organization is not affiliated with any religious tradition, it is open to receiving help from religious leaders for motivation purposes and holds no explicit secular(izing) agenda. It is a practical organization whose main concern is simply boosting voluntary blood donations. If donors' or recruiters' understanding is that God replenishes blood, then so be it. The main thing is that they comprehend that it comes back, whatever the cause.

In more explicitly (bio)medical contexts, however, such understandings may be challenged and cause "epistemological embarrassment." For instance, speaking before an audience at a pan-Indian blood banking conference in Chennai, a medic from Kashmir declared, "We should say [to those reluctant to donate blood] that we have a bone marrow factory. Outside factories have power cuts, but our factory runs with the life force God has given us. When there is loss of blood [through donation], angels bring it back. Blood is the universal life force produced by God's factory." Discomfited, the chair and fellow panelists interrupted and tried to speak over him. But this only caused the medic to raise his voice, awakening audience members from their slumbers to applaud approvingly the Kashmiri medic, thereby provoking the liveliest moment of the day. Similarly, a recruiter in a Delhi government blood bank, speaking to us about replenishment, declared, "I tell them this and I know it is true: blood is continuously destroyed and formed, and it is OK. The fact we are alive proves it comes back. When you tell people that they are formed in the image of God, and this tremendous ocean is there—that you give it and then he gives it back, this force from God—it has a powerful effect on them."

2. Classification

At the same conference in Chennai came a further epistemological embarrassment. Extracted human blood, officially speaking, is defined as a drug, its usage governed and regulated by the Drugs and Cosmetics Act (1940). So, for instance, according to the act, "'blood component' means a drug manufactured or obtained from pooled plasma or blood by fractionation, drawn from donors." At the conference, the deputy drug controller of India gave a keynote emphasizing that it is not only components but whole human blood, too, which falls under the definition of a drug. Another presentation addressed the question "Is blood transfusion safe, or is blood one of the most dangerous drugs in the physician's therapeutic armamentarium?" Toward the end of the talk, a doctor from Karnataka could contain herself no longer. Rising to her feet, she said:

> This Drug Act—it is not a drug! It is not manufactured artificially. It is life force from God. It is not a drug, it is not food, it is not a cosmetic. There should be a life-force authority of India controlling the blood life force. When you put on the *tilak*, there is heaviness there, and this is the area where the gate of God's life force is. So life force and blood donation are totally dependent [on each other]. There are 70 million vaults of energy in one life only. One gram of flesh can light a city for seven days because of the electromagnetic force which is in blood—how can you say it is a drug?

Similarly to the case discussed above, the chair tried to cut her off. Official meanings were under attack in an embarrassingly public forum, in the presence of the deputy drug controller himself, and it was not even a recruiter who had spoken—for being nonmedics, recruiters can be granted some definitional license—but a well-known doctor.

What was in question here, of course, was the supposedly "modern" view of blood as a decultured "biochemical ensemble" (Simpson 2009, 104) that—given its postextraction mixture with anticoagulants and other treatments (e.g., fractionation to separate out plasma)—is considered both bureaucratically and according to medical orthodoxy as simply a drug to be administered. While the above conference interjection disputed the designation of (donated) blood as a "drug" because it eclipses what for the doctor is a more correct understanding of blood as a God-given substance-force, the interruption at the same time constituted a call to remember the human origin of the substance. Her emphasis was as much on the human fleshiness of donated blood as its ultimate divine source—both of which are mocked by the designation "drug," which of course obviates its multiplex human-divine origin.[18]

3. Origin

We turn now to a further calling into question of the human origin of the substance—an origin beyond both the human and divine. We begin with an excerpt from the inaugural address of the 2005 Parliament of Motivators conference,

organized by the AVBDWB and held in Kolkata, which brought recruiters together from across India and the world:

> Human blood possesses no caste, creed, religion, or pedigree. No na-
> tional or state boundaries can keep blood isolated in any domain. It is a
> symbol of unity and service of others. We all know about the revolutions
> of the last five hundred years: the Industrial Revolution, the French Rev-
> olution, and so on. A revolution is a fast change in social circumstances,
> with or without blood shed. We read about these revolutions but didn't
> participate in them. But with blood donation we are a part of it. It is the
> greatest nonpolitical movement that has taken place on our soil. All
> castes took part. No identity or religion was excluded.

While an anthropologist schooled in the many exclusionary layers of blood talk
may encounter many ironies here (see, e.g., Haraway 1995; Williams 1995), it is
not only for the AVBDWB but more widely still in the recruitment world (and
beyond) that blood is figured as a substance of humanism, a kind of cosmic substance of connection. For Drew Leder (1990, 157–73) in his classic phenomeno-
logical treatment of the body, for instance, we form one body with the universe
through blood, and all of nature is consanguineous. Confining ourselves to the
world of blood donation and transfusion, consider a slogan used by WHO and
the International Red Cross in 2004 that posits blood, as a donatable substance,
as that which goes beyond cultural differences: "Many cultures, many nations—
one river of life: blood!"[19] The slogan reflects Viveiros de Castro's (1998) well-
known argument concerning how multiculturalism and mononaturalism are run
together in dominant contemporary Euro-American understandings, with the
former—the "many cultures" of the slogan—overlying a common biological sub-
strate (according to the slogan, blood). To paraphrase Strathern (1995), the nice
thing about blood is that everyone has it: it is multicultural, with its uncontain-
able diverse symbolic associations (Carsten 2011), but also mononatural in that
everyone has it, as exemplified in the way blood groups crosscut caste distinctions otherwise said to be located in the blood.[20] Indeed, for the AVBDWB, that
everyone has it is *precisely* the fortuitous thing about blood. It is this that makes
the donation of blood an action that goes beyond itself—beyond even the invisible stitches holding society together as in Titmuss's (1970) famous account. It
opens up onto the universal—it is humanity at its highest pitch—and as the inaugural address makes clear, in the Indian context it may well be figured as that
which exceeds "caste, creed, religion [and] pedigree." This can allow the blood
donation and transfusion field to be charged with nationalist significance—for
instance, when the AVBDWB organizes blood donation camps deliberately
composed of members of different castes and religious communities—and also

with internationalist significance, such as in the annual camps it organizes in honor of West Indian cricketer Frank Worrell, who donated blood for the captain of the Indian cricket team, Nari Contractor, when he required a transfusion during a tour of the West Indies in 1962.[21]

As will be clear, then, the AVBDWB harbors an ideology of blood donation that feeds it into a political aesthetic of integration—blood donation as a congregative tool. It is little wonder then that some of its members greet the prospect of artificial blood with extreme negativity. Scholars have observed the ways in which the development of bloodless surgery and use of blood substitutes such as Hemopure and Biopure bring into question the model of non-remunerated, altruistic blood donation as advocated by WHO (Lallemand-Stempak 2016, 33) and, famously, Richard Titmuss (1970), who was quite explicit that one of the virtues of the non-remunerated model is the "sense of community" it arises from and fosters (314). For anthropologist Kath Weston (2013b) as well, "the quest for synthetic blood participates in a broader capitalization of nature that promises to domesticate kinship," where we understand "kinship" to stand for a variety of symbolic and substantial ties not limited to the strictly familial (247). AVBDWB members are well aware that research work in this area is progressing, that currently employed blood substitutes have their place, and that development of universally transfusable lab-created nonhuman blood forms might well reduce human suffering. But this is also an organization for which, as we have seen, human blood is exalted as possessing "no caste, creed, religion or pedigree" and is "a symbol of unity and service of others."

Here lies an important conflict between the AVBDWB as a recruitment organization and blood bank medics. While the two constituencies are close allies in the promotion of blood science education and voluntary blood donation more generally, for doctors, unlike AVBDWB members, there exists an intense "professional longing" (Sharp 2006, 211) for the expedited development of viable artificial blood. Such longing is informed not only by a possible solution to safety concerns but also by the difficulties in combatting the general reluctance of people to donate their blood voluntarily. For some medics, the promise of this technology is explicitly substitutive not only in terms of the human blood it will replace, but also in terms of deficits in reason; as one Indian medic puts it, "Indians will never donate their blood [in sufficient quantities]. Our only hope is that sometime, maybe in the next five to seven years, we will not need any blood donors." Thus, if for the AVBDWB blood donation promises political congregation beyond the more practical consequence of aiding medical therapeutics, for the medics the latter is both a more urgent and a more sufficient concern.

We thus encounter competing modes of promise—the promise of a hematological humanism of substantial flows versus a promise of bypassing the necessity for such flows at all. The case may be compared with the introduction of formula milk in the region. If breast milk transmits the suckling mother's love and other feelings to her child and for that reason is highly valued (Van Hollen 2011, 507–8), it can easily be understood why formula milk may be considered a negative (if in some cases medically necessary) presence. Artificial blood, even in its current more and less spectral forms, similarly contains the potential to disrupt the AVBDWB commitment to blood donation as a consummately human practice.

At the aforementioned Parliament of Motivators conference in Kolkata there was a session on developments in synthetic biology (i.e., blood substitutes) in which doctors from blood substitute research teams gave updates on their research. An AVBDWB member in the audience bemoaned the effect that even the prospect of viable artificial blood as a kind of fantasy substance was beginning to have on blood donor motivation: "College students say to us, 'Artificial blood is now available. Why should I donate?'" Another AVBDWB member stood up: "The cost of these substitutes will be so high that in our country they will not be feasible. Even if a substitute is found, blood doesn't cost anything from our bodies." Recalling Weston's argument about blood substitutes constituting yet another front in the capitalization of nature, the audience member's remarks are also suggestive of broader unease concerning how the use of blood substitutes is likely to heighten even further our reliance on pharmaceutical companies (Lallemand-Stempak 2016, 33). Still another member of the audience got to his feet: "There should be no artificial blood!" he shouted. Loud clapping followed. Such statements do not represent the official AVBDWB view, but they do tell us something about the hematological humanism of its members. Artificial blood, indeed, would be the end of the revolution.

Surpluses Out of Place

As will be clear, a central concern of this book is how that which is given is never enough, or alternately, far too much. In moving between the different interlocking proportionalities of blood giving, we explored in this chapter how the "not giving enough" of Indian donors is countered by educational campaigns that project images of a body that in fact has "too much," or at the very least, "more than enough" blood—in fact, virtually an infinite amount. Excess, we suggest, is important because it organizes ways of thinking and acting in blood donation and transfusion contexts in ways that crosscut one another. On the one hand, blood services worldwide are both subject to and must also manage excess—seasonal variations, excessive giving after disasters—as well as the simple need to synchronize incomings and outgoings.[22] On the other, the "more" and the "less" of Indian blood banking consists of, to paraphrase Mary Douglas, surpluses out of place: political overgiving (or posed, corrupt giving as a species of political excess—see chapter 3), blood surpluses in the body that remain *ungiven*, excessive prescription of blood by medics in situations where there is already a severe deficit, and so on. It may at first glance appear paradoxical, even contradictory, to speak of a cultural politics of excess in a situation so obviously characterized by shortages. Nevertheless, this chapter shows the structural imbrication of excess and shortage; for the distribution of blood within the social body to be viable, bodily surpluses must be discursively imagined into being.

Ungiven surpluses in the body, then, are surpluses out of place. As we described, the AVBDWB's aim to produce a perceptual shift from hematologically finite to infinite bodies runs the risk of becoming too successful. In creating the conditions for the making of subjects of reproducible generosity, they seem to simultaneously unmake them—that is, infinite reproducibility undermines the generosity of the act: the gift risks erasure. In this chapter, we have described the imaginative resolution of this conundrum. The use of *dan* by medics and other (non-AVBDWB) recruiters, while principally intended as a culturally sensitive template for encouraging blood donation, has the "side effect" of aiding to retain the sacrificial atmospherics of blood donation. This simultaneous enactment of surplus and sacrifice, excess and loss, has significant implications for how we understand an "Indian" biopolitics. Blood donors do not neatly disaggregate into those who sacrifice and those who can choose not to sacrifice. What emerges instead is a productive enigma, what might be termed *not sacrifice, not not-sacrifice*.[23] The abject-excess binary collapses in the double-negative field of not sacrifice, not *not*-sacrifice. Donor figures simultaneously share a portion of their hemic excess and sacrifice that portion. To be sure, the dynamic entanglement of antisacrificial redescription and sacrificial reactivation will be fitful and uneven. Yet it is possible to see how two seemingly competing messages about the nature of blood giving work with, rather than against, one another.

5

THE BROKEN WORLD OF
TRANSFUSION

Too much, too little: Like the previous chapter, this one concerns activism that both employs and is also about human biological substance. But where the previous chapter focused on how that which is given is never enough, this one concerns perceptions and campaigns concerning how doctors prescribe *too much* of that which has already been given. The proportions of the transfusion, say clinical activists and others, are all wrong in Indian medicine. Once more, then, the focus is on proportionality and on educational campaigning, but here there is a different target: if donors do not give enough because they think they have a deficit when in fact (according to the campaign) they have a surplus, doctors prescribe blood as if they have a surplus when in fact they have a deficit. The irony is obvious, for in so doing, of course, they exacerbate this deficit. Meanwhile, excessive prescription of blood—as if it were a kind of abundantly available tonic—mirrors, at the opposite end of the vein-to-vein chain, the overcollection of blood at religious and political blood donation events—disproportion all around. Once more, excess is at stake, and the different spheres of excess interlock and inform one another. Surpluses must be redistributed, both ideationally and practically. While in chapter 4 we saw how blood donation can no longer be an excessive sacrifice once donors understand they hold an excess of blood, in the instances that concern us here, doctors prescribe too much blood, thereby increasing the already existing deficit. In so doing, they also increase the likelihood that those who legitimately need transfusions will fail to get them.

In the following sections, we track and unpack the ways in which clinical activists take on the problematic specter of doctors' "irrational" and "unscientific" blood prescription. In its stead, they promote "appropriate" blood usage for the better preservation of a scarce resource. As we shall explain, activists' pedagogical practices are underpinned by a number-based "proportional ethics" (Corsín Jiménez 2008). Considering first the single unit transfusion as a figure of particular censure by these activists, we then turn to campaigns to promote the separation of blood into components in order both to better treat patients and to preserve a scare resource. But though understood by clinical activists to be qualitatively and quantitatively necessary, component separation has a dark side as well. The hidden darker potential of component separation forms the focus of the final part of the chapter.

We begin, however, with a troubling case from Rohtak, Haryana. In 2007 a stream of newspapers reported the terrible details of an incident in which medical professors employed at a government hospital in the town took blood from the younger of their two sons for transfusion into the other. The extraction went badly wrong, and the younger son died later in hospital from blood loss. On seeing the disaster unfold, the mother, Promila, tried to kill herself and was placed under sedation in a psychiatric unit. After interrogation of the father, Ashok, it was revealed that the purpose of the amateur transfusion had been to transfer blood from the brighter of the two children to the other, who was about to face his medical entrance exams, having previously failed a pre-entrance exam (one report spoke of the younger brother's "brainy blood"). The reports went on to give a number of curious details about the episode, in particular concerning the possible role of a tantric guru in advising the procedure. In some reports, the guru appeared to Promila in a dream. In others, both a real-world guru and a mysterious figure who appeared in a dream play a part in directing the tragic events. Promila was also reported to be possessed by spirits. Further, the attempted blood transfer appeared to have formed part of a *havan*, the ritual burning of offerings. The reports enumerate the objects found by police in the family house: the ritual paraphernalia of mustard, kerosene oil, and incense sticks, along with blood-soaked syringes and needles.[1] Tantric and hemic excesses ran together.

For commentators, the events were considered to bring to light a number of key issues blighting the medical and educational landscapes. The CNN-IBN news channel brought together a senior doctor from the Indian Medical Association (IMA), a television astrologer and a career adviser to debate "Doctors of death: Science vs. superstition." One of the taglines was "Both doctors—but still did it," and the IMA representative was asked what hope the nation had if even highly educated doctors can fall prey to superstitions concerning the "paranormal," perform "bizarre rituals," and get "possessed by spirits."[2] "Is there a wider malaise?" asked the presenter. "Are there adequate checks on who is able to practice medicine in India?" The doctor agreed that there are not. The astrologer focused on the uncertainty of present times, on how "India's economy is zooming" and on how "in the hurry to reach to the top" everyone "is ready to take any short cuts." "It's not superstition that is winning," continued the astrologer. "It's our own greed." The career adviser was asked, "Do you often see parents putting this inordinate pressure on their children? . . . I mean, these doctors wanted to make their son brilliant—as brilliant as their younger child. They were actually trying to do an amateur blood transfusion from a brilliant child to a not-so-brilliant child so he would become clever. Do you see . . . parents losing their sanity because of the pressure to succeed?" The career adviser responded by pointing to middle class parents' continued neurotic fixation with medicine and engineering as prestigious career routes for their children, and stressing their lack of awareness of diverse and fulfilling opportunities elsewhere.

Pick up any local Indian newspaper, and you are more likely than not to find the tragic story of a young person's suicide attributed to the stresses of exams in combination with parental pressure.[3] For example, several news sources have reported on the cumulative death of about sixty students in the town of Kota in Rajasthan over the last six years.[4] Kota is a famous hub of coaching centers that prepare aspirants for admission to engineering and medical colleges around the country. Lawrence Cohen (1995b, 326; 1998, 137) has written of the production of the "examinable body" in North India. In his Banaras ethnography we meet Sanjay, who is studying for his forestry civil service exams. Concerned at the effects on his memory and vitality of recent intestinal illnesses, he takes a special tonic containing the plant tuber ginseng. Cohen describes the advertising strategies of a number of tonics popular among those facing competitive exams, which play on the projected economic futures of candidates. Given these anxieties—exacerbated by well-known deficiencies in the educational infrastructure—the existence of widespread cheating should probably not come as a surprise.[5] The Rohtak transfusion case seemed to bring together, in a rather unique conjunction, the question of cheating and that of the examinable body; the failed transfusion enfolds elements of both the cheat and the tonic for the production of the elder son's examinable body. Though, of course, it was a very particular occurrence, there are a number of familiar-enough logics that seemed to both precipitate the action and structure responses to it.

The passing on of biomoral qualities by way of contagious contact between persons is a classic theme in scholarship on South Asia.[6] Specifically in the context of blood, we have written elsewhere of the knowledge, spirit, and aspirations that some North Indian blood donors see as contained within their donated blood; resultant patient transfusions are figured by these donors as being as much morally transformative as medically curative.[7] In the Rohtak case, the transfer of "brainy blood" might have been for a less morally uplifting and more instrumental purpose, but in either case forms of knowledge and intelligence are considered transmissible in the hemic transaction.

We begin with this case because its disproportions powerfully draw us into the themes of this chapter, which though they do not operate at such a high pitch, similarly focus on transfusion and excess and on questions concerning the knowledge and reason of doctors. The Rohtak transfusion case is instructive as both an extreme instance of, but also a metaphor for, a wider situation of blood donation and banking characterized by surpluses out of place and the scrutiny of medical reason.

Introducing "Rational Usage"

From the standpoint of clinical activists, there are two main ways in which over-transfusion takes place: through the prescription of whole blood units rather than blood separated into components, and the prescription of single blood units. The single-unit transfusion and the whole-blood transfusion form part of the same complex of inappropriate usage. Doctors are, so to speak, both agents and patients in this situation: transfusion specialists and blood bank doctors seek to educate their fellow clinicians (surgeons, oncologists, etc.) about the perils of prescribing transfusions too readily and in incorrect proportions. Some of this is through "sensitization programs": visiting hospitals and giving talks, organizing workshops, sending out leaflets, developing guidelines, and so on. But they also seek to formally institutionalize the education of all medics about the proper use of blood, most prominently by campaigning to make it a mandatory component of the training of all medics to spend time in a blood bank and for all hospitals to have a transfusion committee for auditing the blood transfusion process. Such a committee would monitor demand, usage, and adverse reactions, and, most importantly, would continually ask the question: Is the right blood product being prescribed for this particular patient? However, there is a problem of authority here that hampers their efforts. Though blood bank medics are skilled doctors themselves, other physicians see their role as simply to provide the goods requested—and certainly not to question or probe the logic of the requisitions that physicians send. Blood bank medics complain that they have no say: "We are not listened to in the hospital." At blood banking conferences, speakers emphasize the need for fortitude: "Lord Krishna used 758 poems in eighteen chapters [in the Bhagavad Gita] to persuade Arjuna to fight. We require that much patience to convince clinicians there is no need for single-unit transfusions."

In seeking to make this intervention, these clinical activists are joined by members of the Association of Voluntary Blood Donors, West Bengal (AVBDWB), which we introduced in the previous chapter. As we shall see, the strategies of these different amateur and clinical constituencies differ somewhat. However, the desired outcome—the "rational usage" of blood by the prescribing physician—is very much shared by them. The AVBDWB was founded in 1980 by teachers and ex-students of Kolkata's Jadavpur University, famed for its nationalist origins. Its first members were educated professionals and intellectuals (and male), though its membership now is much broader. It is proud to have a presence in every district of the state of Bengal. Members each give a few hours every week to help organize camps, write publicity materials, and engage in other recruitment and donor education activities, such as were discussed in chapter 4. Recently, however, it has begun to expand beyond this initial set of activities to campaign for the proper use of blood by physicians as well. "The time has come to educate the blood users," as one member explained to us.

One of the ways the association has done this is to develop special kits on the theme of appropriate blood usage for sending out to every medic in the state whose specialty may give them cause to prescribe transfusions. But if there is a problem of authority for blood bank medics, it is worse still for members of the AVBDWB. One female member told us that though the association knew from the beginning that it was as important to tackle overuse of blood as it was to tackle its underdonation for improving the overall availability of the substance, there was no point in pursuing that, for a simple reason: "Ten, fifteen years ago the doctors wouldn't listen to us because we are not medically qualified. But we have the authority now to approach them." Another member, though, remained quite pessimistic about their campaign: "Doctors are very arrogant. They will not listen to nonmedical people. They fail to realize that anyone can read any book. They may not have a degree, but there is no bar."

While blood bank medics tend to use the expression "rational use of blood" in their campaign materials, the AVBDWD assiduously avoids it. Instead, it prefers the term "appropriate use of the gift of blood." This alternative phraseology is significant in several ways. First, including the word "gift" reflects the AVBDWB's experiences on the front line of blood donor motivation and serves as a reminder of the origins of the product that doctors prescribe—it is a rejoinder to the definitions of donated blood as "just another drug" that we encountered in chapter 4. In recalling to the prescribing physician the sentiment that gave rise to the product now available to them to prescribe, the hope is that it will be treated with greater consideration and care. The word and its placement in the phrase are intended as a deterrent against a hemic commodity fetishism that sees doctors treat donated blood as just another drug. The phrase "gift of blood" is thus meant to excite a particular ethical sensibility or reflexive consideration on the part of prescribers. We can think here of Lawrence Cohen's (2003, 128) invoking of Veena Das's suggestion that the value of drugs should be considered not just in terms of their efficacy, but also in the work achieved in their capacity to be gifted. Both understandings are entirely necessary for the AVBDWB. The efficacy of the treatment, and of the Indian blood donation and transfusion field more widely, is dependent on remembering the origin of the drug as loving offering.

Second, the AVBDWB understands that use of the word "rational" has the potential to needlessly antagonize the very constituency from which it seeks a positive response. It therefore uses the word "appropriate" instead. As one of the members who was central in developing the campaign told us, "'Appropriate' is better than the word 'rational' because it implies current users of blood are irrational." Despite such careful public use of language, though, the campaign inevitably is suggestive of the long history of casting aspersions on the reason of doctors.[8] There is always a particular media outcry when doctors have been deemed to be "promoting superstition," as indicated by the Rohtak transfusion case. The antisuperstition activists with whom we have conducted fieldwork, of whom a good number are themselves medical doctors, reserve particular scorn for physicians thought to have compromised the values of which they are meant to be model upholders.[9] In the cases discussed here, both AVBDWB members and blood bank medics use the word "unscientific" in referring to doctors who in their opinion too readily prescribe transfusions. This work thus joins others that have explored the cultural politics of the (mis)use of drugs in the subcontinent—for instance, oxytocin (Brhlikova et al. 2009), oral polio vaccine (Jeffery 2014a), and psychopharmaceuticals (Ecks 2016). However, our case adds a novel twist, for the drug putatively being overprescribed, in overtly deriving from human bodies, is a very particular kind of drug indeed. Any analysis of blood as a medication, adequately administered or not, cannot but also give an account of the relation between its prescription and its productive origins in the human. Given the situation of hemic scarcity that overprescription both takes place within and contributes to worsening, moderate and informed prescription of blood products comes to mirror, for AVBDWB members, the sentiments that make the prescription existentially possible (i.e., those that inspire human donation), and so to itself look like a form of giving: the appropriate prescription modeled as a kind of gift.[10]

Cosmetic Transfusions

For our first example of inappropriate blood usage, we consider single-unit transfusions. What, for campaigners, is so wrong with them? First of all, they are not medically necessary; no medical benefits to patients will ensue. Second—following directly from the first point—if a patient is unnecessarily transfused a unit of blood, then that person is needlessly placed at risk of contracting a transfusion transmissible infection (TTI). Third, as a therapeutically unnecessary medical event, the single-unit transfusion diminishes further an already precarious blood supply, redirecting blood from those who genuinely need it to those who do not. As an AVBDWB member succinctly put it to us, "Just as when you take one unit of blood [from a donor] there is no difference to their health, if you give [transfuse] one unit to a patient it also makes no difference to health—all that happens is that the patient gets exposed to communicable disease."[11]

We were told again and again by both blood bank clinicians and AVBDWB members that "to reduce the need for blood there must be rational usage," and further that "blood must be requisitioned rationally—only when the minimum need is two units, because a donor can't give that." A female AVBDWB member from Hooghly complained, "Our doctors are not scientific. Our donor motivation techniques have taken the movement to a high level, but the technical side hasn't reached that level." The very particular trope of the medically pointless transfusion that is at the same time potentially infectious and lethal haunts both sets of campaigners: "We must ensure that the benefits of transfusion outweigh the risks," one doctor from a government blood bank in Delhi told us. "A single-unit transfusion is a bomb: it kills patients and puts more at risk." To illustrate the importance of rational usage, campaigners told us moving stories of their friends and family members who on being taken ill with a variety of different complaints—some having little or no connection to blood quantum or quality—were wrongly prescribed single-unit transfusions that resulted in their contracting diseases such as hepatitis C and HIV. AVBDWB members call single-unit transfers *cosmetic transfusions*. As one activist explained to us, "Single-unit transfusions mean nothing in almost every case. Blood from the bank is a foreign body—it must not be transfused unless it is essential. Eighty years ago, Landsteiner said you must not transfuse unless it is lifesaving. The WHO says there should be a transfusion only when the benefit outweighs the risk. Blood donation is a risky venture. It is not like drinking apple juice or some tonic."[12]

We see in the above statement the definitional ambiguity of donated blood. Its status as a drug is on occasion contested, as we saw in chapter 4, but neither must it be viewed as a tonic. In fact, it is precisely its use by doctors as if it were a tonic that is a large part of the problem of its overprescription in single-unit transfusions. Such definitions are something that blood bank doctors themselves can struggle with. A government hospital medic in Delhi told us, "You see we are mentally tuned to thinking this is a drug. It is our training. But sometimes I think, actually, no. This is a human product. How can you call it a drug? But then I started thinking, maybe it's this: When you call it a drug it discourages this notion among physicians that blood is a tonic. That way, it helps against irratio-nal usage." Perhaps this doctor is correct that the drug status of donated blood acts as a guard against its overuse, and the situation would be even worse if it were not classified as a drug. But other products that are perhaps less ambiguous in their designation as drugs—antibiotics, oxytocin, psychopharmaceuticals, and more besides—are also famously overprescribed.[13] Either way, it seems clear enough that use of donated blood as a kind of tonic contributes to the obdurate presence of the single-unit transfusion. We very frequently heard such com-plaints as the following, made to us by a Kolkata blood bank medic: "So often blood is used as a tonic, to boost up your vitality." Patients are often extremely keen to be prescribed a transfusion for the precise same reason that most people are reluctant to donate the substance—they feel they have "less blood" (*khuun ki kami*). We witnessed on numerous occasions how failure to prescribe a transfu-sion could provoke angry reactions on the part of a patient or family members. Even if the specific condition for which the patient has been admitted has no par-ticular hemic aspects, attempts nevertheless may be made to get a transfusion as a kind of "add on." There is the feeling that one has not been treated properly if one has not received a transfusion. If the donation of blood can serve as evidence of commitment in political rallies (see chapters 1 and 3), receiving the same sub-stance can serve as evidence of treatment. Thus, it is perhaps not surprising that some medics prescribe single-unit transfusions "just to make them go away." Clin-ical activists also complain that such transfusions form a kind of shortcut treat-ment that leaves underlying causes in place, especially in the case of women's ane-mia: "They [unreformed medics] give them a unit of blood when they should check the cause of anemia and give iron supplements." Thus, use of the word "cos-metic" is apt in the sense that such transfusions give the *appearance* of receiving treatment, but also in the sense that, like a cosmetic product, transfusions are ap-plied to the bodies of patients to temporarily affect the appearance of their health but not the substance of it.

A further cause of single-unit transfusions, and unnecessary transfusions more generally, comes from some medics' wish to ensure balance in exchange. John Davis (1992, 25) has brilliantly critiqued the way in which anthropologists are wont to cook the books to show "perpetual balance" and "good measure" in exchange—but it is not only anthropologists who do this. Surgeons must predict how much blood a patient will require and, on that basis, ask the patients' rela-tives to donate their blood in order to preemptively replace that which the pa-tient is anticipated to require in a future transfusion. But they are only predic-tions, and a patient may need more or indeed less than relatives have been asked to replace. More frequently they require less, because surgeons perhaps under-standably feel it is a safer bet to overestimate than to underestimate the number of units that might be required for transfusion.[14] We repeatedly heard blood bank medics make complaints such as the following: "[The clinicians] feel that the person's relatives have donated blood and they think, 'Oh, I should give that amount to the patient, otherwise the relatives will say, "Why have I been made to donate blood?"'"

Hence, even if a patient does not require a transfusion, or a transfusion made up of so many units, the patient may still be given one in order to create the image of a "rightful balance" in exchange. In the case of the single-unit transfusion that a surgeon understands to be medically unnecessary and yet politic to give, we find a potentially lethal spin on the "anthropological" cooking of the books: the patient is needlessly exposed to a potentially infectious substance. But we do not want to present an artificial picture of consistent practice here; we shall describe below how other doctors pay no heed at all to images of rightful balance in exchange, instead pursuing an opposite strategy of systematically demanding more replacement units from relatives than are necessary for their family member's transfusion, thereby generating secret surpluses.

There is a final (and from campaigners' perspective particularly confounding) way in which single-unit transfusions find a place in Indian medical practice. To gain a sense of this, we need a working understanding of the numeric and epistemic instability of the unit of blood.

Transfusion of Whole (Unseparated) Blood

In component separation, a centrifuge machine spins the "whole" blood that has been taken directly from each individual so that its multiple components become separated from each other: these are red blood cells, plasma, and platelets.[15] This separation of whole blood takes place because of the accepted medical principle that the sum of its parts is worth more than the whole taken together.[16] On the one hand, it seems to multiply the substance—where there was one "whole" unit there are now three "component" units—and so it makes sense in quantitative terms, helping to compensate for gaps in supply. On the other hand, component separation also allows patients to be treated for the specific ailment from which they suffer. Transfusing a component unit instead of a whole unit avoids treating patients with those parts of blood that are qualitatively unnecessary for their specific condition. Component separation therefore introduces a new particularism into transfusion therapy, and a centrifuge machine is a basic feature of blood bank technology in most of India's medium to large urban centers. The numerical instability of the blood unit that we mentioned a moment ago is an effect of component separation. A unit of blood, if looked at as a whole unit, is a singular unit;

however, it may also be considered as three potential units. Numerical instability is thus at the same time epistemic instability: now one unit, suddenly it is three; but further—three units may just as quickly become one again. Following an analytic that Alberto Corsín Jiménez (2013) has been developing of the reversibility of social forms, we can discern a switching back and forth of the proportions of the unit of blood (one/three, singular/plural). We take pains here to clarify the numeric reversibility and (dis)proportionality of the unit of blood because it has important consequences, as we shall show.

Coming back to the single-unit transfusion, campaigners' two figures of censure—the single-unit transfusion and the whole-unit transfusion—conjoin in what for them is the particularly dismal phenomenon of a transfusion composed of a single unit of whole blood. The perversity of this lies in how the advent of component separation came to make the single whole-unit transfusion a more rather than less compelling proposition for some prescribers. The reason for this lies in the numerical reversibility of the blood unit. In making the single unit simultaneously multiple, component separation can make it seem like three units (and from a particular, subjunctive perspective it is). Prescribing a single unit of whole blood comes to appear like a way of giving the patient a good deal—a kind of three-for-one item. For campaigners, this is perverse because what is meant to be a technology of economy and therapeutic particularism (component separation) ends up making the very practices it is supposed to put an end to (single- and whole-unit transfusions) more attractive.

Part of the problem here is that the processing charges for whole units of blood and component units tend to be roughly the same. So even if from the perspective of campaigners it has severe quantitative and qualitative consequences, one can understand why prescribing a single whole unit might at least appear like a good deal (three for the price of one), and not only that, appear to conform to the protocols of rational usage as a multiple-unit transfusion (three components). As a doctor from a government hospital in Mumbai put it to us, "If something is cheaper, then you go for the cheaper thing. Since fresh frozen plasma (FFP) and red cells are not cheaper than whole blood, then doctors won't use them. Doctors say, 'OK, I will use whole blood, which is three for the same price.'" Patients as well as doctors can assume such an understanding. For instance, parents of children with the severe anemic condition thalassemia, which requires them to receive regular red-cell transfusions to increase hemoglobin levels, sometimes express distress that their children receive merely red cells rather than whole blood. As a father of a child receiving a transfusion in a clinic in Delhi put it to us, "They used to give my daughter whole blood [before component separation], and now she gets only a third of that. This isn't fair!"[17] The attending doctor responded, "We have to explain [to parents] that plasma and platelets are not needed for thalassemia, and that this way we get maximum benefit from one bag of blood." Thus, what to campaigner-doctors appears as a multiplication of substance (one into three) appears to others as a subtraction through division: they are receiving only a third of what they used to.

As we saw in chapter 3, Corsín Jiménez (2008, 186) draws attention to the role of partonomic obviation (hierarchies of part-whole relationships) in transactions: "The part that we give," he says, "is an indication of the whole that is not given— what you see (the gift) is what you do not get (the larger social whole). Gift-giving is thus an expression and effect of proportionality." Partonomic logics extend to the transfusion. As we just noted, for some parents of children with thalassemia, the new arithmetic of component therapy leads them to see the one component their child receives in a transfusion as representing the two they did not get. For campaigners, there is also a partonomic logic to the transfusion, but in reverse: the whole unit that is transfused represents the parts that were not able to be given in other transfusions. What develops is what might be called an exponential arithmetic of ghosts: a transfusion of three units of whole blood, were it given to a child with thalassemia who in fact needed only red cells, would result in the waste of two (component) units per one (whole) unit given—six in total. This is how "wastage" gets quantified: opportunity cost breeds phantom units, always translated by campaigners into lives not saved. Whenever the substance is not multiplied in component separation (i.e., when whole blood rather than component units is prescribed and transfused), a further negative multiplication comes into play of correlative lost lives.

According to Alfred Gell's (1992) schema, opportunity costs are very often of a confirmed magnitude. He asserts that "activities which have high opportunity costs are ones which have highly advantageous, highly feasible alternatives in terms of the map of the field of possible worlds imposed by a given culturally standardized construction of reality" (217). The constructed reality here is that of the transfusion made up of possible desired and undesired kinds of blood unit. The stipulated usefulness of a unit of blood is of course what accusations of wastage rest upon. ("Wastage" is rather a mild term for computations frequently delivered in a vocabulary of *theft of life*.)[18] The magnitude of the opportunity cost is calculable according to the number of patients that might have benefited based on a particular arithmetic of the transfusion made up of separated-out components. For Gell, the concept of the opportunity cost, brought into social theory from economics, is an effective means to bridge the "fatefulness" of subjective time and the objective qualities of time as a dimension (because opportunity cost is both subjective and, to a certain extent, computable). The bridging function of the concept holds for the present case because campaigners' rhetoric of lives not saved involves remarkable projective calculations, which we can see vividly in a scene from a training event for novice donor recruiters in Delhi that we now briefly consider.

The trainer was a blood bank medic from a nearby town who also ran a small NGO promoting voluntary blood donation. He was concerned that blood donor motivation not just be a job for the trainee motivators, but a visceral commitment. Successful motivators were motivators of conviction, he told the trainees. Then began a very interesting procedure of rhetorical mathematics in which he seemed practiced. He went around the room gathering the ages of the trainees and the number of times they professed to having donated their blood. He then wrote these figures on a whiteboard. There followed a kind of ritual public calculation of opportunity-cost figures for each trainee. Knowing their ages allowed the trainer to calculate the maximum number of times the trainees could have donated their blood and then to subtract from that figure the total of actually performed donations in order to arrive at a total number of each trainee's opportunity cost, or phantom, donations. For instance, a person who is thirty-seven years old has been eligible to donate blood for nineteen years—that is, since turning eighteen. Four whole blood donations are possible per year.[19] Nineteen years of eligibility multiplied by four donations per year gives a figure of seventy-six possible donations. The number of actual donations was then subtracted from this figure.

But the trainer was not finished. Component separation, as we know, determines that the number of donations given is not the same as the number of "lives saved." Following from this, in a further dramatic numerical maneuver, the trainer tripled the number of lives not saved by each trainee. For instance, according to the arithmetic of component separation, the trainee whose phantom donations amounted to seventy (seventy-six possible donations minus the six actually given) in fact "failed" to save the lives of 210 patients. The climax came when the trainer added together the ten trainees' individual ghost numbers to arrive at an overall figure of well over a thousand "unsaved" patients. To return to the analytic of partonomy we developed earlier, the trainer spells out the partonomic relation between the given and withheld as an act of criticism, with that which has been given not being subject to acclaim but instead only serving to mathematically underscore that which has not. However accurate or inaccurate this exercise of arithmetical shaming of trainees was, its rhetorical effect was obvious, with several trainees in tears.[20]

A reductive mathematical exercise thus incited visceral, emotional responses, encouraging people to *feel* a particular way. If charity advertisements on television and radio focus less on numbers and more on context and details to encourage people to resonate with the situation at hand, here a hard-rational math exercise accomplishes just that, reminding us of the affective power of numbers. Saba

Mahmood (2005, 106) writes of "micropractices of persuasion," a concept intended partly as a critique of the notion that the pietist movement in Cairo is sustained through "religious indoctrination." Instead of this black-box concept, Mahmood examines the specific (often dialogue-based) practices through which virtue is cultivated and people persuaded "to incline toward one view versus another." In the Indian blood donation and transfusion field, it is noteworthy how frequently numbers are mobilized as a species of rhetorical persuasion and pedagogy (see chapter 6; Copeman 2006; and Copeman 2009a, chap. 2; cf. Maurer 2003, 319), usually—in a seeming paradox—in support of the production of personalization. The trainer's exercise is metaethical (Lambek 2010, 32) in explicitly reflecting on the rights and wrongs of blood donation and interactively seeking to inculcate embodied consistency between role and person on the part of trainee recruiters (see also Reed 2017). In making explicit the possible number of recipients of ungiven donations, the exercise causes an overtly nonspecific mode of donation, via a rhetoric of mathematics and numbers, to become acutely specified in the form of the ghostly magnitude of the unsaved. Through this micropractice of numerical pedagogy, the truths of the urgency of the recruiter's task, and that of the need for constancy in pursuing it, are established (Mahmood 2005, 115).

The whiteboard exercise also serves to demonstrate clearly the way campaigners conceptualize transfusions, both actual and ghostly. The immediate target in this instance was donors and trainee donor recruiters, not doctors. But whether a donation not given, which separated into components would save three, or a requisition demanding whole blood, which unseparated fails to save two, we see that the logic of lives not saved transfers by analogy from undonated units to unprescribed units; from nondonors whose nondonations are made more grievous by the existence of a technology that could have tripled them, to equally, if not more, at fault doctors (since they should be expected to know better) who request whole blood from the blood bank.

A summary may be helpful at this point. We have seen how from the point of view of AVBDWB members and clinical activists, prescribing whole blood is like using the proverbial sledgehammer to crack a nut. If a person with dengue fever requires platelets but is prescribed whole blood, then—in addition to the platelets—they also receive red cell and plasma components—which are qualitatively unnecessary for their particular condition. We have seen how this also brings into view a proportional ethics, since the two medically inessential units might have been used for other patients. These logics are nicely condensed in a poem by a Delhi-based trainee medic that she recites at events staged to educate physicians about rational usage of blood and that is also displayed in an educative space on the website of the Indian Society of Blood Transfusion and Immunohematology:

> Let's understand the need of the hour:
> If you break the handle you don't replace the whole car.
> Transfusion of whole blood if not needed is a mere waste
> Look at the patient's condition, don't be in haste . . .
> Let's make people aware of blood and its fraction.
> A single unit of blood can be used for more and more people's
> satisfaction.[21]

Clinical activists place a greater emphasis on rational usage as a solution to the problem of blood shortages than on motivation of new blood donors, whereas the AVBDWB seeks to approach the problem from both ends of the vein-to-vein chain. As one AVBDWB member put it to us, "We seek to convert a negative situation of nondonors and inappropriate users into the positive achievement of more donors and appropriate users." We can see clinical activists' different emphasis in some of the slogans they use, such as "Separate more, collect less!" Displaying just such a logic, a blood bank medic from Chandigarh, speaking before an audience at an all-India transfusion conference in Chennai, showed a graph composed of data from his hospital in which, in direct consequence of his blood bank's recent introduction of component separation, the number of units available for transfusion goes up even as the number of donations goes down. The latter seemed to be of little consequence to the doctor. He referred to the decline only as a means to more forcefully exhibit the magic of plenty produced by component separation: fewer donations yet more units for transfusion.

In the discussion that followed the Chandigarh medic's presentation, a doctor in the audience compared the technology to tax collection: "We now need only one-third of the donations that we previously needed. I tell people it is like income tax. Less than 1 percent of people are filing returns. You don't need more or higher taxation—just better efficiency. Having only 1 percent fill in returns is the same as not prescribing components." While the analogy's seeming exaltation of the cold reason of efficient processing as the answer to shortages certainly reflects a difference in emphasis between clinical activists and the AVBDWB, the latter organization, though it would avoid this medic's means of argument, would not disagree with what he argues *for*—namely, greater economy and care in the treatment of donated blood. But rather than an outlook that sees more careful usage as something akin to a *replacement of* the gift (or a means of causing fewer donations to be necessary for the same number of transfusions), AVBDWB members instead view careful usage as a mode of *fidelity to* the gift: careful treatment of donated blood honors the sentiments that give rise to it. Members explained to us: "Donors donate for compassion and love for human beings. Therefore, it is important that the blood is used in an appropriate and effective manner"; and

"People show their love by giving this gift of love; it comes from compassion and a love for humanity. People are not donating a commodity but their love, so we must respect this and use it properly."

Fidelity to the gift means allowing the logic and sentiment of the offering to seep into the manner of its usage. In this view, using blood with caution and care—treating it reverentially—is a kind of philanthropy since, first, it evidences an attitude informed by, *affected* by, the sentiment that gave rise to it, and second, in abjuring single and whole units, the saved units can save others. Careful usage itself takes on the form of a gift, and a gift in two directions at once—to those who can be helped by careful usage and back to the donor whose sentiments are honored. What the AVBDWB seeks through its campaigns in this area, then, is to ensure that the gift remains animated with the spirit of its giver, reminding doctors that donated blood is not just another drug. This is quite unlike the position put forward by the doctor we cited earlier who, in wondering why donated blood is legally classified as a drug, suggests that the purpose of such a classification might have been in order to act as a prompt to medics to avoid treating it as a tonic and in consequence overprescribing it.

This, perhaps, is how the *hau* subsists in the blood donation and transfusion world—not in any straightforward way striving to return to its original giver (Mauss 2016 [1925]), but ensuring the gift's proper use, and so both giving back to the giver and giving relief to patients, and more broadly to the broken world of the transfusion. Neither a drug nor a tonic, donated blood is to be treated as an honored guest. Taking care of donated blood between its initial donation and its eventual transfusion, the blood bank must offer it proper hospitality. Concepts of gift, hospitality, and proportionality converge here. Treating it correctly according to its true proportions is to allow oneself to be animated by its *hau* and so to be a good host. Recent anthropological engagements with hospitality, however, have noted the tensions that concepts of hospitality so frequently embody between reciprocity and calculation, and between generosity and parasitism (Candea and da Col 2012). Let us now consider the potential for parasitism that component separation unleashes, where it is not the guest that is potentially parasitical upon the host but the host who is potentially parasitical upon the gift and its giver.

Concealing Separation

In the previous chapter, we conveyed how medics continue to communicate mixed messages about the nature of blood donation: is it metaphorical kin with Shiva's drinking of poison, or is it a perfectly safe mode of transfer involving so little loss as to barely register even as a gift, never mind a sacrifice? Just as the unit

of blood is itself epistemologically unstable, a further set of unstable and conflicting messages attaches to component separation. The question arises: *Should the
technology be disclosed to donors?*

Part of the reason that the practices and messages of blood banking in the
country are shot through with contradictions is that there is no single system, but
a set of competing institutions and varieties of donation: voluntary, replacement,
and paid (usually in the guise of replacement). We have written elsewhere about
how some blood banks actively publicize component separation as a means to
generate more voluntary blood donations.[22] The logic of such publicity, we argued, lies in its priming of knowledge of spiritual returns: give one blood donation, and get three portions of technologically mediated *punya*—component separation not only as an efficient use of blood but also as an efficient means for the
blood donor to maximize spiritual incomings for minimum outgo. So to ask if
the technology should be disclosed to donors might appear meaningless—the cat
is already out of the bag. But publicity is unevenly effective and its targets differentiated. For some blood banks, as we shall now see, it is convenient that donors
remain ignorant of the separation of their donated blood into components. The
present work therefore joins others that have explored the withholding of information and purposeful concealment of key medical processes from both patients
and donors of biological materials in medical contexts in South Asia (e.g., Pande
2014; Vora 2015).[23] As is also the case in Bärnreuther's (2018b) excellent study of
egg and sperm donation in Delhi, we are centrally concerned with how a dearth
of information—specifically, in our case, practices of invisibility—can produce
a surplus in the clinic. We do not take issue with the critical tone struck in some
of the works just mentioned, since these authors undoubtedly encounter elements
of profiteering and economic exploitation in their field sites that warrant exposure and censure. We do, however, take up a position that allows for the possibility of ethical ambiguity and different competing concerns with respect to withholding information in the ethnographic contexts we explore.

There are, then, two contradictory and, on the face of it, mutually canceling
strategies in place with respect to publicity concerning component separation:
one that makes it a central feature of voluntary blood donation promotional campaigns, and another characterized by purposive nondisclosure. What lies behind
this divergence? Part of the answer lies with the voluntary blood donor card. It is
standard practice in the country for voluntary blood donors to receive a "credit
card" that entitles them in the future to receive for themselves, or their close family
members, a quantity of blood equivalent to that which they have donated.[24] In
theory this means that, should they need them, voluntary blood donors can expect to receive in future "for free" and without having to provide additional replacement units an equivalent number of units to those which they have hitherto

donated. However, in practice blood banks may well decline to honor the card and demand replacement donations regardless, a situation that contributes significantly to generalized distrust within the Indian blood banking setup.[25] The key problem that arises with component separation, though, is that the technology makes ambiguous the seemingly neat equation between units given and units eligible to receive. A further question arises: How much *does* a donor donate in donating their blood—one unit or three? If donors become aware that their single donated unit subsequently is divided to make three units, then they may expect this fact to be reflected in the quantities of blood that they and their relatives are eligible to receive for free if and when they require them; and, of course, giving out blood "for free" is not an attractive proposition for blood banks. Not only does it mean giving blood without getting a replacement from relatives (diminishing stocks), but it also means foregoing the processing charge attached to each unit of blood (diminishing funds).[26]

The motivation for concealment or nondisclosure of separation thus becomes clearer: it is in order to prevent donors from seeking to take credit for the multiplicity generated by component separation, and so the proportional reversibility of the unit of blood again becomes evident. If medics are encouraged by clinical activists to see one donated unit as three, donors are encouraged by many blood bank medics to maintain a view of the donated unit as singular in order to thwart the multiplication of expectations. But it is in the context of replacement blood donation that questions of parasitism, entitlement, and possible exploitation become most acute.

We were sitting in the back of a Delhi government hospital blood bank office where the medic in charge that afternoon was negotiating with a male schoolteacher who, along with several of his colleagues, had donated blood to replace that which was required by his maternal aunt, who had earlier been admitted to the same hospital with severe anemia. The schoolteacher also happened to be a Hindu, the significance of which will become clear. He said to the medic, "I have given one unit from which you have made three portions. So out of that, only the red portion [i.e., red cells] was given to my aunt, and the other two white portions [i.e., platelets and plasma] were not given. So are those two still there in my account?" The man, who was probably already aware of component separation technology, had come to realize that his blood had been separated because the blood bank does not pass blood directly to the relevant doctors but to the patients' relatives, who then carry it to the ward. The schoolteacher had noticed that he was carrying a lesser quantity and a different color of blood than that which he had donated, correctly concluding that his blood had been separated/multiplied. At issue for the medic was the fact that the man now sought "credit" for the other two units as well. If he had donated three-in-one but only one went to his aunt, then should he not have two remaining units "in his account"?

After the medic had brushed away the schoolteacher's argument and the schoolteacher had departed the office, the medic—herself a Hindu—told us, "You know, they [Hindus] are not the type to keep donating without getting something in return. This is the psyche of the Hindus as far as I am concerned. It is better they don't know about component therapy, otherwise you see what happens?" Laughing at her own lack of political correctness, she continued: "The problem with [the schoolteacher]—he was too educated." She went on to discuss the possibility of using hospital porters to convey blood to wards instead of patients' relatives in order to keep the latter unaware of the technology. She returned to her consideration of communal differences between blood donors:

> My mother-in-law will visit the temple because she wants salvation for herself; my father, he goes to the temple for his salvation, to be closer to God. We Hindus do not have a community type of feeling—you rarely hear of our temples feeding the poor, teaching people. Only those sects that came out of Hinduism like the Arya Samaj or Sikhs—they don't just think of their salvation, you know: "Oh, I've given the *pandit* so much that I reach God." . . . People in these organizations are more prone to donate. It is very difficult to make Hindus into donors. They will only give for their brothers, their mother. They come and they say, "*Card me to yeh likha hai ki yeh mere is ko milega*" [They say it is written in the card that my blood will go to my own]. They will never say, "It is *dan*. I'll just donate and forget about it." They will always say things like that man [the schoolteacher]: "I have given one unit from which you have made three [i.e., in component separation]. Now give me the credit for that."

First, then, there is the question of just who should get credit for the three transfusable units produced by one donation. The species of politics at stake here is one of causation and entitlement. Donors are indeed indispensable in producing such an outcome. But they are, of course, not the only cause. The "extra" two units are "made" (*baneye*) by blood bank technicians and the developers of the technology. Physicians are clear that it is they who are responsible for the three-ness of the donated unit, not donors. It is medics' labor that counts.[27] Yet as we mentioned earlier, some blood banks publicize the technology precisely in order to encourage donors to take credit for the multiplier effects of component separation—not credit in terms of units entitled to receive but a kind of "informational return" (Konrad 2005, 116) of the proportions of their gift's effects that may be translated into an idea of spiritual return: not just blessings or *punya* in the singular, but *many* of these "spiritual" rewards.[28] So we see that entitlements, returns, and credits consequent on component separation are to be encouraged and primed, but only when they are of the spiritual kind that costs the blood bank nothing. Here, then, it is convenient for medics fleetingly to recognize the labor of donors as precipitating a mode of return (a spiritual one) that might motivate them to donate *for free*. When one needs blood for oneself, or a relative, such credits are clearly not going to be much use. Yet one can see how the grooming in donors of an appreciation of the amplified spiritual or informational returns consequent on component technology may well undercut a further message about how donors must not harbor analogous enhanced expectations of entitlement to blood consequent on the same technology.

Second, the doctor raises the related issue of *dan*. The classification of blood donation as *rakt-dan*, or less frequently *khun-dan*, performs all sorts of significant cultural and practical work for blood banks. Voluntary, non-remunerated blood donation—as opposed to the still prevalent modes of paid and family-replacement blood donation—is the international standard as advocated by global health organizations such as WHO and the Red Cross for reasons of safety. Like voluntary blood donation, *dan* is archetypally a gift given anonymously for which no return should be countenanced, with its origins believed to reside in Hindu law. Hence, characterizing voluntary blood donation as *dan* has allowed blood banks to make the asymmetry and anonymity that voluntary donation requires seem less like an outside imposition than an appropriately Indic way to conduct blood donation. In articulating her complaint about donors' expectations of (material) returns consequent on their knowledge of component separation, the medic asserts that (Hindu) donors "will never say 'It is *dan*. I'll just donate and forget about it.'" This brings in still further associations of *dan*, specifically the matter of its alienability. Parry (1986, 461) puts the matter plainly: classically speaking, *dan* "is alienated in an absolute way, and the very definition of the gift is that it involves the complete extinction of the donor's propriety rights in favor of the recipient." In other words, it is not the blood donor's place to worry about what happens to their donated blood. As a mode of *dan*, once it has been offered it should no longer be the donor's concern; they can have no further claims on it.[29] Good blood donors forget they have even made a donation. In light of this, concealing separation is legitimate, even advisable; medics "help" donors maintain the highest standards of *dan* in not disclosing component separation to them. While nondisclosure may be in blood banks' interests in order to forestall claims for additional credits, it is also good for the donor whose donation becomes more virtuous—assisted *dan*, so to speak. (It also seems clear that part of the reason doctors complain so much about donors' grasping demands for credits is that the label "*dan*" creates impossible expectations of donor-virtue.)

But once again we must return to the question of the mixed messages sent out by blood bank medics. Replacement blood donation is explicitly an exchange, and a forcible one at that: relatives donate blood so that their family member may receive it. Moreover, even if voluntary blood donation resembles classical variations of *dan* more closely than replacement in being given anonymously and without immediate reward, it too contains the element of an entitlement: that of future blood equivalent to what has been donated in the past. It is blood banks themselves that offer the entitlement in voluntary donation and set up the (seeming) like-for-like exchange in replacement donation, and then it is the blood banks that complain when donors contravene the highest principles of disinterested *dan* in engaging in the exchange-like behavior that blood banks have set up.

It is not difficult to see why donors would seek the assurance of additional credits consequent on component separation. Sitting in the back of a blood bank office in Chandigarh, we witnessed a similar interaction to that which we described above. A middle-aged female had donated her blood in replacement for a distant relation of her husband. (It is worth noting that bride-giving families are frequently expected to provide replacement blood units for even distant members of bride-receiving families who are in need of transfusions. Blood units thereby come to form a hematic supplement to the practice of dowry giving.)[30] The donor, having come to understand that her donated blood had been separated into three component units, wondered aloud why her donated unit only counted as one with respect to what her husband's relation was due to receive. Moreover, she inquired, if her own close family should require blood in the future, would the two additional units made from her one donated unit "reflect" and "count"—that is, be made available for free for her family without further replacement? In this case the medic was more sympathetic, making a few reassuring noises if no firm promises. Upon the donor's leaving, the medic reflected to us:

> You see the mindset? Yes, we say it is this *dan*, that *dan*, oh it is such a pure and altruistic *dan*, the highest *dan*! But it works with only a handful of donors. She wanted those units [made from component separation to be present] on her account. You see, it's a vicious cycle of shortages which leads to this type of behavior. They get panicky because they were made to run about and they were forced to donate. "It's your patient, you have to bring, you have to bring" [say blood bank staff]. She's so scared of the situation, she wants to have something for the future to be posted to her account so next time she won't have to run about.

But as we have seen, blood banks emphatically wish to post the multiplied units to *their* account, not the donor's, even if in this case the doctor is more ready than other physicians to empathize with the situation of donors and understand just why they might wish to secure credits and entitlements.

Unknown Excesses

We briefly return to *dan*, for *dan* now comes into focus not just as a "cultural support" to help bring about blood safety but also as a means for medics to take for free that from which they may profit. Component separation and its concealment, of course, exacerbate the matter: in voluntary donation, one now takes for free that which may become three transfusable units. In replacement, for a transfusion made up of four component units, relatives must provide four whole units, which separated out into components become twelve. Monica Konrad (2005, 134) reports similar practices of replacement and separation taking place in Britain under the euphemistic name of "egg giving." In this scenario, ova are donated by future recipients of IVF treatment as a condition for receiving that treatment. And very much like in component separation, extracted ova can be separated out, resulting in multiple implantable entities from a "single" donation. Thus, asks Konrad, "Does not the semblance of a 'like' for 'like' gift exchange obscure what, in certain instances, might be the occasion for systematized profit-making?" (134). Writing of semen donation in the context of Delhi, Bärnreuther (2018b) draws attention to how the language of *dan* can on occasion form an explicit part of the business strategy of reproductive clinics in the capital: "The term donation [assists clinics] in keeping the buying costs of semen samples low and deriving profits from its sale." The same language also serves to "conceal the fact that donated reproductive substances eventually enter market relations."

The ideology of *dan* would appear to perform a similar function with respect to blood donation: for replacement, it justifies the nondisclosure of component separation to donors (donors are behooved to just give and forget); for the voluntary mode, it greases the process of obtaining units "for free" that upon separation triple in value—the donor all the while being given "credit" for only one. We are a long way here from the medics, discussed earlier, who even if it is not medically necessary transfuse patients in recognition of their relatives' preemptive replacement donations. In the cases under discussion here, physicians may *present* relatives with an image of measured equilibrium in exchange while nonetheless generating secret surpluses. Once more, the unevenness and variance of blood prescription practices is evident.

We also come to see how component separation renders the term "replacement donation" a misnomer. Relatives of a patient who requires a transfusion are asked—without being made aware of the fact—to provide far more than a mere replacement for what is required by their family member. When a blood bank receives a requisition for a six-unit transfusion, family members must donate six units (and pay six processing charges) in order to secure the release of the necessary six units. But factoring in component separation, the blood bank de facto takes eighteen (six times three) units; thereby attaining a "profit" of twelve (eighteen minus six) units. This is how practices of invisibility produce surpluses in the blood bank. The "like" for "like" of replacement is misleading. Family members who are already likely to be troubled and anxious about their sick relative are made to donate far more than is necessary: six units, when only two donations (two times three) would have accounted for the number of units needed for their relative's transfusion. We must also recall here the acute fears most people in the subcontinent have concerning the procedure (see chapter 4). Medics, then, systematically demand more from donors than they actually need to replace what is required for a given transfusion. If the reversibility of the blood unit's proportions is to be made to work in favor of the blood bank in this way—donors continuing to view the donated unit as "one," medics viewing it as "three," and donors donating more than they think they are donating—then evidently, from the standpoint of doctors, the technology must be concealed from donors. Though we are a world away from the "tantric" transfusion with which we began this chapter, replacement donation comes to form a parallel with it as an excessive extraction on its own terms. This is of course far from being a transparent or ideal state of affairs; there is the suggestion of a kind of secret parasitism on the part of blood banks. But while we do not wish to avoid a moral accounting (L. Cohen 2011a, 33), sweeping terms such as "exploitation" and "profiteering" are often used when more specific and nuanced forms of inquiry are warranted. We recognize with Vaibhav Saria (2016) that "failure to follow the imperatives of medical protocols and global health may not necessarily be the failure of the logic of care." So we now consider the reasons medics give for concealing separation.

We asked a medic at a government hospital blood bank why component separation is not used by doctors to reduce the burden on the families of patients—for instance, if a six-unit transfusion is required, why not ask relatives to donate just two units? After all, we added, we have heard other doctors use slogans such as "Separate more, collect less." The physician responded with candor:

> Yes, we [i.e., his blood bank] practice 100 percent component separation, but still, whole blood is a useful fiction [to maintain for donors]. Luckily for us, the community is not fully educated. That's good for us;

otherwise we would not be able to assist these people. We say to someone having a bypass, "OK, we need a minimum schedule of eight units."
In a bypass there will, for instance, be two red cells, four platelets, two
plasma [required]. Since we separate components from the whole and
use only what is needed, nearly everyone gives us more than what is required by them. This is good, because we use this [i.e., the hidden sur-
plus] for those who cannot generate replacement automatically. If they're
very alert, they'll ask how many red cells have you used . . . you know,
and then we'll be in trouble.

Recognizing the illicitness of the way in which his blood bank generates surpluses, the medic nevertheless defended the practice as being in the service of hematic redistribution. When he mentioned "those who cannot generate replacement automatically," he was referring to transfusion patients whose relatives and/
or friends are unable or unwilling to donate their blood in replacement. *Unwilling*: It is certainly the case that when asked to donate blood in replacement for a
family member, many relatives vanish into thin air (or, if they have the financial
means, pay "professional" donors to impersonate them). *Unable*: The argument
is entirely plausible: migrant workers in Delhi who require a transfusion but whose
families reside in far-off places do often face serious difficulties in finding replacement blood donors. At the time of our fieldwork, construction workers on the
Delhi metro formed a particularly large constituency of migrant workers in the
city, with many of them hailing from Bihar, Rajasthan, Uttar Pradesh, and places
further afield. Transfusion-necessitating accidents were not uncommon (see
Sadana 2010, 80), but frequently no family members were present—the workers
were on their own in the city. It is on such occasions, suggested the medic, that
the secretly generated surpluses are deployed in a kind of robbing from the "kin
rich" to pay the "kin poor."

A medic at an NGO-run blood bank spoke to us in similar terms. She admitted to demanding six whole donations from families when only six components
were required: "There is no harm in that. The blood bank is merely taking another donation, more donations. Why? Because we want to give the leftover to
other patients." Concealment of separation is justified, she argues, because what
is covertly taken from donors is going to help others. She went on to spell out the
arithmetic: "Two donations gives me six components. I take a donation for each
component, so I take six donations. That gives me eighteen components. I don't
think I am doing anything wrong." Multiplication upon multiplication.

The technology of component separation is naturally allied with neither ex-
ploitative nor redistributive practices. The technology produces a multiplication,
or an excess, and different things can be done with that excess. During the months

that we spent attending a government hospital blood bank in Delhi, there was a policy of dispensing platelets without the need for replacement donation. This was possible, we were told, because of the secret surpluses it had been able to generate from component separation: the forcible deal of replacement blood donation was deactivated for some by virtue of the blood bank's covert extraction from others. One NGO-run blood bank that is well known for charging lower processing charges than other blood banks in Delhi was able to do so (as we were informed by its staff) because component separation allowed it to take three charges for one donated unit. But a potential for profiteering is obviously also present. Donors and recipients have to trust that the processing charge for donated units merely covers service costs. Charges vary widely between blood banks. Staff at corporate hospital blood banks put the high cost of units at their blood banks down to the superior testing technologies and equipment at their disposal. "Our blood is the safest available in Delhi," we were told—by a number of different corporate blood banks.

The scenario approaches a Derridean one: the gift unknown in its giving is the purest of all (Derrida 1992, 14). In terms of *dan*, as we saw, the gift should be completely alienated, the donor having no further claims on it. Blood bank physicians instrumentalize this understanding of *dan* in seeking to explain their own behavior. But, of course, the donated blood that donors do not know they are donating is later charged for: in the same instant that the technology multiplies units for transfusion and possible spiritual fruits, it also multiplies processing charges. To modify David Harvey's (2005) classic diagnosis of the workings of late-era capitalism, what we find is accumulation through *unconscious* dispossession. Our use of the word "unconscious" should not lead us to consider the practice impalpable or without consequences for these *involuntary* donors: in fact, they are made to donate more than they need to in situations that are often already ones of extreme anxiety. This of course is where the darker potential of the technology is located. Yet even accumulation through unconscious dispossession resists binary moral accounting if the covertly produced excess is channeled to redistributive ends. In such instances, secret accumulation in an agonistic world of deficits and divergent norms and practices of giving, treating, and receiving blood becomes a way of negotiating outcomes that sustain vulnerable life.

Hematic (Dis)proportions

The nightmare image of a donation of blood gone wrong—an excessive donation that does not end until the donor is entirely drained of his or her lifeblood—figures notably in the reasons that people in India provide for declining to donate their blood. One reluctant Delhiite's statement—"The needle will burst my skin. Everything will spill out. It will never stop"—can stand here for the many we heard during fieldwork that expressed similar sentiments.[31] Yet we also came across the reverse: devotee blood donors actively seeking to donate more than once, who, frustrated by a blood bank's refusal to accept more than a single donation, would threaten to go and donate again elsewhere. Discussing what he takes to be the Euro-American view of a person's excessive devotion to one or other particular mode of exchange as a sign of mental imbalance, John Davis (1992, 45) gives blood donation to excess as an example: "A blood donor who donates all his blood is clearly mad." Coming back to the image of blood donation gone wrong—but now intentionally so—the 2011 Danish-Swedish television crime drama *The Bridge* spectacularized the fantasy of medical blood extraction as an inexorable emptying. One of the several victims of a villain who counts his murders as protests against a varied assortment of social maladies is bled to death via an apparently expert use of medical equipment. The scene resembles a blood donation, but one that continues beyond when the standard 450 milliliters of fluid has been reached. The slow emptying—steady and controlled in a medical setting resembling blood donation (apart from the straps that tie the victim down)—is streamed live on the Internet, to cease only if the villain's demands are met (they are not).

This chapter has explored both excessive donation and excessive prescription of blood. The Rohtak transfusion incident, with which we began, combines elements of each. In examining campaigns to reduce unnecessary transfusions and so preserve a precious resource, we have focused in particular on disproportions between the donated unit of blood and the transfused unit of blood, which throw the balance of exchange off-kilter. Epistemologically unstable, blood units oscillate between different proportions, leading to productive confusions (for the accumulative blood bank). This instability is especially evident in replacement donation, where most donors simply do not possess the technical knowledge to know when, if, or how to call it quits (Latour and Callon 1997). The excess of their donations remains unknown to them. Further, the voluntary blood donor card entitles the donor and his or her immediate family to receive future quantities of blood "equivalent to the amount donated." But just what *is* the amount donated? The numeric reversibility of the blood unit—now one, now three, back to one again—results in opacity.

In the previous chapter, we drew on Alberto Corsín Jiménez's work (2013) in developing an idea of "spillover hematology." The medic we quoted earlier who takes whole donations to replace single component units "because we want to give the leftover to other patients" is explaining to us how the benefit of maintaining the fiction of "like" for "like" replacement lies in the way in which the excess can be made to spill over to assist other patients. But of course for this strategy to work, it must not be disclosed. This makes it markedly different from the species of spill-over hematology we considered in the previous chapter in which, for the AVB-DWB, the body's productive activity of providing "more blood than it needs" means that it can be made to deliver its "goodness" beyond its original catchment area (130). At the same time, the two modes of spillover form part of the same wider complex in which "surpluses out of place" must be pushed into the "right" places.

We have suggested that the surplus and redistribution of donated blood can provide a novel window on debates about overprescription of drugs in the subcontinent and elsewhere. When the drug is derived from human biological matter, different questions are raised about care and hospitality for the drug that might help impede its careless disbursal. For AVBDWB activists in particular, fidelity to the gift of blood must mean abjuring overprescription of it. In other words, AVB-DWB activists argue that the logic of the usage of donated blood must come to be permeated by the sentiment that informed the initial donation. Care for the gift, to be measured by the extent to which medics refrain from prescribing single- or whole-unit transfusions, itself takes on the form of a gift. That is, care for the sentiment underlying the original gift results in a surplus that may be gifted to an extra few *and* back to the donor whose sentiments are honored when the treatment of the gift remains animated with the spirit of its giver: the *hau* of prescription. The nature of the blood unit as partonomic again comes into focus: the whole unit that is transfused represents the parts that were not able to be given in other transfusions. The micropractices of persuasion we have explored here employ just such an arithmetic of ungiven units whose ghostly existence is negatively called into being by single- and whole-unit transfusions. Indeed, as we saw, with the proportions of the transfusion all wrong, clinical activists develop a proportional ethics to counter excessive prescription and the deficits it exacerbates. A numerical pedagogy of phantom units is central to the practices and arguments through which virtue-as-appropriate-prescription is cultivated and doctors are persuaded to incline toward a view of blood other than as a tonic in abundant supply. Requisitions for single or whole units are thus translated into a numeracy of "lives not saved." In evoking the role played by questions of therapeutic secrecy and excess, and the indeterminate numeracy of the gift, we come to see how each of these, in turn, informs the reason and form of the transfusion.

BLOOD IN THE TIME OF THE CIVIC

In her important work on modern social time, anthropologist Laura Bear (2014a, 27) uses the term "modern time of the civic" in reference to a particular Durga Puja *pandal* (religious pavilion) in Kolkata. Images of thwarted futures and ruined pasts converge in the time-space of the *pandal*, along with the redemptory cosmogony represented by Durga. The goddess appears in Bear's analysis as a mediator whose presence ensures the continued productivity of the city.[1] On a day marked by the collapse of an anticipated industrial future,[2] it is her care and authority that would ensure, despite the collapse, the continuation of "the modern time of the civic" (27). The layered, conflictual, overlapping nature of the temporal images and experiences at the *pandal* can be understood as a synecdoche of modern social time more generally, which is irreducible to time economy and speed, as (over)emphasized in much existing scholarship (Bear 2016a, 488).

In this chapter, our focus is on blood in the time of the civic: our object of analysis is blood that is donated voluntarily as a dutiful contribution to civic life that in turn ensures the continued efficacy and productivity of transfusion medicine. These voluntary donations take place according to a seemingly simple time map—namely, repetition, ideally at three-month intervals. This is in contrast to apparently less civic-minded blood donation modes: the potentially dangerous commercial transaction of "professional" (the vernacular for paid or commercial) donation, and the one-time mode of "replacement" donation, performed in order to release blood for the benefit of one's immediate family member in need of transfusion. These modes of donation, as we shall see, are characterized by different temporalities. A routine of dutiful, repetitive bloodshed structures voluntary blood donation's time of the civic. Institutional medical demand for blood is continuous: the iterative presumption of a single voluntary blood donation in time is that it forms one of a series (Strathern 2017, 201). In Kockelman and Bernstein's (2012, 322) terms, voluntary blood donation foregrounds temporality as metricality: "the repetition of tokens of a common event type."[3]

Importantly, we find intersecting temporalities even at the basic level of the ideal, routinized repetition. If routinized blood donation is a mode of social time, the biological time of cellular production is the major determinant of the biomedically mandated three-month gap between donations. The time regime of the repeated voluntary, social donation emerges from and is mapped upon the lifetime of blood cells. This time regime of routinized replenishment might be compared to labor routines, which similarly rely on the temporality of biological replenishment. Returning to donate blood every three months depends on blood being a renewable resource, with the rejuvenation of one's blood over time equivalent to the rejuvenation of the worker overnight: "Just as the length of the working day poses a limit point to the extent to which the vitality of the worker must be renewed on a daily basis so that he or she might continue to labor, blood can also be subjected to this logic of marginal utility" (Anagnost 2006, 523). To assume the social role of blood donor is to be ready to treat one's body as a producer of blood (Berner 2010, 198). Repetition (of donation) in time is intertwined with the time of production.

In the next two chapters, we examine the different temporal registers and representations that structure and compete within the field of blood donation and transfusion in India. While the following chapter focuses on engagements with and imaginings of the future in this field, the focus here is on how blood in the time of the civic—its repetitive excorporation over time for (bio)medical purposes—is reliant on and structured by a remarkably diverse set of temporalities. Further, revealing these multiple temporalities complicates the notion of the three-monthly repetition of donation as simply a biomedical or biologically based routine. Instead, the time of the civic comes into view as being "secretly" supported by an array of temporal structures and irruptions that are incognizable to biomedical reason.

Thus, we show how blood in the time of the civic is made possible by overlapping temporal registers and reckonings. We will see, then, that the temporality of metricality is not only that but also a temporal achievement based on all sorts of nonroutinized times. The first part of the chapter focuses on the divergent rhythms of blood donation. We then explore the dimension of astral time as a determinant of the ideal, repeat voluntary blood donor. In the final part of the chapter, we turn to inheritance and memory as ambivalent enablers of routinized repetition in the Indian blood donation and transfusion world.

Too Often, Not Often Enough: Donation Rhythms and the Time of Kinship

Each mode of blood donation possesses a different rhythm, consideration of which is key to understanding that mode. At the same time, overlaps exist between these distinct rhythms that, as we shall see, can cause the modes to appear to have a Russian-doll-like relationship to one another.

As we noted in chapter 4, the ideal rhythm of voluntary blood donation is that of repetition over time, and repetition is possible because of the biological rhythm of cellular production and destruction: the blood given is replenished and re-formed. As we saw, educational campaigners endlessly communicate the facts of replenishment: seventy-two hours after a donation for the quantity to return, six to eight weeks for the quality. Ideally, then, a voluntary blood donor donates his or her blood every three months. This is understood to ensure both the continued health of donors—important, of course, as a condition of repetition—and a continuous supply of blood for blood banks. Moreover, such blood is not only repeatedly donated but repeatedly tested, in theory enhancing safety for recipients.

Medical authorities therefore have a favorable view of the voluntary blood donor who donates blood many times and often. But, recalling the (dis)proportionality of donating and prescribing witnessed in the previous chapters, it is possible to give too many times: that is, if the stipulated time lapse between donations, which is three months, is not respected.[4] This concern is motivated by the allegedly poor quality of blood that results from professional blood donors donating once or twice a week. Paid donors are said to mask low hemoglobin levels by consuming iron tablets. The iron supplement is a kind of time-tricking device (Moroșanu and Ringel 2016), since it makes it seem as if three months have passed since the previous donation. But iron supplements are not foolproof: evidence of the number of times a professional donor has given in the recent past may be read on their skin through fresh venipuncture marks. The pathologically speeded up rhythm of professional donation is understood to endanger the health of both donors and recipients. In comparison with repeat voluntary donation, paid donation embodies an *uncivic* temporality.

Professional and replacement donation are often spoken of in the same breath, particularly by campaigners for voluntary donation for whom both forms of donation are deviants to the mode they seek to promote. In particular, replacement donation is considered frequently to encompass the paid variety, since relatives too fearful themselves to donate may pay others to donate in their stead. Both modes are alleged to encourage prospective donors to lie about their fitness to donate, thereby endangering recipients. In the case of paid donation, donors might lie in order to be accepted for donation and hence be remunerated; in the case of replacement donation, the lie facilitates treatment for their family member. (Recall that replacement is not a direct donation that makes up the relative's transfusion, but one that travels to unknown others. Lying may endanger recipients, but not *their* specific family member.) In temporal terms, however, these modes are binary opposites: if professional blood donors donate blood too often, replacement donors do not donate often enough, for replacement donations are by their nature one-time donations made for a specific purpose. Temporally speaking, the modes are differently deviant and disproportionate.

Replacement also possesses a temporally conflictual relationship with voluntary donation. The time of replacement does not emerge from, nor is it mapped onto, the biological time of cellular production, as is ideally the case with voluntary donation. Rather, replacement intersects with a different tempo altogether—namely, the "overdetermined" reproductive time of kinship, since in replacement one donates in order to avert a threat to the "long-term continuity of kinship affect and obligation" (Bear 2014a, 8, 19).[5] In fact, the reproductive kinship time of replacement not only is not mapped onto the biological time of cellular production that structures voluntary donation, but it conflicts with it. This is because a person may be asked to donate in replacement once or many times, depending on the frequency with which their family members require transfusions. The voluntary and replacement modes coexist in a mixed system of procurement as temporal antagonists, since those with experience of donating in replacement come to have a compelling reason to refrain from ever donating blood voluntarily. This is because if a person is called upon to donate blood in replacement for a family member but has donated voluntarily within the previous three months, then they will be ineligible to do so again, potentially disrupting their family's ability to facilitate the transfusion required by their ailing family member. "OK, you are asking me to donate my blood now," said a middle-aged man, with incredulity, to a recruiter at a mall in south Delhi where a voluntary camp was being held. "My brother has bypass surgery [scheduled for] next month [when he will need replacement donations], so you tell me, how can I donate [now]?"[6] In this way, the long-term continuity and affect of kinship time conflicts with the ideal rhythm and repetition of voluntary blood donation. If the voluntary, paid, and replacement modes are on a continuum of regular, too regular, and irregular, this case shows how these different regularities come into conflict.

Put another way, we can say that the conflict is one between abstract and concrete temporalities. The four-time yearly rhythm of voluntary blood donation, though based on a biological tempo of cellular production and destruction, is abstract because it is ideal: rarely adhered to or concretely actualized. This ideal was instituted by the Indian government's National Blood Policy in 2002 and remains an ever receding target, still in the process of being instituted ten years after replacement donation was meant to have been phased out. The actual, concrete temporal experience of blood donation for most Indians remains the erratic rhythm of replacement. Moreover, it is not just that the rhythms are different, but that they are in conflict (Bear 2014a). The time reckoning of voluntary blood donation remains abstract and unrealized precisely due to people's concrete experience of the episodic, unpredictable rhythm of replacement donation. Ensuring that one is available for replacement donations and therefore able to help safeguard the continuity of kinship ties can mean, quite reasonably, eschewing the ideal of voluntary donation. In practical terms, the phased discontinuation of replacement is problematic because what results is not a "best of both worlds" mixed system, but one in which the different modes actively undermine each other due to the different temporal imperatives informing them.

Retemporalization

Yet the story is not only one of conflict. We suggested earlier that voluntary blood donation's metrical temporality, when actualized, is an achievement based on different kinds of nonroutinized times. We now consider ways in which blood banks seek to harmonize the replacement and voluntary modes, making the former into a resource for constructing the latter. Though the "one-time" nature of replacement sees it arise, as a necessary action for relatives, out of specific medical-familial situations, it is also, of course, a repeatable act. A family member's illness may be long-term and require repeat transfusions and therefore replacement donations, or different relatives may require replacement donations on different occasions. Similarly, voluntary donation is only routinized in ideal terms. It is perfectly possible to give voluntarily only once. We examine here exhortations that replacement donors should be temporally reformed, or converted, into repeat voluntary donors. We also examine how, in order to achieve the metricality meant to characterize the voluntary mode, that mode may be made to resemble a one-time donation that is repeated (i.e., a replacement donation). The answer, in other words, is to make the voluntary and replacement modes more like one another: Russian-doll temporalities.

Replacement donation can be compared with Harvey Whitehouse's (2000) definition of the imagistic mode of religiosity, which he describes as being constituted by sporadic and intense bursts of religious activity that may in later life induce "flashbulb," or delimited episodic memories. Traumatic initiation ceremonies are an example of the imagistic mode (Laidlaw 2004, 4). This mode gives rise to a concentrated solidarity among those involved, but such people are likely to be small in number and limited to specific locations. The emotionally extreme circumstances of replacement donation, taken together with its infrequency and family-centeredness, we can equate with the imagistic terrain of Whitehouse's schema.

In the doctrinal mode of religiosity, on the other hand, worship is routinized, formulaic, and heavily repetitious. This kind of activity—consisting typically of regular ceremonies with sermons, hymns, and readings—gives rise to schemas of semantic memory within which the contexts and persons involved in transmission are cognitively marginalized. The resulting solidarity is thus diffuse and large-scale, but contrary to imagistic experience, largely impersonal. We may thus equate voluntary donation—in ideal terms—with the doctrinal mode of religiosity. In a voluntary system, the model donor gives blood every three months (i.e., four times a year), without specific reason, with no one particular in mind, and indeed should be completely devoid of preferences in this regard. Voluntary donation is thus a universalistic mode of donation, a status it shares with doctrinal modes of religiosity (Whitehouse 2000, 160–89).

As we have explained, the irregular episodic temporality of replacement donation is lamented by voluntary blood donation recruiters, for the simple reason that blood banks require a constant supply. Much rhetoric therefore concerns the need to convert replacement donors into voluntary ones—a project of temporal reform (or "retemporalization" [Chua 2011]). As Safe Blood, a Delhi-based NGO, states in its publicity materials, "Education and motivation techniques need to be devised to convert nondonors into donors and one-time replacement donors into repeat donors." The global problem of irregular voluntary donation forms a parallel with the persistence of replacement donation in India. For instance, the Austrian Red Cross has published a poster with a picture of Santa Claus and this caption: "Nowadays Santa Claus doesn't just appear at Christmas time, but also in spring, summer, and autumn when he brings a gift of life by donating blood himself! Four times a year!" A second shows a picture of a woman drinking beer alongside the caption: "*O'zapft* is an expression from the Munich beer festival when the first barrel is tapped and beer flows like water. Blood should not flow only on one special annual occasion—but four times a year!"[7] Attempts to retemporalize the giving practices of blood donors are thus hardly unique to India. In India, however, doctors proclaim the direct equivalence of one-time voluntary donations and replacement donations. As one Delhi-based blood bank medic put it to us, "Giving blood once at a camp is only as good as a replacement donation. You call it a voluntary donation, but it is a one-time donation, and risks come from one-time donation, whether done [voluntarily] at a camp or as replacement." Though some statistics appear to dispute the equivalence (Nanu et al. 1997), and one-time voluntary and replacement donations certainly arise out of very different situations and emotional circumstances, the insufficiency of the singular donation is underscored in both cases. One should give repeatedly over time, always looking forward to the next donation. "One can give one's kidneys once, and one's other organs only once, but blood donation is special . . ." said a medic from NACO at a solicitation function in front of schoolchildren before concluding, "Don't evaluate the past; speak only of future donations."

Safe Blood's call for conversion from replacement (imagistic) to voluntary (doctrinal) donation is important, for instead of denigrating replacement and seeking its elimination, replacement is here proffered as a condition that needs to be generalized. Gillian Cohen's (1989, 114–15) proposition that "semantic knowledge is derived from episodic memories by a process of abstraction and generalization" is pertinent here for helping describe the sought-for temporal relation between replacement and voluntary modes of donation. Such proponents of the voluntary, doctrinal mode seek to structure, discipline, or generalize irregular, episodic outbursts of donation activity, with the doctrinal mode coming to consist of imagistic events pulled temporally closer together. We thus encounter the incorporation of the imagistic mode into the doctrinal one as a means of securing repetition: voluntary blood donation on the emotionally charged occasion of a guru's death anniversary, a politician's birthday, or for the specific object of an imagined thalassemic child.[8] The replacement and voluntary modes come to appear less temporally antagonistic.

The AVBDWB (see chapters 4 and 5) in particular has been active in mobilizing Indian nationalist cyclical (calendric) time, identifying everything from National Teacher's Day to the birthday of freedom fighter Netaji Subhash Chandra Bose (see chapter 2) as days for blood donation events. For the former they will approach teachers, for the latter the nationalist leader's present-day adherents, and so on. Thus, they transform the conflictual temporal relationship between replacement and voluntary donation by sublating the temporal features of replacement within the voluntary mode. Spontaneous, or impulsive, acts of giving have long been framed in contrast to routinized, rationalized charity, with charities sometimes deprecating the former and seeking to bring it under rational control (Bornstein 2009, 623). From one perspective, the bid to secure routinized repetition of blood donation recalls just such a Weberian scenario of seeking to discipline irregular charitable action. But insofar as the voluntary variant emerges from and retains temporal features of replacement, we can see that things are not quite so simple; voluntary blood donation's temporality as metricality is built upon nonroutinized imagistic traits associated with the replacement form. The time of the civic is thick and layered, enmeshed with rhythms of kinship, religion, and politics.

But if the imagistic nature of replacement donation is abstracted and generalized in the voluntary mode as the solution to a particular temporal problem, the solution has resulted in new temporal problems. First, annual repetition (for instance on a guru's death anniversary) is still insufficient for securing a regular blood supply. This is mitigated in supply terms in part by the mobilization of many different days of significance across the yearly calendar. Yet the ideal of the regular repeat donor remains unrealized; in donating at events at their places of work (as in the example of teachers) or worship (e.g., on the guru's birthday), most voluntary donors end up giving just once rather than four times a year. Moreover, blood donation camps organized by guru movements and political parties rouse the emotions of devotees and party members to produce spectacular collection figures on a particular day—to maximize media coverage, surpass world records, glorify the guru, and so on. As we described in chapter 3, this is at odds with the continuity of demand.

A particular problem with the devotional one-time camp at which large collection figures are sought is how it clashes with the durational time of blood cells. While plasma can be frozen and kept indefinitely, red cells have a thirty-day refrigerated shelf life, and platelets have just five days. Receiving massive quantities of blood at a single point in time is not consistent with the continuousness of demand, for the limited cellular durations of units means that many of them will expire before they can be transfused. Such camps therefore compromise the synchronizing function of blood banks in which the elements to be synchronized are not durable and thus are dependent upon the correct temporal as well as spatial coordination of each to the other (recipient body and excorporated blood). Blood banks seek to persuade guru organizations to stagger and routinize their camps—to bring the episodic temporality of devotional time into line with the ongoing time of supply—but with only limited success. The Sant Nirankari devotional order's multiple camps spread out over the summer months is a notable, but somewhat isolated, success story here.[9]

In the specific case of the Dera Sacha Sauda megacamps that have several times obtained world record status for most blood collected in a single day, there arises still another temporal clash. The dominant temporality at such events is that of rush (Ssorin-Chaikov 2006): donors and organizers are up against a time limit, since the world record they seek to surpass is that of most blood collected in a single day. Numerous medics report pressure being put on them to collect smaller quantities in order to speed up donation times and so collect more units. In such cases, rather than successful sublation of replacement temporalities within the voluntary mode, further temporal conflicts arise: spectacular annual or one-off voluntary events in devotional or political contexts may produce (1) too many units, such that many of them expire, and (2) "speeded up" units, such that many of them are substandard.

There is a second temporal sublation of replacement within the voluntary blood donation mode, which relates to family and generation. We earlier framed a contrast in temporal terms between the repetition over time of voluntary donation (founded on cellular time) and one-time replacement donation (founded on safeguarding generational time). But just as repeat voluntary donations come to be figured by recruiters as abstractions of one-time replacement donations, concepts of family and reproductive time reappear in the mode of donation that is seemingly antithetical to them. Recruitment posters emphasize that affect-laden kinship time in the form of family relationships will be sustained courtesy of voluntary donations (e.g., the image of a child and the text, "My mummy is back home because you donated blood"). Such posters suggest to the donor that the patient who is saved may be someone who sustains a family, so saving the patient is in effect a gift forward. Further, in potentially saving a person yet to produce children, this gift may directly facilitate future reproductive kinship time (e.g., the common rhyming slogan "A part [*ansh*] of your blood can save somebody's generation/family line [*vansh*]").[10]

Such imaginings depict voluntarily donated blood as a profound force of genealogical continuity and potential just as much as family replacement.[11] In so doing, voluntarily donated blood comes to appear almost as a reproductive gift in the same category as ova, sperm, and embryos—that is, not only sustaining a life in peril but also engendering new lives and familial forms. Voluntarily donated blood comes to be charged with a power of preservation and generation that extends beyond recipients per se to include their dependents and descendants, both actual and future-conjectural. This, then, is the second way in which the temporal sublation of replacement within voluntary donation occurs: what in replacement are concrete experiences of family and reproductive time reappear in voluntary donation contexts in the form of time representations used to motivate donors. It is now not one's own family relationships and generational potential that are at stake, but those of unknown and unknowable others.

Quantified Donors

We turn now to a further way in which the ideal of routinized repetition comes to be secured by means of "other" temporalities that may not, at first glance, seem consonant with it at all. Specifically, we turn to astrological time reckoning, which features in the field of blood donation and transfusion in several quite distinct ways.[12] The question that concerns us here, and that animates recruiters influenced by astrology, is one that is fundamental to the voluntary blood donation project as a whole: Just who will give repeatedly over time according to the ideal rhythm of voluntary blood donation? The answer is not obvious. Routinized repetition comes to be treated as an astrological problem. Recruiters ask: Can astrological significance be read into the number of times people give blood, and if so, might there be some degree of motivational economy in focusing recruitment efforts on those whose horoscopes will make them more likely to be responsive to the cause? In other words, what is the relation between the time and date of birth and the number of times a person repeats the act of blood donation?

Mahesh Trivedi, from Ahmedabad, is not representative of all or even most blood donor recruiters in being preoccupied with the astrological significance of blood donation. But his investigations into the matter, and those also of the handful of other blood donor recruiters we met, is indicative of how new terrains of application are continuously being found for astrological theory. It is indicative also of the diverse forms of creative thinking that inform voluntary blood donation solicitation efforts, and of a form of time-reckoning in the blood donation and transfusion field in which causality and fortune hinge on the cosmic order. We met him a number of times at blood donor recruitment conferences in different Indian cities. Mahesh's business card states, "Centurion Blood Donor and Hon Sec, Indian Red Cross Soc, Ahmedabad." "My true qualification is I am a centurion blood donor," he tells us. Borrowing from cricket, this is his way of saying that he belongs to that rare category of person who has donated blood more than one hundred times. (He also told us, "We have in Gujarat the first woman centurion donor—we will get Jayalalitha [the iconic former chief minister of Tamil Nadu] to present the award to her.")[13] He is honorary secretary of the local Red Cross Society on account of both the number of times he has donated blood and his dedicated voluntary blood donation solicitation efforts performed over decades. The latter have particularly focused on the plight of thalassemic children and their regular requirement of blood for transfusion. Now in his sixties, he is no longer eligible to donate his blood, but he continues his strenuous campaign efforts. Increasingly he seeks to combine his involvement in blood donation with his interest in astrology.

He showed us a letter he had written to prominent blood banks across the country detailing his preliminary findings and also requesting their help in identifying other centurion donors whom he might contact and ask to undergo an astrological consultation.

> I am very happy to inform you that I have given my centurion blood on 12.2.95 in Ahmedabad. . . . I have always been apprehensive as to why I preferred to tread on a humanitarian path. Many of my friends, as they

say, preferred to join such a noble activity for the reason that they felt the need for their religion or the society or the nation at different occasions, which prompted them forcefully to take up such a noble cause whereas in my case I personally cannot come forward with such a reasoning, even after scoring a century. Now after scoring a century I think I must search for the impulse, which might have led me to score a century. There ought to be some.

One of my astrologer friends . . . concluded that the influence of Mars in my life has prompted me to take up this noble and humanitarian program. He provided me with many other remarks, which need comprehensive study for coming to conclusive remarks. . . . Honorable Shri B J Divan Retired Chief Justice of Gujarat High Court and a veteran blood donor has quoted that many of the judges are found to have the influence of Jupiter as per their horoscopes.

It seems that there be some such relation or the influence of the star and other celestial objects on our lives which can be examined by compiling the data. . . . With this in mind, I request you to kindly provide me the detailed information of veteran donors registered in your organization to whom I can address this letter and get basic data concerning their horoscope and details of blood donation which may provide me an opportunity to study and prepare a research which may guide any works and students in the field of astrology, medicine, blood donation and related sciences.

About twenty blood banks wrote back, and Mahesh was able to compile a study of sorts.[14] Of his findings, he told us, "When I examined the horoscopes of centurion donors, I found Mars (related to blood), Venus (strength), Sun (leadership), and Jupiter (a balanced mind, continuing with assurance, the guru part—your preacher and teacher for the right path) to be powerful. I have these in good position. At the time of my birth, my horoscope led me to do good specifically with my blood."

A female recruiter who operates in Delhi also cited to us the influence of Mars and Venus in her horoscope as determining hers and others' commitment to blood donation. Recounting the fiftieth time she had donated blood, she told us: "I thought to myself it must be written by God—this is your destiny to go on doing this with no consideration. Mars is related to bloodletting, and Venus is your strength, and if these two are powerful in your horoscope you will be guided to give blood, and Jupiter makes you carry on with no consideration. They will guide you to do it—it is your destiny. Such people we must focus on."

Other voluntary blood donation recruiters, and a number of astrologically aware and inclined donors besides, made similar suggestions to us concerning the practical sense it would make to focus recruitment activities on candidates whose horoscopes might make them predisposed to the cause. Few details were given about how this might be accomplished—one recruiter spoke of seeking access to relevant census data—and we found no evidence of blood banks actually focusing their solicitation efforts in such a way (and in the specific case of Mahesh, his research seemed more a theoretical than a practical exercise). Rather, it is indicative of a way of thinking about blood donation. The suggestion is that were blood banks to take prospective donors' times of birth into account, it might take less time and effort to encourage blood donation: the time(s) of astrology—the specificity of the date and time of birth as a means of forecasting or gaining knowledge of the future—potentially offers recruiters temporal and logistical economy. Linear "workday" time might be economized by bringing a seemingly quite other time reckoning into the picture. If the role of astrology in facilitating "fast-time religion" has recently been suggested, especially on TV news channels (Udupa 2016), for some blood donation recruiters, astrology has the capacity to assist in fast-time motivation.[15]

But it is not only a matter of saving time and of the astral time of birth. If pursued, such a strategy might eventuate the "dream of repetition in time" (Bear 2014b, 78): the repeated blood donations of the model (veteran or "centurion") voluntary blood donor, who gives time and time again. The dutiful repetition that makes up blood donation's time of the civic thus comes to be understood as inseparable from the time of birth, the power of Jupiter to establish continuous assurance (in donating), and the time of astrological prediction more generally.

Rhythms and Potentials

For Mahesh Trivedi, donation repetitions cannot be thought of separately from their counterpart, transfusion repetitions. Transfusion, too, might be considered rhythmically. For a heart operation, one may require just a one-time transfusion, whereas someone with thalassemia may require a transfusion every few weeks. Mahesh donated his blood repeatedly over time precisely because people with thalassemia require repeat transfusions. "A friend of mine has received 450 units in her life so far for her survival," he told us. "I donated my blood 117 times. So you see, we need five or six centurion donors to put their lives' contributions together for the life of just one person with thalassemia. What pride I had for being a centurion donor has gone because I could not save one person with thalassemia." Mahesh thereby turns the usual rhetoric of solicitation on its head: rather than saving 117 lives, he has saved not even one. The proportions of repetition are min-iaturized (see chapter 5); emphasized, instead, are the disproportions of ongoing thalassemic requirement.

The proportions of donation and transfusion are to be measured not only by quantity but also by frequency. The logic of phantom (ungiven) units, discussed in chapter 5, declares that one person, donating regularly, can save many people. In Trivedi's reversal, many are needed simply in order to save one person. In chap-ter 5, we saw how a trainer mapped phantom units according to a set of tempo-ral particulars: the trainee recruiters' times of birth and current ages were mea-sured against a rhythm of four possible donations per year. Units remain ungiven *in time*. For promoters of voluntary blood donation, the voluntary mode parto-nomically enacts the temporal critique of replacement donation, which stands, for them, for the units that could have been donated if repeated over time accord-ing to the voluntary ideal. If voluntary blood donation enacted represents the "actualization of the potentials that are virtually present in our lives" (Mazzarella 2010, 723), replacement represents the extinguishing of such potentials.

Part of what makes Bear's work such a useful guide in documenting the tem-poralities of the Indian blood donation and transfusion field is her emphasis on both productive agency and conflict in time. The reproductive time of kinship—safeguarded by replacement donations—can conflict with the rhythm of volun-tary donation and its harnessing of the death and regeneration of blood cells. Med-ics and recruiters must labor to align the family-centeredness of replacement with the more abstract nature of voluntary blood donation, thereby emphasiz-ing the generative potential of the latter. They must also find ways to produce the continuity meant to characterize voluntary blood donation through manipula-tions of the one-time nature of replacement. Voluntary blood donation is com-posed of family time even though, in some respects, it is also opposed to it. Rhythms are always composed of other rhythms. For some recruiters, astrologi-cal reasoning promises to unlock the secrets of repetition. The existence of cen-turion donors—those who have repeated the act of blood donation one hundred times or more—seems to call for explanation. Such hematic commitment, as re-vealed by a particular attitude toward time (a will to repeat), has itself a temporal explanation (time of birth). Different times once more interlock in enabling ways.

Repetition as Violence

In chapter 2 we discussed Mohandas Gandhi's condemnation of logics of "blood for blood" in the context of Jallianwala Bagh. For him, demanding blood for blood was not just a contravention of the ethics of nonviolence, but also a sign of weakness to be overcome in the practice of *satyagraha*. The phraseology of "blood for blood" possesses a fraught history in the region as a sign of, and call for, violent bloodshed, often in the context of communal riots. After the assassination of Prime Minister Indira Gandhi in 1984, along with slogans such as *Tumne hamari ma ko mara hai* ("You have killed our mother"), the inflammatory phrase *Khun ka badla khun* ("Blood must be avenged with blood") was chanted both as a precursor to, and during, the devastating attacks on Sikhs that took place in Delhi and elsewhere (Das 2007, 153; Dalrymple 1993, 28). A variant of the phrase also played a part in the worst communal violence since the Ayodhya riots of 1992, which took place ten years later in Gujarat after fifty-nine Hindus were killed on a train returning from Ayodhya. In retaliation, at least seven hundred Muslims were massacred. Inciting the subsequent massacre of Muslims the day after the train killings, two Gujarati daily newspapers carried the headline "Avenge Blood with Blood."[16]

The negative reciprocity of retaliatory bloodshed is, of course, a form of repetition: the phrase "blood for blood" incites vengeful repetition. However, blood donation has had a special role in refusals to countenance such a politics of vengeful repetition. This is most notably so in the case of the assassination of the Sant Nirankari guru Baba Gurbachan Singh in 1981 by militant Sikhs, following which Nirankari devotees demanded violent revenge. We quote devotees recalling these events: "The people went to Baba Ji to say we should take revenge (*badla*)," "The [devotees] all said [to the successor guru], give us an order. Command us to do something [violent] so we may also have the sentiment (*bhavna*) of sacrifice (*tyag*)." The successor Nirankari guru, Baba Hardev Singh, the son of Gurbachan Singh, is reported to have responded, "We will definitely take revenge, but by love (*prem*). Our revenge is to donate blood for the needy persons."[17]

As we noted earlier in this chapter (see also chapter 2), the Sant Nirankaris are now prolific providers of blood in Delhi and beyond, with the devotional movement collaborating with the Red Cross blood bank to collect as much as 20 percent of the capital's voluntarily donated blood. At every camp, the movement's exhortatory slogan that "blood should flow into veins (*nari*), not drains (*nali*)" is uttered, thereby repeatedly underscoring not only a contrast between nonviolent and violent modes of bloodshed but also how the former emerged from—and is even a form of—the latter. Nirankari blood donations are not only a response to violence but are themselves a sublimated form of it: such a mode of revenge possesses a peculiar kind of inclusiveness (it is participatory). Moreover, it is also repeatable. Indeed, both revenge for and reenactment of the guru's sacrifice seem to be fused together in Nirankari blood donations. As the public address system announced at one Nirankari camp we attended, "After He [Gurbachan Singh] had sacrificed his life, *lakhs* [hundreds of thousands] of people wanted to be included in the sacrifice. They all wanted an opportunity to do something. Baba Ji [Hardev Singh] said [of Nirankari blood donation], 'You are talking of one Baba Ji [i.e., the predecessor guru, Gurbachan Singh], but I have produced thousands of Baba Jis for you.'" What should be clear by now is that in repeating both their former guru's sacrifice and in revenging it over and over again, the Sant Nirankari mobilization of blood donation as an act of memory and sacrificial repetition comes to structure and enable what at first glance appeared like the very simple time map of voluntary blood donation at three-month intervals. The menacing logic of "blood for blood," reworked thus, comes into view as a positive force and a mode of repetition capable of supporting the time of the civic.

Public blood donation events that make reference to bloody deaths are not the preserve of the Sant Nirankaris. Just as the first blood donation camps conducted by the Sant Nirankari Mission took place in response to the death of Baba Gurbachan Singh, the Dera Sacha Sauda's first world record-breaking donation camp was conducted on the death anniversary of its preceding guru. Meanwhile, the Youth Congress holds camps on the death anniversaries (sometimes also the birthdays) of Indira, Rajiv, and Sanjay Gandhi, respectively. The two most prominently remembered politicians in such camps are Indira and Rajiv Gandhi, both assassinated and remembered as martyrs who shed their blood for the nation.[18] Though less mythologized than the Nirankari engagement with blood donation, such political camps are no less repetitions of prior excorporations.

Relatedly, voluntary blood donation events are conducted, perhaps more than any other occasion, on days of bloody nationalist significance, such as on Martyrs' Day (23 March), the day on which, in 1931, Bhagat Singh and his fellow freedom fighters were hung by the British and cremated in Ferozepur, Punjab. Similar events that precipitate nationalist bleeding reenactments are the death anniversaries of Bose and other revolutionaries.[19] Consider, for instance, an RSS (Rashtriya Swayamsevak Sangh) blood donation camp held in Amritsar on Martyrs' Day. At this camp, donors received on their foreheads a *tilak* of dust that had been brought in a *kalash* from Bhagat Singh's cremation grounds on the bank of the Sutlej in Ferozepur.[20] The dust materially embodied the ashes of the martyrs. In chapter 2 we discussed Gandhi's remarks about how "the holy blood of innocent people" sanctified the land of Jallianwala Bagh. The *tilak* of dust from the cremation grounds contains something of this, especially in light of RSS writings concerning its claim of how in 1947 the organization was instrumental in restoring Jammu and Kashmir to India. Many RSS volunteers, they say, were killed: "One feels a wave of sacrifice in one's mind while wishing to touch the blood-red soil of Palandhari where the soldiers and the RSS workers shed their blood. Repeated salutes to such brave sacrifices."[21] As we noted in chapter 2, a blood donation camp in 2009 was staged in a spatiotemporal conjunction saturated with nationalist significance: Jallianwala Bagh on Mohandas's Gandhi's birthday (Gandhi Jayanti). The camp's organizers stated that its aim was "to awake the government from deep slumber to grant the status of freedom fighter to the martyrs killed during the massacre of 13 April 1919."[22] Nationalist materials— blood, ashes, and soil—coagulate as tributary mimetic repetitions within a "material timescape" (Bear 2017, 143) of memory. Such variant recodings of "blood for blood" highlight again how the repetition as dutiful routine demanded by voluntary blood donation incorporates—is constituted by—quite other modes of repetition besides.

Inheritance as Repetition

We turn now to a related but different mode of repetition. We have already detailed the mimetic quality of Nirankari blood donations as repeatable copies of the prior guru's bloodshed. In chapter 2, as well, we considered Ravi Chander Gupta's blood excorporations as a kind of injunctive mimesis and reanimation of prior nationalist blood sacrifices. Consider now some of the mimetic ways in which gurus come to succeed one another. Incorporation, writes Judith Butler (1998, 727), may be understood as a kind of psychic miming. If legitimate guruship requires the claimant to partake of prior gurus and other divine forms, then a whole array of mimetic techniques can come into play as part of a methodology of incorporation. Thus, a Mumbai-based guru who claims to be the reincarnation of Shirdi Sai Baba adopts mannerisms and accoutrements said to be characteristic of the forbear guru, while the son of a deceased guru in Gwalior, soon after his father's passing, began uttering unexpected remarks of the sort formerly made by his father (Gold 2012, 253).[23] Was the father-guru now acting in and through the son? Whatever the case, it is clear that a certain mimetic proficiency can be helpful for gurus or would-be gurus in matters of succession and incorporation. Let us bear this in mind as we explore an episode that complicates still further the layered repetitions that go into making voluntary blood donation's metrical temporality.

In 2007, the guru presiding over the Haryana-based devotional order the Dera Sacha Sauda (henceforth the DSS) stood accused of publicly copying—in the manner of his dress but also ritually—Guru Gobind Singh, the final living Sikh guru according to orthodox Sikhs. Photographs depicting the imitation—initially published in local newspapers but soon in massive circulation via electronic media—provoked sustained civil unrest in areas of Punjab, Rajasthan, Haryana, and Delhi from May to June 2007, with the loss of several lives. In 2008 there was even an attempt to assassinate the DSS guru. We have drawn out some of the mimetic properties of the event and its aftermath elsewhere; here we want to exclusively explore the role of mimetic repetition of bloodshed as a guru's means for claiming the mantle of a tradition.[24] We suggest that the mimetic significance of the episode lies not just in the ritual and sartorial imitations contained in the photographs themselves, but also within a much larger-scale, longitudinal, and differentiated mimetic complex of blood and sacrifice that structures the relations between orthodox Sikhism and a number of ambiguously connected-yet-separate devotional orders, predominantly in the *sant* tradition, whose turbaned spiritual masters appear "as if" Sikhs and, indeed, frequently hail from Sikh backgrounds.[25] We shall see how mimesis as inheritance of spiritual tradition—mimesis in the mode of "sacred repetition" (Mann 1981, 49)—becomes absorbed into and constitutive of the seemingly quite "other" time of routinized repetition.

Newspaper reportage focused on the DSS guru's imitative dress—his turban (*dumala*), decorative plume (*kalgi*), dress (*chola*), and waist belt (*kamar-kassa*)—which was reminiscent of Guru Gobind Singh as he is represented in popular religious (or "calendar") art. But the alleged copying went beyond the merely sartorial. The guru is seen distributing a pink liquid substance (said to be a mixture of water, milk, and Rooh Afza *sharbat*) to devotees in an action strikingly similar to the distribution of *amrit* (baptismal nectar) at the Sikh baptism ceremony, though the substance is tellingly renamed "*Jaam-e-Insaan*" ("Wine of Humanity") in the DSS appropriation.[26] Moreover, just as, at their baptism, Sikhs take the name "Singh" or "Kaur," thereby obliterating (at least in theory) their caste identity, texts accompanying the images as they were first published declared that baptized devotees of the Dera Sacha Sauda were now to shun their family names and take instead the name "*Insaan*"—"Human." Sikh protests against the imitation and the DSS defense, which we outline below, thus point to contestation about rights of representation—about who can represent the likeness of a particular guru and in what way. Indeed, one way of framing the events is as an infringement of ritual-intellectual property, as acts of plagiarism.

Concentrating on Internet attacks on the DSS guru, and responses by DSS adherents, we shall see that blood donation and other modes of biological gifts are mobilized by adherents as a very special kind of copy: what we call "copies that usurp." This kind of copy is a corrective copy, for it implies the deficiency of that which is copied. The suggestion is that DSS adherents seek, in their acts of corrective mimesis, to revitalize the neglected ideal and thereby become better Sikhs than Sikhs themselves—copy as usurpation. We can see such effects, for instance, in the DSS usage of "Insaan" as a critical commentary on the persistence of caste discrimination within the mainstream Sikh community. The bestowal of "Insaan" is no doubt a copy of the "original" Sikh substitution of "Singh" and "Kaur" for family names, but it is a corrective copy, for it insinuates the failure of that which is copied.

Following from this, a common response to Sikh attacks on the character of the DSS guru by his devotees is to expound upon the great charitable feats enacted by the DSS. The argument, on the face of it, is simple: DSS charitable endeavors indicate the true and saintly nature of the movement and that it does not deserve the opprobrium heaped upon it. But there is another subtler implication here: DSS charity is framed as the sacrifice Khalsa Sikhs are no longer willing to make. We provide two examples:

> It was the true saint Gurmeet Ram Rahim Singh ji who has prepared [his devotees] to help people in times of disasters. Check out the history of last 10 years, and you will find that anywhere in India, if at all there has been any natural calamity, the Dera Sacha Sauda Master and the followers have been the key helping persons, without whom the affected people would have been left to suffer infinitely!!! Such an institution and its followers are only and only worth respect and praise for all their sacrifices and noble deeds.[27]

> *babe ne 3 hospital bhi kholen hain jahan garibo ko free medical facilities milti hain, babe ke sangat puri INDIAN ARMED FORCE ke monthly blood requirement puri karte hain*, WORLD RECORD IN BLOOD DONATION, TREE PLANTATION, ORGAN DONATIONS, HELPING IN EARTH- QUAKE, DROUGHT, FLOOD AFFECTED PEOPLE AND LAKHS OF OTHER SOCIAL UPLIFTMENT PROGRAMMES [Baba has also opened three hospitals where the poor receive free medical facilities, and his followers fulfill the monthly blood requirements of the Indian Armed Forces . . .] . . . *jo great deeds ho rahi hain proof ke sath voh aapko dikh nahi rahi?* [Can't you see that these great deeds are proofs of his saintliness?][28]

Charity in capital letters and with exclamation marks is thus central to DSS devotees' defense of their guru, providing authentic "proof" of his true character. But in addition to the use of charity as an idiom of defense, there are grounds for conceiving of DSS supercharity as a critical means for the DSS, more offensively (in both senses of the word), to stake a claim on the devotional real. We quote again from the writer of the second quotation, who is responding to a Sikh discussant's reference to allegations of rape made against the DSS guru: "Sir, please also comment what good you have done for society? May be then we start worshipping you. YOU MAY ACT SIKH BUT YOU ARE NOT SIKH, SIKH IS LEADER WHO HELPS." The writer of the first quote, referring to Sikh persecution of the DSS, also asks, "Where was the police when the so called True Sikhs were setting the Deras in Punjab on fire, beating people and trying to kill them as well????"

The DSS has attained several world records for its feats of blood donation, and we have argued elsewhere that the devotional order has been at the forefront of exploring the expressive possibilities of this medical practice.[29] What is significant here is that DSS devotees donated their blood in direct response to the initial Sikh attacks on the movement in May 2007, as a form of protest. At the height of these tensions, a DSS blogger wrote, "The followers of DSS are expressing their dissatisfaction by donating blood but bad-tempered people are flowing the blood of innocent people. Sikh protesters are forgetting . . . that Respected Sri Guru Gobind Singh Ji has given the swords for saving [the] helpless, not to make the blood shed out of helpless people. These terrorists have taken the lives of many innocent people in the last decade when there was demand of Khalistan . . . whereas on the other hand DSS devotees are proving themselves to be real sikhs by donating blood, by giving their kidneys, bone marrow and eyes after death for the sake of humanity." The writer thus suggests that the DSS's protest in the form of service of humanity makes it really Sikh, whereas the violent nature of the orthodox Sikh response represents a perversion of true Sikh principles.

The claim is also implicitly made that DSS devotees' donation of body parts reanimates a consecrated template laid down by Guru Gobind Singh in a way that orthodox Sikhs fail to do. As is well known, at the foundation of the *khalsa* in 1699, Guru Gobind Singh "through a dramatic hoax, demanded the ultimate test of loyalty to his person as a holy man" (Gold 1987, 21). Gold (176–77) draws on Macauliffe's account:

> Guru Gobind Singh had summoned his followers outside his tent, and when they had all assembled he asked if "any one of his beloved Sikhs [were] ready to lay down his life for him?" . . . All grew pale . . . A third time he spoke in a louder voice, "If there be any true Sikh of mine, let him give me his head as an offering and proof of his faith." One disciple finally accepted the challenge and entered into the tent with the guru. Outside, the assembled followers heard the sharp thud of steel cutting through flesh, and the guru emerged alone, his sword dripping with blood. One by one, four more volunteers came forward. Four more times

the thud of the sword was heard, and the guru displayed it soaked in blood. Finally, the guru revealed that his demands for a disciple's life had only been a test: the disciples were still alive and goat's blood was on the sword.

Blood donation appears nearly always to take place within a larger field of extractions with which it can form powerful analogies.[30] The analogy here is evidently between Guru Gobind Singh's call for bodily sacrifice and the DSS commitment to donate blood and other body parts. In fact, the latter may be understood as a kind of mimesis of the former, but it is a *corrective* variant of mimesis, for it draws attention to alleged unwillingness on the part of so called True Sikhs to engage in extractive service. The blogger argues, along with other DSS adherents, that it is only the DSS that fulfills Guru Gobind Singh's teachings in this respect, with its plentiful corporeal offerings "for the sake of humanity." The contrast thus becomes one between "Sikhs" and *Real Sikhs*—as defined (or revealed) by those who are willing to excavate their bodies most deeply. Moreover, DSS blood donation forms a similar test of devotion to the offering of one's head at the formation of the *khalsa*. We may refer here to the profound fears devotees must overcome in order to donate (see chapter 4). For most followers, blood donation is understood to be a dramatically unhealthy activity; that they nonetheless donate is indicative of the spiritual benefits they assume will derive from willingness to undergo the test of devotion.[31]

This demonstrates the extent to which claims to the devotional real are made through the idiom of sacrifice. Sikh Internet discussants seek to deflect the DSS claim on the devotional real with statements that emphasize the exemplary, un-replicable sacrifices of Sikhs: "I don't think any of [the DSS guru's] followers would give *their* heads for him." The DSS argument, on the other hand, concedes the point that Sikhism centers on a foundational sacrifice, while suggesting that "so called True Sikhs' have disavowed this critical tenet, which is at present properly fulfilled only by the DSS. So who then now are the *Real Sikhs*?" DSS donations, thus, are critically partonomic in the sense we described in chapter 3: the part which is given over by the DSS illuminates an apparent gap between that which is given (by DSS devotees) and that which is withheld (by Sikhs). This gap becomes the basis not only of critical social commentary but also of a claim to what we are calling the devotional real—of true succession. Blood donation is again an expression and effect of proportionality with a critical function.[32]

Blood donation as mimesis, then, is highly ambivalent here: it forms a sacred repetition of sacrifices foundational to the Sikh *khalsa* that at the same time serves as a partonomic critique of present Sikhs' "failure" to uphold such principles. To inherit, of course, is a temporal relation: it is to "receive or be left with (a situation, object, etc.) from a predecessor or former owner."[33] DSS donation repetitions enact the order's claim to a spiritual inheritance. The DSS movement (its devotees claim) abides by the principles formerly associated with those who now attack it. This claim to succession, unlike the example we gave earlier, is not by way of spirit possession. It was made in part through performance of ritual and by the bearing of particular accouterments—but not only that. Blood donations as sacred repetitions formed part of the claim, and in so doing succession politics and the temporality of inheritance come to inform and provide ambivalent support for blood's time of the civic. We say ambivalent, for as we have already intimated, from the point of view of medics the DSS approach to blood donation is materially and temporally disproportionate: its collection of a massive number of units on specific days can clash with the durational time of cells, and the rush to collect world-record-surpassing quantities can result in units of insufficient quality. However, though DSS blood camp repetitions may be irregular and not accord flawlessly with the ideal of the three-month time lapse between voluntary donations, they are repetitions nonetheless—repetitions that connote a rough synchronization between divergent temporal imperatives and that are symptomatic of a key form that temporality as metricality takes in the Indian blood donation world. The specific episode of DSS blood donations as a means of protesting against Sikh attacks embodied a particularly layered timescape: in addition to enabling a claim to inheritance (in forming a repetition proper to, but neglected by, Sikhs), its framing as a response to Sikh attacks on the movement also bore traces of the logic of repetition as sublimated violence ("blood for blood") as described above in reference to the Nirankaris.

But here is another mimetic repetition laying claim to a contested legacy. We have so far been concerned with an act of alleged mimicry performed by the DSS guru. In a striking act of countermimesis, however—a counter claim on the real, so to speak—the Sikh temporal body, the Akal Takht, issued a call in February 2009 for Sikhs to congregate on the festival of Hola Mohalla to donate blood in such quantities as would surpass the existing world record, a record held, of course, by the DSS. In other words, it was now orthodox *Sikh* organizations who were copying a DSS strategy of public self-representation in a kind of mimetic power struggle. We quote from the *sandesh* (message) of the Akal Takht (translated from the original Punjabi):

> The *Khalsa Panth* of the Guru is the successor to a great tradition where our ancestors have set historical accomplishments by sacrificing their lives for the betterment of the society. The Gurus established such magnanimous examples by sacrificing their own lives that the Sikhs have felt

privileged in doing the same for spreading happiness in the society. . . . The message of Sri Akal Takht Sahib for the entire Sikh *Sangat* is that in addition to other forms of social service, the service through blood donation, organ donation and eye donation should also be made a part and parcel of our lives. Every Sikh should donate blood at least once in the memory of the martyrs of the Sikh faith. To commence this noble task, the day of Holla Mohalla (10 March 2009) has been chosen by various Sikh organizations under the umbrella of Sri Akal Takht Sahib. The blood donation will take place at Sri Anandpur Sahib at a very large scale. This is the sacred place where Sri Guru Gobind Singh Ji bestowed us with a spiritual life through the Nectar of Amrit. Being His Sikh, it is our duty and responsibility to offer our contribution in this noble cause for the support of our society and to save someone's life. The Sikh *Sangat* is requested to volunteer with whole-hearted dedication in this cause.[34]

With references to the historical sacrifices of Sikh martyrs and a call to donate blood in their memory, this appeal has the sense that the event formed part of an attempt to reanimate a principle of sacrifice that the DSS accuses mainstream Sikhism of misplacing. It is also significant that the event was staged at Sri Anandpur Sahib, where Guru Gobind Singh is said to have demanded the heads of five of his devotees: land and soil, once again, bind together sacrifices located in different temporal moments. The suggestion of sacrifice is made even plainer in a poster advertising the blood donation event that depicts the bloodied heads of Sikh martyrs impaled on spears, a reference to a particularly violent period of Sikh persecution in the early eighteenth century. Beneath the impaled heads lies the Punjabi text: "To give blood in order to protect honor (*laaj*) / That is our faith (*eeman*) / May it always fly high / Our symbol of Khalsa." And below that, in English: "We are what we *repeatedly* do. . . . It's not an act but a *habit* for Sikhs. . . . Excellence in saving humanity! Let's *prove it, again*" (emphasis added).

The "honor" that must be protected, we suggest, is the honor called into question by the DSS with its techniques of corrective mimesis. The exhortation to "prove it, again" likely alludes to Guru Gobind Singh's demand for bloody proof of devotion but probably most pertinently connects with a desire to fortify the public representation of Sikhism—to prove, in other words, that Sikhism is *still* animated by its foundational principles of sacrifice. The "again" points to the repetitive nature of the event: the slogan explicitly frames the event as a repetition of prior Sikh sacrifices in another form—a form now seemingly defined by the DSS. The Sikh retort constituted an act of corrective mimesis, then, in two ways: first, it sought to correct the DSS insinuation of there being a disconnect between founding ideals and current practice; and second, unlike other (i.e., DSS) blood camps that are merely an "act," this is blood donation *for real.*

The DSS's claim to the devotional real, via sacrificial blood and body donation, was thus met in kind, demonstrating how Sikh authorities had begun to play by DSS rules in seeing blood donation as a contemporary analogue of the *khalsa*'s founding sacrifices. That the event was meant as a rebuke to the DSS was not mentioned in the Akal Takht *sandesh*, but it was widely interpreted in such a way in newspaper articles and discussion forums. "Sikhs Give Blood to Defeat Dera Sacha Sauda," ran a *DNA* newspaper headline. According to the article, "Sikhs gave blood, literally, to defeat the Dera Sacha Sauda on Hola Mohalla. . . . Their idea was to displace the Dera from the Guinness Book of World Records where it holds the envious record of having organized the largest-ever single blood donation camp in the world at Bapu Ji village in Sri Gangananagar."[35]

The reference to displacing the DSS from the *Guinness Book* is telling. Consider now the following comment from a Sikh discussion forum focusing on the Sikh world record attempt: "Great effort and something good to unite youth on a common platform and help make them better citizens. But do we know the reason behind this and how it started? The whole reason is that someone came across Dera Sacha Sauda's record in the Guinness Book and *they decided to break it and remove his name.* All I am trying to say is that it started as something to surpass someone else, but not as a *seva* to humankind" (emphasis added).[36] In other words, as in the potlatch system among the Indians of the American Northwest Coast, what results from these charitable potlatches is the literal vanquishing of names. In this system, "competitive feasts and contests in wealth-destruction were held in order to validate claims to highly valued nonmaterial possessions: to ancestral names, titles, totemic crests and special prerogatives in the main cycle of rituals, the winter ceremonial. Wealth was only a means; the ultimate goals of actors in the system were to obtain ritual prerogative" (Harrison 1992, 236). We have suggested that high-profile charitable expenditure forms part of a DSS strategy to lay claim to ritual forms and, on the part of Sikh institutions, to wrest them back. Expenditure "is economic activity in which the loss must be as great as possible in order to certify a claim on ultimate meaning" (Chidester 2005, 4). The expenditure of the charitable potlatch, we argue, stakes its claim in a similar way—ritual property and the devotional real contested via how much (blood) one can give away.

Donate blood "at least once," demands the Akal Takht. Indian voluntary blood donation is composed out of the many times of the "at least once." "We are what we *repeatedly* do. . . . It's not an act but a *habit* for Sikhs. . . . Let's prove it, *again.*" Laying claim is composed of diverse modes of sacred repetition. One such mode is blood donation, which becomes a critical means for the mimetic habitation of prior forms. Repetition as proof of inheritance both enables and *is the form taken by* the repetition of voluntary blood donation: repetitions made out of (other) repetitions.

Disruptive Enablements

It is time to come back and donate.

—Letter sent to registered voluntary blood donors in Canada (cited in Smith and Charbonneau 2016, 231)

We thus see how repetitive enactments of blood donation as memorialization, as derivations of the astral, as sublimated responses to the demand of "blood for blood," and finally as mimetic claims and counterclaims to inheritance coagulate in the service of the routinized repetition of voluntary blood donation. Thus, the constitutive rhythms of astrology, politics, and religion disruptively enable the metarhythm of voluntary donation. For as we have noted, sporadic protest donation events (as in the case of the DSS), or even annual blood camp repetitions (e.g., on a guru's birthday or death anniversary), are not obviously congruent with the predictable regularity of blood supply as desired by proponents and promoters of voluntary blood donation. But this is how voluntary blood donation's temporality as metricality is pieced together: a differential multiplicity of irregularities made to form effects akin to a patterned regularity. Recall the NACO medic's demand for repetition before schoolchildren in Delhi: "Don't evaluate the past; speak only of future donations." Yet as we have seen, blood donation as memorial reenactment is precisely conditional on an engagement with past sheddings of blood. To adapt Kierkegaard, blood is donated forward despite—in these instances, *because of*—being understood backward. The idea of repetition as *recollection forward* (Kierkegaard 1983, 131) never seemed so apt.

HEMATIC FUTURES

This book has presented a number of ways in which blood might be considered a substance that exists in the subjunctive mood. To be in the subjunctive mood—"usually signified in verbal language by auxiliaries such as 'might,' 'could,' or 'should,' by the substitution of 'would have' for 'had' and by the use of 'if' clauses" (Zelizer 2004, 163)—is "to be trafficking in human possibilities rather than in settled certainties" (Bruner 1986, 26). Veena Das invokes this mood in reading and listening to the narratives of her ethnographic interlocutors, which reveal points of reflection and unfulfilled potentialities, as well as actualities (Das 2015b). To speak of *blood's "as if"* is to recognize how frequently the substance flows in bodies, tubes, and thoughts in states of hopeful uncertainty. Here we revisit some of these flows, both smooth and disrupted, and consider some supplementary ones in order to gain access to and convey the differentiated nature of hematic possibility in India.

We use the term "differentiated" advisedly. Laura Bear (2014a, 3) has recently questioned what she sees as the overly narrow anthropological focus on the future as either evacuated, nostalgic, or radically uncertain due to conditions of precarity. Such renderings are not necessarily inaccurate, but they tend to be understood and portrayed singularly, with too little attention paid to the differentiated and overlapping modes of temporal thought and action that factor into the visions and experiences they describe. Similar to the singularizing accounts Bear finds in anthropology, we find in studies of biopolitics and biotechnologies a particularly dominant rendering of biopolitical futures that pictures attitudes toward them as ever more risk averse and amenable to the involvement of new forms of capital and governance. Indeed, when futures are invoked in prevailing analyses of biological exchange, they tend to be certain neoliberal futurities that are emphasized—for instance, the forms of individualized insurance they may engender. Such accounts often cite Rose and Novas (2005, 452) on how contemporary forms of governmentality encourage citizens to foster an "active stance toward the future." For example, Brown, Kraft, and Martin's discussion of umbilical-cord blood banking points out that blood stem cells "are saturated with metaphors of banking, saving, investment and insurance, the deposition of biological assets that should accrue value and worth over the passage of time, as the twin futures of medical progress and disease risk are drawn nearer to the present" (2006, 315). As Marilyn Strathern (2009) explains in her account of the work of analogy in Catherine Waldby and Robert Mitchell's discussion of cord blood banking (2006, 125), such practices often gain their validation and support "from beyond medicine, from the world of personal insurance and personalized risk management. Private blood banking is a form of 'biological insurance.'" Strathern suggests that in forming such descriptions, Waldby and Mitchell borrow from finance in the same way as those they are giving an account of.

Like Bear, we have no interest in dismissing such accounts of biopolitical futures, which in many cases have been extremely persuasive. We do want to suggest, however, that these might not be the only futures on offer and that even where such metafutural accounts possess merit, too little recognition is given to the multiple, layered chronotopes of modern time that constitute them. In this book, we have taken a step back from the world of biotechnological possibility and novelty that is the main focus of the aforementioned accounts. Unlike the forms of biological insurance described by Rose and others, blood donation and transfusion are longstanding technologies that, in their basic form, are no longer at the frontiers of biomedicine. Notwithstanding the possibility of profiteering through secrecy (see chapter 5) and the persistence of paid donation (chapter 6), neither do they entwine capital with the politics of life in the same way. The anticipatory logics of blood and blood donation that we trace here thus cause us to be in sympathy with Marsland and Prince's (2012) critique of how the focus of Rose and others on biotechnological subjectivities is skewed toward Euro-America and away from biopolitics at the margins in resource-poor regions of the world. Focusing on flows of blood in the margins, we see how biopolitical imaginations of speculation and futurity may be at least as varied as impressions and durabilities of the past.

To give a preliminary sense of our approach, let us briefly revisit our discussion in chapter 5 of the case of a "tantric" transfusion gone seriously wrong that resulted in the death of the donor child. In India, as elsewhere, medical doctors are considered not just to be exemplars of progressive modernity but also its midwives. So it was all the more shocking that the parents of the young boy, whose blood was "donated" to their elder son, allegedly on the advice of a tantric priest, were doctors. The purpose of the transfusion was reported to have been to transmit intelligence ("brainy blood") from one brother to the other in advance of the latter's medical exams. Unsurprisingly, subsequent reflection on the event formed an occasion for journalistic cliches about the juxtaposition of the medieval and the modern in India (Pinney 2004, 202) and for "feudal accusation" (L. Cohen 2008, 45). Blood flowed from the *younger* to the *elder* son, but the blood flowed too *quickly*; it was meant to enable a hopeful future for an allegedly unintelligent child—to form a kind of quick fix—but in fact caused a break in time and the radical curtailment of the other son's future. Recall the words of the TV astrologer who sought to explain the case in the light of the promise but also uncertainty of the present national moment: "[With] India's economy . . . zooming . . . in the hurry to reach to the top . . . [everyone] is ready to take any short cuts. It's not superstition that is winning, it's our own greed."

To reiterate: we do not take issue with arguments that emphasize the significance of neoliberal futurity in biomedical and biotechnological domains, but we suggest that the undifferentiated conception of the future they tend to offer can only account for a small part of the complexity of biomedical future-scapes (cf. Bear 2017, 143). The above episode shows this well, for indeed, it appears that a quest to access future economic gains, as narrativized by the government and all forms of media, might well have been important—the transfusion a kind of hematic speculation. But feudal accusation, thwarted modernity, rush, and speed in the form of both time representations and modes of labor in/of time, also formed constitutive presences. The case might stand as a metaphor for the heterochrony of the Indian blood donation and transfusion field—its layered, conflictual forms (Bear 2014a, 25) and its vitality (Vora 2015) and danger.

Blood's "As If"

If the younger son's blood was thought to carry his knowledge, it also carried the hopes of the boys' parents. In the disastrous denouement, however, its excorporative flow came to signify the persistence of the time of the feudal in contrast to the "linear, progressive, homogeneous and forward-looking" time that, in spite of Gandhi's dreams of Ram Rajya and continuing millennial strains of political thinking (Devji 2004), remains the "official" temporality of the modern Indian political scene (P. Banerjee 2013, 2). Indeed, blood all too often exemplifies this persistence of "backward" time. Studies have underscored the significance of caste-based purity of blood in the perpetuation of a kin-based system of blood procurement in Pakistan (Mumtaz, Bowen, and Mumtaz 2012) and have shown the continuing significance of caste (as "agnatic blood") in contexts of donor insemination and adoption in metropolitan India (Bharadwaj 2003), while strategies that attempt to forestall the occurrence of mixing in transfusion underscore the persistence of perceptions of the dangers of mixing. For instance, members of Hindu right-wing groups in Mumbai have been reported to avoid the dangers of intermixture that the possible future need for a transfusion would necessitate by stocking their own blood for their own future use (Heuzé 1992, 2261).

In chapter 6 we discussed the slogan "Blood for blood" as a menacing call for mimetic repetition of bloodshed in situations of communal tension. We also described Hindutva calls for mimetic bloodshed as a rejection of historical appeals for communal harmony, also in the idiom of blood (i.e., the different yet overlapping Gandhian and Nehruvian invocations of blood-mixing as an index of communal solidarity). A prevalent Hindutva hematic framing suggests, "The blood flowing in the veins of Indian Muslims is the same as Lord Rama and Krishna. . . . In a true sense, both Lord Rama and Krishna are ancestors of Indian Muslims."[1] It is part of a common political parlance that stresses—*insists* upon—inclusiveness.[2] Former Indian defense minister George Fernandez (a Christian), for example, declares, "I look at a Pakistani as the flesh of our flesh and the blood of our blood. We are two different nations but one people."[3] A former leader of the BJP similarly asserted that "Muslims are the flesh of our flesh and the blood of our blood but they never got their rightful share in the nation's development nor have they been able to join the national mainstream to play their due role in nation-building."[4] Of course, such inclusive rhetorical moves insinuate that were Muslims not of the same blood as Hindus, then it might indeed be legitimate to discriminate against them. Inclusion slips easily into accusation. After the catastrophic communal violence of 2002 in Gujarat, the VHP (Vishwa Hindu Parishad, "World Hindu Council") leader, Praveen Togadia, is reported to have declared, "India's Muslims should submit to genetic tests. Since the forefathers of Muslims are Hindus, how can the blood of Arabia flow in their blood? I advise all Muslims to get tested for their Hindu origin."[5] Echoing the blood mysticism of earlier prominent Hindutva ideologues such as Vinayak Damodar Savarkar, who lay extreme emphasis on "the racial inheritance of Hindu blood" (Bhatt 2001, 95) and for whom, notoriously, "the blood in [converts'] veins . . . [cries] aloud with the recollections of the dear old ties from which they were so cruelly snatched away at the point of sword" (Savarkar 2007, 95–96), for Togadia, religion ceases to refer to belief or practice but simply to blood: the blood of Arabia does not flow in Indian Muslims' veins; they are "mere" converts. It is a kind of nationalist version of what has been identified as the medicalization of kinship, where a connection must exist "irrespective of choice": "Biomedicine insists on uniting those who may not choose to be connected" (Finkler 2001, 239). Blood, in such conceptions, holds and fixes a set of connections, with the VHP leader turning to biomedicine and blood tests in order to attempt to enforce co-ercive inclusion. In a discussion of conceptual "male" and "female" interpene-tration, Judith Butler (1993, 50–51) is interested in ideas that set limits on "re-ceptivity" and that make it imperative not to "depart from one's own nature" in spite of interactions with alterity. Similarly, Hindu-right activist rhetoric relies on the idea that one cannot be displaced from one's original "nature," located in—revealed by—blood. In the appeal made by the VHP leader to blood as con-summate repository of indisputable knowledge, the body appears paradoxically as both prior to and locus of "religion"—"prior" in the sense that biomedical ex-amination of the bodies of Muslims is what will reveal that they are not Muslims, and "locus" in the sense that it is in bodies that religion is nonetheless to be found.

Biotechnological time "mixes frames and registers" so that "now" can appear simultaneously as "then" (Strong 2009, 187). Global genetic-mapping schemes, justified as the key to securing future health care benefits, may serve as well to both naturalize and pathologize "archetypal" caste distinctions (Egorova 2011); Togadia's call for genetic tests enrolls a signifier of modernity and promise in an attempt to give new force to a well-worn form of hate speech that calls on blood (see, e.g., Hansen 2001, 84). According to the linear, progressive, forward-looking model of time, blood—in the examples we have just given—is principally a sub-stance of the past, of backward time (it is perhaps less that blood is "modern-ized" in its association with genetic testing but that genetic testing is "blooded" in the encounter [Franklin 2013]). But it is in part because of such "negative" as-sociations that blood can work powerfully in the subjunctive mood to help cre-ate realities that hold out "the hope that life could become other than it is" (Das 2015a, 53).[6]

For instance, in chapter 2 we described how Mohandas Gandhi came to an un-derstanding of blood purity based on how the blood shed by different religious communities formed one "mingled stream" that, in its very mixing, sacralized the land on which it was poured. Intermixing, under the sign of nonviolence, puri-fies the body politic even as—*because*—it transgresses communal boundaries. Anxieties about the mixing of substances are positively repurposed. Here, for Gan-dhi, lay blood's potential. Consider as well the case of artist and provocateur Shihan Hussaini as well as the Bhopali activists, whom we met in chapter 3. There we described how both used blood as a tool to persuade political figures to do their bidding. If in those cases portraiture and blood writing were employed for instrumental purposes, there is another side to communicating via blood that un-derscores the performative role of mixing in blood's subjunctive mood.

In Hussaini's case, such mixing was achieved in the space of the portrait itself. Planned, enacted, and then subject to commentary, this was elaborated, reflexive mixture. Indeed, Hussaini was keen to explain to us uses of his portraiture that went beyond the "profane" side of politics of personal gain and that instead touched upon the politically sublime or utopian (Hansen 2001)—for instance, his use of blood portraiture in 1994 during Chennai's Ganesh Chaturthi festival. The Ganesh festival features an array of pandals (pavilions) and the construction of large statues of the god, which are taken in procession and placed in the sea. The festival's history of stoking communal tension is well known (R. Kaur 2001). According to Hussaini, these tensions became particularly acute during the early 1990s because of a dispute about the route of the procession through a predominantly Muslim area in the Chennai neighborhood of Triplicane. Every time it ventured through the area, stated Hussaini,

> Muslims prayed in silence. There were meant to be no drums, but the festivities [nevertheless] became very loud, and miscreants would throw firecrackers, and the Muslims [would] throw stones. Every year there was bloodshed, and I said in 1994 I'd do something to influence all Hindus and Muslims, and in a huge hall I brought Muslim and Hindu students and mixed their blood and drew a huge portrait of Ganesha, and I drew Muslims and Hindus stamping on weapons. . . . After 1994 the rioting stopped and now there is peace.

Whether or not his portrait of Ganesh had the effects he implies, the episode forms a further example of blood's subjunctive potential: performative mixing in order to effect a desired (politically sublime) outcome. It is, of course, a highly moral image, the commingling of bloods forming a depiction of the possibility of an undivided community in liquid form. Hussaini himself married a Hindu (i.e., had a "mixed marriage"). As is well known, there is an oft-posited logically implied sequence between intermarriages, substance transfers, and communal harmony (Carsten 2007). Unlike the mixed community marriages described by Veena Das (2010, 397) in Delhi, which engage the life of the other on the level of the everyday, thereby coming to form a challenge to the solidity of oppositional identities, Hussaini presents commingling as a spectacle. Rather than the everyday enactment of "nextness" (377), Hussaini "stages" such a state as the image of a future community that it might also, in some small way, help to achieve: a prefigurative politics of substance.

Mixing is central to Marriott's (1989, 18) ethnosociological modeling (see chapters 1 and 3) as a pivotal dynamic process and variable alongside unmarking and unmatching (purity is said to lie in being "matched," "unmarked," and "unmixed"). One of Marriott's key postulations here is that mixing is "nonreflex-ive." Though what he means by this term is not necessarily straightforward (a kind of mathematical property), he is clear that he perceives a general "rarity of reflexivity" in "the Hindu world" (19). We can, of course, point to cases such as Gandhi's commitment to and elaboration of hematic intermixing (chapter 2), to the Bhopali enunciation of the political via blood writing (chapter 3), and Hus-saini's performative imaging of the same as highly reflexive engagements with the hematic "mingled stream." No doubt Marriott might reply that these cases are hardly representative. But the explicit reflexivity and staged nature of the Ganesh painting allows us to return to our argument in chapter 3 concerning the reflex-ive operationalization of Marriott's schematic categories in order to produce par-ticular effects. There we showed how Nirankari devotees seek to restore a lost symbiosis of substance-code (Marriott 1976) via blood donation as a kind of dis-tribution mechanism: a key category within Marriott's schema (substance-code) is made to persist precisely by way of a reflexive intervention that highlights a fail-ure in a putative norm. For a range of actors in this book (including Gandhi, Nirankari devotees, Hussaini, and Bhopali activists), mixture is enacted as a tool of inventive intervention. We are entirely in sympathy with Lawrence Cohen's (1995b, 328–29) critical observation concerning Marriott's models—namely, that they discount "nonHindu, nonuppercaste, and antinomian experience . . . ; the messiness of life is neglected to fit it to a triune model; and the projected desire of the theorist . . . for a coherent, predictable, and rule-bound universe remains unquestioned." Yet if we unfix the variables—allow the variables to themselves be variable (and manipulable) and, critically, treat them as products of history—their productivity can come into focus. When thrust into the messiness of life, detached from an exclusively Hindu world, treated reflexively with antinomian aplomb, and transformed into critical methodologies, these processes can con-tinue to carry purchase.[7]

Resonating with the Ganesh portrait, in chapter 4 we discussed the AVBDWB's conceptualization of voluntary blood donation as holding out the hope of a he-matological humanism of substantial flows beyond caste and religion. Blood as a substance, together with blood donation as a kind of ritualized frame for action, images for members of this vanguard organization a shared "subjunctive . . . 'as if' or 'could be' universe" (Seligman et al. 2008, 7) in which we come to realize the consanguinity of humanity. But this "could be" universe is in conflict with a different "could be" universe. "Our only hope," as one medic put it to us, "is that sometime, maybe in the next five to seven years, we will not need any blood do-nors." It is in connection with the technoscientific aspiration to substitute blood with an altogether new substance that the world of blood donation and transfu-sion comes closest to the biocapitalized and optimized futures we discussed at the beginning of this chapter. But even if blood products were to reach such a fully pharmaceuticalized form, inequalities in access and the niche and exclusionary markets likely to develop around them mean that they are unlikely to herald the kind of hematological revolution envisaged by technoscientific hype.

We have already seen that blood's "as ifs" are differently multiple. A further example was offered in chapter 2, in which we elaborated Ravi Chander Gupta's emotive blood portraits. These portraits are also, of course, in a subjunctive mood, "expressing wish, emotion and possibilities rather than actualities" (V. Das 2012, 137). Indeed, their relation to actualities remains opaque. Depicting freedom fighters (mythologized actualities) whose blood was shed in the past, Gupta hopes they will stimulate willingness on the part of their patriotic viewers to shed their (and others') blood in the future in service of the nation. The pictures express sanguinary aspirations. Like Hussaini's portrait of Ganesh, they also embody a hoped-for precipitative force; one could say they collapse the imperative into the subjunctive. But unlike Hussaini's portrait, it is willingness to shed blood—not a willingness to cease shedding it—that is wished for and prompted. Since these portraits, encoded with a hope for "future bloodshed," are also literally composed of blood as their material medium, we can say that they form a case of the "enacted subjunctive" (Sutton-Smith 1997)—"the world where possibilities are acted out" (Thrift 2008, 119).

In chapter 3 we explored how Sant Nirankari blood donations imagine new kinds of relations. Like Gupta's portraits and Hussaini's depiction of Ganesh, their offerings both express and seek to eventuate a particular wish: the creation of ties of humanity (*insaniyat ka rishta*) based on an expansively redefined code (in Marriott's [1976] sense), which are attainable through generalized diffusion of substance via blood donation as distributory mechanism. Blood donation offers the movement a world of hematic possibility. As we explained, an image is formed of donated Nirankari blood circulating outward, mixing with many other bloods to both reformulate and restore a lost unity of substance-code.

Following from this, let us briefly return to Togadia and Hindutva blood rhetoric to again show how Marriott's schematic categories can remain productive and useful if (and only if) they are detached from a rule-bound and exclusively Hindu universe. In 2002 the *Milli Gazette*, which styles itself as Indian Muslims' leading English newspaper, prefaced an interview with Togadia with an intriguingly positive take on "blood ties" as the locus of a hopeful future:

> Dr Pravin Togadia comes from the noble profession of healing and professes to be a believer in the nobler ideas of Hinduism. Yet, he would not pause for a moment before making uncharitable remarks against Islam and Muslims. He holds Indian Muslims responsible for atrocities

in Pakistan, Bangladesh and, in the same breath, Kashmir. That, to him, is justification enough for the two-month-long Gujarat carnage. Distribution of a million trishuls at kumbh, followed by similar trishul-distribution campaigns at other places in India, fire arms training to Bajrang Dal cadres and repeated attacks on Muslim passengers in Sabarmati Express (pre-designed to provoke a dangerous conflict) by VHP storm-troopers in days preceding Godhra, which have brought the country to the precipice, do not bother him at all. However, there is still a silver lining in the darkness of hate: *Dr Togadia does recognise the shared ancestry of Indian Muslims and Hindus. All of us know that blood is thicker than water, and a day might come when this burning rage fuelled by angry people like Dr Togadia would cool down and blood ties would reassert themselves.*[8]

Recall Togadia's statement that India's Muslims must have their blood tested to demonstrate that "the blood of Arabia" does not flow within them. What is divisive in his speech—a means of underscoring a putative Islamic aberration (deviance from blood) as a justification for persecution—is instead taken by the editors of the *Milli Gazette* as indicative of a divorce between code and substance that *may only be temporary*, for "a day might come" when "blood ties would reassert themselves." Marriott states that code and substance "cannot have separate existences in [the] world of constituted things as conceived by most South Asians" (1976, 110). But as in the ethical vision of the Nirankaris, as also in the worlds of many of the actors discussed in this book, the problem foregrounded in the editorial preface to Togadia's interview is *precisely their separate existences.* The present scenario (the piece was written soon after the Gujarat massacres) is marked by bloodshed, not blood ties. The editors' hope in these times of political division and abjection is that substance and code might be tied back together: the moral-substantial blood tie. For all that "ties through blood—including blood recast in the coin of genes and information—have been bloody enough already" (Haraway 1995, 265), hematic visions of substantial community retain their power, even amid, and in part because of, devastating bloodshed. Yet the editors' vision of reuniting substance and code is undercut by Togadia in the interview that follows the preface: "All Hindus and Muslims should accept one reality—that we are ethnically and culturally the same. No one from the Hindu-Muslim society must suffer German-Jew paradigm. Each and every Muslim of India emanates ancestorily from the gene, RBC, bone, blood and flesh of a Hindu." The *Milli Gazette*'s reconciliatory gesture toward a "silver lining" future—where substance and code may be reunited—is compromised by Togadia's assertion of the "prior" purity of Hindu flesh and blood, a norm from which Muslim blood can only descend or deviate.

Also in chapter 3 we explored another possibility: that blood donation as a political style (Nandy 1970) might allow political actors to appear to move beyond the critique of political signs. However, if such witnessed, apparently incontrovertible blood extractions once held out an elusive promise of erasing past mistrust and regenerating political communication, we described—by way of numerous illustrative cases—how it equally provides new possibilities for political dissembling. This is where blood and blood donation's "as if" enters a negative space. What Congress activists offered at the fake blood donation camp discussed in chapter 3 were *as if* blood donations. If the "as if" of fabrication and counterfeit is a particular species of the subjunctive, it reminds us that "noetic space"— an "imaginative space teeming with alternatives to the actual" (Amsterdam and Bruner 2000, 237)—does not necessarily contain alternatives that are either moral or desirable. "As if" blood donations were also a focus of chapter 5, which elaborated on ways in which the unactualized potential of the ungiven (and so untransfused) blood unit was imaginatively called into being by clinical activists as a figure of censure. The Bhopali activists' sarcastic gift of paper hearts to the Indian prime minister, through partonomic obviation, similarly called attention to the assistance for survivors of the Bhopal gas disaster that was promised by the government but remained and remains ungiven (chapter 3).

We offer a further example now of how political blood donation events form sites of potential—of hope, liminality, and possibility—rather than certainty (Barnett 2015, 413, 421). In chapter 6 we explained how voluntary blood donation's temporality as metricality is stitched together out of "other" repetitions, such as annual memorial blood donation camps at which donors mimetically repeat the blood shed by the remembered person. Rajiv Gandhi's death anniversary is a case in point. In 2003, the Congress Party sponsored nationwide blood camps to commemorate his death. These events draw attention to the political capital the party aspires to, but they are also risky: "Because the outcome cannot be known in advance, success and failure . . . are contingent" (Howe 2000, 67).

Asserting that "the best way to pay tribute to Rajiv Gandhi [on his death anniversary] is to follow his path in nation building," the Andhra Pradesh Youth Congress (APYC) attempted to surpass all previous records in blood donation.[9] In 2002, according to APYC president Venkata Rao, they "managed to gain an entry in the *Limca Book of Records*, but it was rejected by the *Guinness Book of Records* for lack of proper documentation. . . . This time, the YC had taken care to file all the documents, affidavits, videos and photos of the blood camps."[10] It seemed that in 2003 everything had been done to militate against the "risk of incorrect performance" (Howe 2000, 69) so that due recognition would be granted to the organization's blood collecting feats. The key ritual props of affidavits, videos, and photos would aid proper inscription of these acts and thus not inhibit due recognition as their absence had done the previous year. Collection fever was also manifested on the national level. It was claimed that "blood would be collected from 35,000 donors all over the country, which would be a world record. From Karnataka, blood would be collected from over 3,000 donors."[11] Specifying the precise intention prior to its carrying out, however, leaves little room for innovation or for explaining away results that may differ from the stated intention.

Newspaper articles that emerged in the week following the camps stated that the APYC "has recommended action against its presidents in five districts for not properly organizing blood donation camps on Rajiv's death anniversary." A spokesman said that the Khammam and Anantapur Youth Congress wings "failed to organize even a single blood donation camp despite reminders."[12] The Karaikal Youth Congress leader was suspended for failing to participate in the party's blood donation program.[13] A scheme that was meant to enhance the status of the party, to show its commitment to society and nation and its ability to mobilize its activists, ended up resulting in inglorious and rather humiliating headlines such as "Karaikal Youth Cong. Leader Suspended" and "Youth Congress for Action on Its Presidents."[14] Rather than mobilizing and motivating the nation for a noble cause, the party failed even to mobilize and motivate many of its own local leaders to organize donation camps; the party became its own opponent and was symbolically toppled by the forces that it itself had released.[15]

In memorial blood donation camps more generally, the past event of political assassination is reinvented as sacrifice in the present—a form of creative remembering and mimetic repetition that seeks to instantiate desired political futures. The thwarted hope of the 2003 camps, which ended up putting the organizers themselves on trial, is of course consonant with the wider debased state of political blood extractions discussed in chapter 3. But what we also argued in that chapter is that even in the face of a perceptual-ideational shift concerning political blood extractions from ritual of verification to spectacle of dissembling, they do continue to retain a certain communicative force. Blood, as a political material, likewise continues, in spite of everything, to be laden with hopes, wishes, and possibility: a subjunctive substance.

Here we return to our earlier discussion of transitivity. The subjunctive mood accompanies *transitions* (S. Srinivas 2016, 144; Turner 1982), and blood, of course, is a substance that transits ("transit" and "transition" both derive from the Latin *transitio*, from *transire*—"go across"). Marriott (1989, 16, 21, 27) models time as a form of substance in Hindu thought and experience. Blood flows as a movement in time; it is *the* spatiotemporal substance. It transits within bodies and in multiple ways outside of them as well. We may recall here Hoeyer's (2013, 7) definition of excorporable body parts as *temporal relations*—"a step on the way from having been part of a body to not being so anymore"—rather than entities.[16] It is perhaps in part because of blood's propensity to movement (as a temporal relation)—its transitioning around and between bodies and between insides and outsides, its flowing "elsewhere"—that it becomes a subjunctive substance, freighted with potentials and possibilities.[17] In Marriott's conception, time is a kind of substance. With respect to blood we might agree, but put it in reverse: substance is a kind of time.

Other Futures

Zero-Sum Futures?

In the future, according to Regalia Mason, a character in Jeanette Winterson's novel *Tanglewreck* (2006), "Wasted Time will be a thing of the past. Parents will have more Time to spend with their children, children will live longer happier lives. There will be no need to rush and race. There will be enough Time" (Winterson 2006, 333). How so? In part, because of time's substantial zero-sum transmissibility in the form of the "Time Transfusion."

Winterson's novel uses science fiction to explore how we have arrived at a moment where it is seemingly permissible "to harm some bodies when attempting to prolong the lives of certain others" (McCormack 2012, 179). The novel renders commoditized time in starkly biological terms. Trading time as a commodity, a company called Quanta offers Time Transfusions; infinite life is possible, but only at the expense of others' lifetimes. Cut to an almost empty ward in Bethlehem Hospital. The door sign at the entrance says "GIRLS 8–12." The heroine Silver has crept into the otherwise secure space of the hospital unseen. Wondering at the seeming lack of any activity on the operating floor, she finally hears a heart beating, "unmistakable, like on a loudspeaker." She sees a young girl lying peacefully inside a capsule: "Silver watched her, and saw something very strange start to happen; the girl began to age. Faint lines appeared on her face. Her skin grew redder and coarser. The lines deepened, her hair thinned and turned grey. Her skin wrinkled. She was old."

In another cylinder close by, however, lay a woman who "was beautiful but not young, or rather she was getting younger every second. Her skin began to smooth out. Her cheeks plumped. The crow's feet under her eyes disappeared and the lines on each side of her mouth vanished. Her hair was thick and blonde and her face was radiant. She was in the prime of her life" (Winterson 2006, 323–25). The recipient—who is none other than the CEO of Quanta, Regalia Mason—later eats cheese and scrambled eggs: "'Protein is essential after a Time Transfusion,' she said" (332). It is in extolling the benefits of the procedure that Mason tells

Silver that wasted time will be a thing of the past. When Silver points out that the procedure also steals time, causing people to die, Mason responds, "Quanta has been instrumental in reducing the world's surplus population."[18]

Science fiction uses the future as a metaphor for the present (Chozinski 2016, 58) to enact (often critical) commentary on contemporary times. Winterson's account, which makes explicit the asymmetrical temporal flows of many kinds of present-day biological exchange, allows us to see clearly how flows of biological matter are simultaneously flows of commoditized time. Nancy Scheper-Hughes (2000, 193) famously noted how the black-market flow of organs "follows the modern routes of capital: from South to North, from Third to First World, from poor to rich, from black and brown to white, and from female to male." To Scheper-Hughes's unequal extractive dyads of poor/rich, black/white, and male/female, Winterson adds that of young/old: the young girl's future time visibly drains from her, even as it is transfused into the villain who decreases in age before our very eyes.

Marx's critique of capitalist commodification is famously filled with metaphors of bodily violation, mobilizing imagery of the extraction of young blood: the factory night shift "only slightly quenches the vampire thirst for the living blood of labor," while apologists for industry insist that "British industry . . . vampire-like, could but live by sucking blood, and children's blood, too" (Marx 1990, 367; see also Healy 2006, 6–7; Anagnost 2006, 510). Metaphor "travels back" (Franklin 2014) with present-day literal organ and blood selling now providing the backdrop to rereadings of Marx's foundational critique of capitalism. In her work on organ transplantation in the United States, Lesley Sharp (2006) notes that the majority of brain dead organ donors in the United States are young men killed by guns or in traffic accidents, while Ishiguro's dystopian novel *Never Let Me Go* (2005), which was also made into a film, features cloned children whose purpose is to provide organs to service the "normal" population until, after several donations, they undergo "completion." In the HBO show *Silicon Valley*, Gavin Belson—the emblematic tech-titan—attends startup meetings while connected to his youthful "transfusion assistant," extolling the virtues of the pseudoscience of wellness parabiosis. Young blood, and the buying and selling of youthful futures, remain figures of apprehension both in scenes of biological exchange and wider discourses of present-era capitalism (e.g., Comaroff and Comaroff 1999).

The temporal effects of diverse modes of biological exchange are usually explained in terms of asymmetrical exchange. Quite simply, the securing of recipient futures is at the expense of donor lifetimes—that is, finite lifetime is transferred from one to another, usually from donor to recipient. Sharp (2006) highlights a species of time that she calls "salvational": transplant recipients declare that they have been "born again"; a language of conversion and renewed faith is employed by both recipients and their families, who also celebrate annual *rebirthdays* (110). But, of course, the recipient's rebirthday is, at the same time and inescapably, the day on which the donor's future was cut short; it is a day of tragedy for another family. Meanwhile, in his work on kidney selling and family planning operations in Chennai, Lawrence Cohen (1999; 2001) explains how kidney sellers are sold the promise of a better future through surgery that will enable them to cancel past debts. But instead he documents thwarted promise and endangered vital time. This is because (1) the debilitating effects of the surgery compromise future work prospects, (2) the initial conditions of indebtedness remain, and (3) being known to reside in a "kidney belt" area can make lenders quicker and more aggressive in calling in debts. Sellers become more vulnerable to future indebtedness and ill health. Cohen's devastating conclusion is that they give up a part of their future in order to have a future at all. Donor and recipient futures are in a zero-sum relationship, where the rights (to a future) of the latter are privileged over those of the former.

What we find in the Indian blood donation and transfusion field is a set of understandings about time extraction and reincorporation that both parallel and diverge from the zero-sum futures discussed above. A remarkably pronounced time representation in the field publicizes transfusions as transmitting time in a way that is not at all dissimilar to that conveyed by Winterson in *Tanglewreck*, but with a crucial difference: blood banks emphasize that time is indeed transmitted and received, but at minimal cost to donors who "spend mere minutes" in donating. In other words, the directionality proposed by blood banks here directly counters the extractive flow of life-material from donor to recipient we have discussed above; the cost to donors is represented as minimal and nonexistent, and not life-threatening or depletive (cf. Vora 2015). At the same time— and recalling the zero-sum finitudes of Cohen's and Sharp's ethnographies, reluctant prospective donors do not accept this reconfiguration at all. They fear that their donation would curtail their own reproductive futures in the form of infertility and/or impotence ("I can't donate—I'm getting married next month") and vital time in the form of debilitating illnesses: blood donation as "defuturing" (Fry 1999).

Recruiters' retemporalizing of the act of donation seeks to make a virtue of necessity in attempting not just to neutralize a damaging time representation but also to attract potential donors through emphasizing an enchanting temporal economy that sees the minutes it takes to donate translate and transform into whole recipient lifetimes. According to this time representation, not only are the minutes it takes to donate not "taken" from donors, but they are granted *to* them as a kind of gift. Meanwhile the figure of the child is mobilized not as an entity from whom time is stolen, but as the beneficiary of transfusion-enabled futures.

We return here to the question of proportionality, for it is the dramatic disproportion between time given and time received that is mobilized by recruiters as a micropractice of temporal persuasion. After Corsín Jiménez (2013, 77), we might call the process one of (rhetorical) temporal aggrandizement.

To be sure, time remains a commodity in the sense that recruiters recognize people's time as a competitor—hence the emphasis on "taking beds to donors," with "bloodmobiles" traveling to peoples' places of work, study, and worship for donation events. Similarly, economy remains central to recruiters' time representations. An AVBDWB activist in Kolkata, in comparing blood donation to education, characterized blood donation to us as an act of extraordinary temporal economy: "Where else can you save a life in a quarter of an hour? For giving someone literacy you have to spend an hour a day for four months, and they will forget easily if they don't continue afterwards." Minimal temporal contributions by donors potentially result in immense temporal consequences for recipients.

Such time representations are strikingly prominent in publicity materials that aim to motivate donors on account of the drama of the escalation between temporal income and outgo: "A minute of yours could mean a lifetime for another" says a poster in Delhi's Red Cross blood bank. "It only takes a few minutes to save someone's life," says another in Chandigarh. "Donate blood. It means a few minutes to you . . . but a lifetime for somebody else," says one in a Delhi government hospital blood bank. "Would you give a few minutes to save a few lives? Please walk in. Donate blood. Experience the joy of giving," says another. Yet another is particularly emotive: beside a photograph of a newborn baby are the words "I thought I had no time to give blood until I held a baby with no time left without it." A motivational song, set to the tune of a *bhajan* and sung before schoolchildren in Delhi, goes: "Oh youth, listen to us. Through blood is this life, through blood is this time (*rakt see hai zindagi, rakt se hai yeh sama*)."

On another poster, an egg timer is transformed into a "blood timer," with an image of drops of blood, not sand, passing through it. The Bengali slogan accompanying it asserts that time is not merely tricked; it is defeated: "Time is defeated by blood donation. If you spend only 5 minutes you can save a whole life-time (*Samay tumi har menecho raktadaner kache pancht minute karle kharach ekti joban banche*)." Moreover, many posters feature thalassemic children—those with the most future time to lose if blood is not received. This further rhetorically enhances the temporal proportions of the gift of blood.

This time representation is often coupled together with a politics of rush and discourse of urgency and crisis. The former president of a voluntary blood bank in Delhi stated in a newspaper interview, "It is a tragedy that in a city of 15 million people there is a shortage of 75,000 units of blood. Every minute someone, somewhere dies for want of the right type of blood group, whereas donating blood takes only a few minutes and can make a difference between life and death."[19] The website of a Chennai blood bank likewise employs together a temporality of aggrandizement and an affective language of urgency: "Make blood donation a way of life. Please do not wait for a call from any blood bank. Walk in and donate blood. Blood banks need time to test your blood after donation. Spread the message that donating blood is safe and simple. Your donation of blood can help save up to four precious lives. It takes less than the time spent on an average telephone call. Someone might need blood today. You have the power to save. We can stop the crisis. Will you help?"[20]

The temporal proportions of the blood gift are thus mobilized by recruiters as a means of recruitment-by-enchantment. The "concrete time of human finitude" (Bear 2016a, 492) is outwitted (tricked) and overcome (defeated) through blood donation. In Alfred Gell's formulation (1999, 167), enchantment is achieved by objects in their necessary referral to the technical means of their coming into being. In referring to prior dexterity, objects objectify past action while in their present-ness they render that action "in progress." However, in the main, the virtuosity that is objectified is consigned to imaginings of its creation in the past. Blood donation reverses this technology of enchantment—it is enchantment with a futural orientation. The task of recruiters is to enchant prospective donors with regard to a set of procedures that they have the power to set in motion and for which they are configured as being ultimately responsible. Of course, the doctor or technician usually refers to donors as merely providers of "starting material" (Faber 2004). In chapter 5 we saw, in reference to replacement donation and component separation, how medics have an interest in claiming it is their own labor of extraction, separation, and testing, and not the labor of donation, that counts. There we described a kind of proportional politics of the gift: If component separation creates units out of units, then who should be allowed to take credit?

The proportions that are at stake here, of course, are those of time. Donors are figured as forming time out of time—as enacting dramatic escalations of it in an almost alchemical process where it is not transformation in kind that counts (since what donors give is figured as being also what recipients receive) but of proportion (since the small quantities donors give are received as whole *lifetimes*). Size and scale are again at issue, with the relation of magnitude (Corsín Jiménez 2013, 36) between that which is offered and that received—the disproportion between them—forming part of a temporally oriented marketing strategy in tune with the time representations described in chapter 6 in which recruiters charge donors with being able to save and generate family reproductive time.[21] The partonomic features of the gift differ from those discussed in chapters 3 and 5.[22] Here the relation between the given and the withheld is not invoked as the basis of moral commentary. The partonomic relation of note is that which exists between the "same gift" located at different moments in time. What you see (the donation in time) is what you do not get (that which is received—aggrandized time); a small "part" of time transforms into a "whole" lifetime.

We underscore that these are time *representations*. More practically what recipients receive is tested and treated blood components, usually from several different sources, which may or may not help them to recover. There is rarely a singular identity between a particular donated unit and a transfusion, so it is poetic license to say that one donor's few minutes is subject to alchemical aggrandizement into a whole lifetime saved. Further, it takes time to receive a transfusion—several hours usually—with transfusion usually forming one part of a treatment regime, along with drugs, consultations, rehabilitative exercises, and so on. Together, these may assist in patient recoveries and help extend the concrete time of human finitude. Blood donations are laden with diverse temporalities, and the effects of receiving them include effects of a temporal nature. But recruitment by enchantment, which extols the way in which time is created out of time, is a conjuring trick. Its purpose being to boost medically useful blood donation, it is, perhaps, another lie told without mendacity (see chapter 4)—a "politics of the gigantic and the exaggerated" (Corsín Jiménez 2013, 76–77).

In exploring temporal proportionalities here, our purpose has not been to criticize existing commentaries on biological exchange in which donor and recipient finitudes are argued to be in a zero-sum relationship—there is much to suggest that such commentaries are all too accurate for the situations they describe—but rather to enlarge the discussion with another case that foregrounds how a time representation that is damaging to the project of voluntary blood donation comes to be countered by another that temporally reproportions the donation of blood and its projected effects in a new rhetoric of temporal persuasion.

Astral Futures

We discussed in chapter 6 possible relations between the date, time, and place of birth; the number of times a person donates blood; and the time of the workday. We turn now to a second astral proposition: that blood donation may be employed in order to manipulate the future events allotted to persons according to their *bhagya*. We cite a representative example of this line of thinking from the *Tare Sitare* (Stars) section of a national Hindi daily by astrologer-columnist Pandit K. K. Sharma:

> Why does a person become involved in accidents (*durghatnaon*) again and again (*bar-bar*), and why do they suffer death-like pain again and again? These questions are answered by his horoscope (*janam patrika*).

In an accident, along with bodily injury the person also loses blood, and blood's owner is the moon, and if the moon becomes polluted by Mars, then that person's blood keeps getting regularly polluted. When the moon is weak in a person's horoscope, their blood is not dispensed correctly. [The] manufacturing of blood is controlled by Mars. This is how we can conclude that production of blood and maintenance of the body are done by both Mars and the moon. . . . Big operations [and illnesses] like [or concerning] appendicitis, cancer, pleurisy, tonsils, high fever, death, red marks on the body, surgery, bleeding (*khun behena*), wounds, accidents, murder and bloody skirmishes (*khun-kharaaba*)—all of these are studied under Mars. . . . Those persons whose horoscopes have inauspicious (*ashubh*) combinations of Mangal (Mars) and Shani (Saturn) and who suffer from accidents again and again, can do the following remedies (*upaays*): Such people should do regular blood donation (*niyamit rakt daan*). This is the only way to protect them and their bodies (*shareer*). By regular (*niyamit*) blood donation, you can avert (*talna*) the accidents which are due to occur in your horoscope. They can also do *mahamrityunja paath* (a Shiva-related prayer recitation). Or the regular *paath* of Hanumanji's Sankat Mochan. Regular recitation of Mohammad Rasool Allah also protects (*hifaazat*) such people.[23]

In her work on astrological consultations in Banaras, Caterina Guenzi (2012) notes that the astrologer is not only a specialist in identifying auspicious and inauspicious moments in time, as suggested in many existing analyses, but that he also "identifies and calculates the material and symbolic 'lots' to which his clients are entitled, and, according to their wishes and needs, he elaborates strategies aimed at increasing, saving, or investing shares of wealth" (40). But this can work both ways: one's "astral store" may contain misfortune, in which case a kind of reverse or remedial astrology is practiced: "Although it usually indicates goods or wealth, the concept of *yog* [the astral configuration used to indicate the moment in which the good allotted to the person is available to them] may sometimes refer to a loss or to a danger, as when a person has the '*yog* for accidents.' In this case, rather than potential wealth, the *yog* indicates the 'risk' of getting one's share, and the astrologer will prescribe some remedial and protective measures in order to avoid the risk" (49).

With respect to blood donation, it is of course remedial astrology and the "*yog* for accidents" that is at stake. Pandit K. K. Sharma suggests that blood donation can act as a kind of preemptive strike against the potentially catastrophic blood loss that occurs in "accidents" (*durghatnaon*); if *ashubh* blood must be spilled, better that this be in the controlled manner of medical blood donation than in an accident. Recitation of various devotional formulas may also help, but blood donation is the preeminent prophylactic identified here against accidents. Moreover, it is *regular* blood donation (*niyamit rakt daan*) that is recommended—a strategy well in keeping with the dream of repetition in time that is the ideal rhythm of voluntary blood donation. Once again astral time (as preventative routine) appears to be at least approximately in synch with the officially sanctioned donation rhythm in which giving blood is routine. The *Pandit*'s recommended course of action for the person whose *bhagya* foretells accidents takes blood donation as a prophylactic "time tricking" (Moroşanu and Ringel 2016) device that aims to inoculate the donor against his or her foretold future. The word "inoculate" is germane since the procedure involves the agentive introduction of an infective agent (i.e., moderate bloodshed) into donors in order to immunize them (against immoderate bloodshed).

In response to audience questions to Indian TV astrologers concerning their future life chances (in marriage, work, and so on), solutions are offered that often involve moral prescriptions such as Vedic chanting or donations to the underprivileged (Udupa 2016, 16). Blood donation is not infrequently mobilized as a technique for the management of the donor's allotted share. Pandit Priyasharan Tripati, in an episode of his morning astrology show on the news channel IBC24, laid emphasis on the nature of blood donation as a form of *dan*: "It's such an important *dan* that the nation truly needs. It can save somebody's life; it is *pran-dan* (life donation). You should cooperate with us in this great mission (*maha-mission*)."[24]

Yet, to paraphrase Derrida (1997, 144) in his discussion of Baudelaire, for Tripati, to donate blood is to do a good deed while at the same time making a good deal. As Tripati explained: "In this way you can do good for the society and country and also do good for your planets. Blood donation appeases the planets (*grihashanti*), so one moves from bad luck (*amangal*) to good luck (*mangal*). Blood is red in color so if you donate blood it completely removes the *mangal dosha* (fault in Mars). If the *mangal* is with *ketu* it protects you also from the need for surgery (lit. 'scissors')." The astrologer goes on to explain how blood donation also calms tensions, anger, and worry caused by the influence on the horoscope of Mars.

Blood donation as *pran-dan* is both part of a larger *maha-mission* and a remover of the donor's inauspiciousness, but there is little sense here of the latter passing on to transfusion recipients. Säävälä (2001) has shown the continuing relevance of ideas concerning the removal of inauspiciousness through gift giving in urban life (specifically, in Hyderabad). Through such means, she argues, low-caste families can maneuver themselves into secure middle-class identities. According to Säävälä, the ejection of inauspiciousness by one party need not dictate that it is transferred to another, as is understood to happen in the contexts explored in the classic works on *dana* by Parry (1994) and Raheja (1989). In the cases Säävälä documents, families seeking to remove inauspiciousness through giving simultaneously *accepted* gifts as an important feature of the process, indicating that "the dynamics of ritual gift-giving cannot be summed up simply as the passing on of evil influences through giving *dannam* [unreciprocated gifts]" (2001, 314). Similarly, manipulating one's future through blood donation toward auspiciousness and away from accidents, and so on, does not seem to entail a willed transferal of evil influences to transfusion recipients, which would indeed be a scenario seemingly quite at odds with Tripati's emphasis on blood donation as a *maha-mission* for society and nation.

Prophylaxis and Insurance

Blood's relation to the planets helps to form the future; blood donation as a labor in and of time (Bear 2014a) inoculates the donor against an undesirable version of it. Blood donation as prophylaxis is not the province of astrology alone. It is also practiced by the devotees of a charismatic guru, Aniruddha Bapu, based in Mumbai.[25] Bapu foretells a time of disasters. Devotees voluntarily donate their blood—as a humanitarian gesture, to be sure—but also to inoculate themselves against a great forthcoming bloodshed: "If you donate blood for me once," says the guru, "you will never need to take blood, and neither will your next seven generations." Inoculation and insurance are intimates in that both are oriented toward future uncertainties and provide protective measures against them—both are anticipatory logics—but they are usually distinguishable as separate actions and modes of reason: whereas inoculation seeks to prevent possible eventualities, insurance provides protection against the effects of those eventualities when they come to pass. But blood donation in millennial time combines the two modes of preparedness: "Soon there will be rivers of blood flowing so we are donating to get ready for that. . . . So many people are going to die, and we can't help that. But those who survive can take our blood." *Inoculation* for the donating person and *insurance* for others are held together in such donation acts. The time of the civic—voluntary blood donation's metatemporality composed of repetitions over time as dutiful contributions to civic life (see chapter 6)—folds together rational and millennial times in relations of disruptive enablement. Hematic futures are differentially multiple.

In chapter 5 we described a less cosmic insurance mode: the voluntary card offered to donors after they have donated. As we explained, this card entitles them or their family members to receive blood should they require it in the future. The card is a locus of dissension in Indian blood banking circles for several reasons.

Chief among them is that it makes the blood bank too banklike in the most primitive sense of a system of deposits and withdrawals. Of course, any blood bank contains features of such a system, but the card individualizes and privatizes those features (cf. Strathern 2009, 15). For many blood bankers, the passbook function of the card and future expectations it seems to engender make it a kind of Trojan horse undermining the larger project of constituting a donor base that gives with no sense of entitlement or expectation. As a Mumbai recruiter put it to us: "A lot of donations are not voluntary in the real sense because they are looking for something they get out of giving blood—a lot of donors give because they want the assurance they will receive it whenever they want it in the future. The card system is very retrograde. Some day we will have to wean them off it because you're creating blood depositors. [The card] is a matter of the psychology of donors—it is to get them to donate."

Does the card reflect a psychology of expectation on the part of donors, as this recruiter suggests, or does it rather create such a psychology? Slogans such as "Be a donor, not a depositor," prominently displayed in Mumbai, for instance, reflect this recruiter's wish to wean donors off the cards they are currently given. From the point of view of donors, however, the picture is confusing and disheartening: blood banks give them cards entitling them to receive free blood should they need it, but if they seek to utilize them they are criticized for failing to donate their blood without expectation. Indeed, blood banks may not honor the cards. Blood banks appear to call into existence a certain conception of morality but also destroy the grounds for taking it seriously (Poole 1991, ix). Different futural imperatives compete with one another: a utopic future in which voluntary donations will be made "without expectation" and a more practical one in which one's family members will be able to obtain blood should they require it.

Blood banks' refusal to honor the cards they dispense represents an attempt both to limit their liabilities and to stabilize the gift as a gift. Such stabilization attempts only underscore the scandalous alterability of transactional forms. The card is more than just a marker and creator of expectation and provider of protection against the effects of possible eventualities. It is in reference to the card that we can see most clearly how what was supposed to be a series of linear transitions between transactional forms, from those classed as dangerous and obsolete (paid and replacement) to another classed as safe and modern (voluntary), is in fact a domain of transactional simultaneity and reversion: voluntary donation, if a card is involved, may be viewed as "paid donation in kind." Moreover, that card—already an "in kind" payment—may itself be sold. But the offering of the card also (and again) brings to light the closeness of replacement and voluntary donation. They are temporal inversions of one another. In one case the donor must replace that which is needed for his or her transfusion-requiring relative; in the other, the blood bank replaces for the donor's transfusion-requiring relative what was previously taken from the donor. In its temporal arrangement, voluntary donation is made visible as a preemptive, or nonimmediate, mode of replacement. An ideal-typical voluntary donor donates for anybody who is in need. But rationales of specificity accompany this outward movement: the donor card entitles specific people to benefit (i.e., those known to the donor or the donor's immediate family); a donation for anyone is therefore simultaneously a narrow-focused protective act. In replacement donation the rationale of specificity is reactive and immediate; in voluntary donation it is preemptive, a kind of forward planning. Thus, the narrow specificity of replacement is not eliminated in the successor transactional form but rather repositioned: it comes into play in a different moment, with the abstracted gift for anyone in part facilitated by the entitlement it provides for someone. This is not to suggest that donors' motivations are in either case deallike; neither would we wish to overlook the key experiential differences between the forms but would rather point out the structural similarities and reversions between the transactions that are the source of the dissensus and controversy attached to them. When we also consider the ways in which the rhythm of replacement informs the pattern of voluntary camps (see chapter 6), voluntary donation comes to appear positively possessed by the replacement mode it was meant to supplant, the relation between them not one of succession but sublation—an economy of Russian dolls.

Bloodscape of Difference

Let us now return to our analytic of a bloodscape of difference by reading back through it the different thematics of this book. Recall that the bloodscape of difference, in our characterization, is composed of interrelations between temporalities, proportionalities, and sovereignties, each of which itself, critically, is differentially composed.

Different temporalities: Mimetic bleeding is bleeding that refers back to and reenacts a prior bleeding; it is also, therefore, a form of repetition. The repetition is never isomorphic with that which is repeated; it is separate and different. But the mimetic repeat may also *extend* that which is repeated, make it endure, and open it up to a new sphere of actions and relationships. It may constitute a form of, or claim to, inheritance (DSS bleeding as a mimetic extension of Sikh bleeding; see chapter 6). It may in turn serve to contest that inheritance (Sikh bleeding as a mimetic extension of DSS bleeding as a mimetic extension of Sikh bleeding). It may reenact, make fresh, and form a response to nationalist bleeding (chapter 2) or other sacrifices (chapter 6). It may call for its own mimesis (chapter 2). Acts of bleeding "quote" other acts of bleeding (chapters 1 and 2). Voluntary blood donation's temporality as metricality is a composite of these and other repetitions. The nonhuman repetition of cellular death and regeneration allows the movement, examined in chapter 4, from a conception of the act of blood donation as irreversible and nonrepeatable to an act that is reversible and therefore repeatable. "It is time to come back and donate," says the blood service. The donor can only "come back" because blood comes back.

The rhythms of blood donation are multiple and conflicted, and the time it takes to give, the time it takes to receive and the time that is "enabled" are in complex relation. Institutionally speaking, the transfusion, which itself embodies "a temporality of second chances" (V. Das 2007, 101), is a remarkable spatiotemporal achievement—a product of many different actors' labor in and of time across the vein-to-vein chain (cf. Berner and Bjorkman 2017). As we explained above, blood is a substance of time in its own right, its futures inclusive of but not reducible to the speculative claims of promissory biocapital. The wishes and hopes it carries are linked to its transitivity.

Different proportionalities: Drawing on Corsín Jiménez's innovative work, we have employed a proportional lens to trace substances and exchanges in and out of balance, and suggest that such a lens is indispensable for studying bloodscapes of difference, since rightful hematic balances (both within and outside bodies) are rare in the extreme, with whole economies and rhetorical and campaign apparatuses coming into existence in order to correct them (see chapters 4 and 5). We emphasize again, however, that proportionalities, temporalities, and sovereignties emerge together and in dialectical relations within bloodscapes.[26] For instance, temporalities of repetition may be disproportionate, as when a paid donor gives too frequently, or a replacement donor not frequently enough (chapter 6). The figure of the phantom or ghost unit (chapter 5)—an "as if" blood product belonging to virtual time—is calculated by subtracting the actualized part from the potential whole: whether blood donors (chapters 3 and 5) or blood prescribers (chapter 5) form the target, morally charged proportional logics may be mobilized as means of pointing out failings and inducing reform.

The "sizing up and down of descriptions" (Corsín Jiménez 2013, 2) is a scalar property of a blood economy that is in large part formed out of attempts to move surpluses that are out of place into the "right" places (chapters 4 and 5). Excesses can be useful if properly located (distributed). The excess of sacrifice, we suggested, is not eliminated but redimensioned. This is in spite of AVBDWB efforts to make the only hematic excess that matters the one that is held within all human bodies. In this regard, and again following an insight from Corsín Jiménez, we suggested the term "spillover hematology." The *gift share* identified by AVBDWB

activists—flowing over its originating biological province to help others as well—
is political because it is a field of contestation. Consisting of the surplus within a
person's lifeblood that can be safely donated, it is made to stand against depictions of a selfishness biologically determined, for it now looks as if human bodies were *made to give* (pro)portions of their blood to others (chapter 4). A darker
spillover hematology was described in chapter 5: another kind of surplus is secretly generated in the blood bank. This is possible due to the epistemological in-
scrutability of the blood unit, the proportions of which are productively reversible: one, now three, and back to one again. Component separation redimensions
the unit of blood—it is a technology of (dis)proportionality.[27] How will the effects generated by the resizing of the blood unit be channeled—redistributively
in order to help the "kin-poor," or acquisitively?

A proportional politics is also evident in the way in which gifts may be mobilized as a particular species of criticism: in chapter 3 we elaborated the partonomic
gift that foregrounds proportional relations between the given and not given, with
that which is given underscoring (and thereby critiquing) that which is not (i.e.,
deficits and absences of care and concern). The Sant Nirankaris display just such
a logic in critiquing (and redressing) fallen familial forms; the Bhopali activist-
children who donate paper hearts to the prime minister do likewise.

Different sovereignties: Relationships between excess and sovereignty are
fascinatingly explored by Sheila Ager (2006). The particular immoderation she
is interested in is royal incest in the Ptolemaic dynasty in which the breaching of
limits produced and displayed power. We have explored a connected dynamic:
immoderate bloodshed in political contexts as claims to authority and legitimacy
(e.g., the Shiv Sena's contested mega blood donation camp on Maharashtra
Day and the discussion of "substances of the civic" [chapter 3]), and inheritance
(chapter 6).

Blood donations and blood paintings perform bodily political commitments.
Apparently less easy to simulate than fasting, blood extractions may, in fact, be
just as deceptive. If one focus of chapter 3 was discussion of a fake blood donation camp taken as a species of political corruption, blood is also donated to protest, precisely, corruption. Indeed, this book has held together and moved between commentaries and campaigns *as* and *about* bloodshed. "City Youth Donate
Blood for Corruption-Free India," states a headline from 2011.[28] We see that
though such performances may "quote," or mimetically repeat, other bleedings,
they are often, at the same time, enacted in the subjunctive mood. "'It is another
war of freedom (from corruption) for which we decided to donate our blood just
to express our solidarity to Anna [Hazare],' said Vipulendra Pratap Singh, a research scholar of Hindi department." Donating *to* the future, these Banaras Hindu

University students' blood extractions also express a wish about it (that the future nation be corruption free). Yet the donations also form mimetic repetitions of the blood shed by nationalist freedom fighters: two wars of freedom—one from colonial rule, the other from corruption. Blood—a substance of time—flows between times, connecting and separating them. In this case its flow connects past and future sovereignties.

Many of Gandhi's hematic reflections were also of course made in the context of an anticolonial politics. Moving from his personal concern to maintain proper circulation and blood pressure—in complex biomoral relation with external events—to delineate a hematic politics of sovereignty, the scalar specter of corrupt blood and locating the means to purify it were once more matters of concern. We encounter different blood purities and ways of thinking about hydraulic equilibrium. In particular, the blood mingled in martyrdom comes to be thought of as a process of purification. This commitment to intermixing comes to define a new set of criteria for the purity of blood in the body politic—the equidistant relation of several religious groups to the possibility of its sacrifice. A marker of abhorrent violence, ex-sanguination may yet give cause for celebration if performed unwaveringly in the face of the corrupt blood of a sovereign power. It is in this sense that blood flows between violence and nonviolence, connecting and separating the two misleadingly polar poles: demonstrating their mutual implication. As we saw in chapter 3, it also possesses a double valence in the case of menstrual activism. Indian feminist activists recognize the polyvalence of blood to connote violence and enforce segregation, yet they are also able to make it flow differently as a mechanism of exposure and medium of truth: blood's *as if*, here, refers to a future sovereignty of bleeding, which will exist beyond the province of purity and pollution in newly remade substance-code relations. The substance flows: relations between substances and social order are not static.

The following was posted on Facebook on 18 August 2016 by "Blood Donors India": "#Hyderabad ONLY Kamma Caste Donors, O+ve blood needed at Max Cure Hospital. 3 yr old CHILD. Pls call [. . .]." Blood Donors India subsequently disowned and deleted the post, declaring it to be a fake, but not before many with Indian-sounding usernames had commented:

> is this a joke? It's a 3 year old child and thy r looking for caste here?

> Group of mad people

> Shameless

> And in India even freaking blood needs to be caste proofed. Pathetic how perfect idiots still exist in India. Time to call and ask the joker how does the caste matter for blood for a baby.

I will be happy if they dont get blood group accordingly to their caste preference and their loved one dies.

I am a non kamma, want to donate blood, save the child and kick on the parents' ass till they bleed to death.

The hoax, as Fleming and O'Carroll (2010, 58) put it, "lies in order to tell the truth." Hoax or not, the post certainly did occasion revealing anxieties and accusations. The reversibility of the substance: from a hematic utopia of the "mingled stream" and flows across difference comes a quick return to caste-based purity and passionate denunciation. Caste politics may indeed witness rapid degenerations of hematic utopias. We quote from a poem by Varavara Rao that was written in response to upper-caste protests against the Indian government's move to institutionalize affirmative action in higher education and public employment (original in Telugu).[29]

> We stand in hospital queues
> To sell blood to buy food
> Except for the smell of poverty and hunger
> How can it acquire
> The patriotic flavor
> Of your blood donation?

Like the Bhopali children's gifts of paper hearts, the words of the poem are laced with irony. Yet here the gift *not* given critiques that which *is*. We suggest that it is not that the model of partonomic critique is destabilized by the example of Rao's poem, but that it is made flexible: the proportional elements of transactions can be pejoratively valued as surfeits and deficits and become subject to moral judgments. The given and the withheld, so to speak, comment on one another: the given upon the withheld, or indeed, the withheld upon the given.

This book has illustrated that blood donation is now an established mode of public protest throughout India, and this has included blood donation in order to protest caste reservations. For instance, in 2007 trainee medics in Bangalore fasted, conducted numerous boycotts, formed a silent human chain, and donated blood in protest against proposals to reserve 27 percent of places in elite medical institutions for so-called Other Backward Classes.[30] In a riposte to the special privileges claimed by pro-reservation campaigners, protesters sought to occupy the modernist-integrative high ground in protesting charitably (the beneficiaries being pointedly *no one in particular*). For all the poetic license taken in Rao's poem (as if all low-caste people had to sell their blood to survive), the point is compellingly made that one has to be of a certain socioeconomic status to even begin to consider voluntarily shedding one's blood as a means of political expression. The "we" of the poem—laborers, those of nonelite status who might qualify for reservations—are hardly likely to consider that they possess the surplus blood necessary to shed it in order to form political statements. (They are far more likely to consider their bodies to contain a deficit.) Thus, that which is *not* given—that which indeed may be sold—thus dramatically highlights the self-serving underlay of the "integrative," "charitable," and "patriotic" protest blood donation and its class basis. The bloodscape of difference contains other substances besides. The drama of the mediatized blood gift, suggests Rao, all too easily deflects attention from other ungiven substances of the civic and bare survival: food and water.

Notes

1. BLOODSCAPE OF DIFFERENCE

1. https://www.facebook.com/ArchanaPathology/.

2. "On November 8, 2016, Indian Prime Minister Narendra Modi, in a stunning surprise announcement, declared that 500 and 1,000 rupee notes were to be demonetized (i.e., removed from circulation as legal tender). In the interest of eliminating tax evasion by targeting so-called black money and monetary fraud, he set a 50-day target for exchanging the old notes for new ones" (*The Diplomat*, 5 January 2017). On surgery as political rhetoric, see Cohen (2011b). We also briefly discuss surgical strikes in chapter 2.

3. *Times of India*, 10 January 2017.

4. We borrow the term "political hematology" from Anidjar (2011, 2).

5. Indeed, this work is in some respects an updating of Ashis Nandy's (1970) stocktaking of "national political style[s]."

6. This is a paraphrase of Spencer (2008, 626). See also Mukharji's (2014) fascinating historical analysis of "serosociality," caste and "sanguinary" identities (c. 1918–1960) in India. We note here that serological surveys also held out a utopic promise "in inverse proportion to their capacity to actually generate any conclusive insights. . . . What contributed to the growing appeal of sero-anthropological surveys was precisely its inability to distinguish. Its promise to submerge all visible difference into a deeper sympathy and commonality of blood . . ." (164).

7. *Thaindian News*, 16 December 2007.

8. Shore's (1999, 27) remarks about the "promiscuous techniques and messy encounters" of qualitative research are borne out.

9. We took inspiration from Strathern (2014, 66).

10. For perspectives on figures and practices of "recruitment," both recent and historical, see the work of Mathangi Krishnamurthy (2018) and Radhika Singha (2011).

11. For a full description of how a camp functions, and the nature of the camp as a contemporary social form, see Alter (2008b), Copeman (2009a, chap. 1), and L. Cohen (2011b).

12. See Copeman (2009a).

13. See Copeman and Quack (2018) for a fuller account of bi-instrumentalism.

14. See Copeman (2009a, 9).

15. We also attended a handful of camps in Kolkata and Mumbai.

16. Youth Congress is the youth wing of the Congress Party. Under Indira Gandhi's son Sanjay in the 1970s, it was a "delinquent boys' club" (Khilnani 1997, 47). Now it conducts social service activities and campaigns for the party.

17. "She sacrificed her family" is a reference to the fact that Sonia Gandhi's husband and mother-in-law were both assassinated.

18. See D. Mines (2002) and M. Banerjee (2014) on political uses of public spaces in the subcontinent.

19. The prominent subgroups of the ICJB are Bhopal Gas Peedit Mahila Stationary Karmachari Sangh (Bhopal Women's Gas Victim's Stationary Labor Organization), Bhopal Gas Peedit Mahila Purush Sangharsh Morcha (Bhopal Men and Women's Gas Victim's Struggle Forum), and the Bhopal Group for Information and Action.

20. Indira Gandhi was India's third prime minister, discontinuously in power for fifteen years between 1966 and 1984.

21. The Emergency was a period of twenty-one months from 1975 to 1977 when Prime Minister Indira Gandhi declared a rule of emergency and suspended civil liberties and press freedom. See Tarlo (2003, 27–28) and V. Das (2007, 173).

22. *Hindustan Times*, 4 January 2011.

23. The Indian Youth Congress was formed in 1952 but "was really activated in 1970 under the leadership of Mr. Sanjay Gandhi who gave it a constructive program of tree-plantation, slum-clearance, blood-donation, family-planning and literacy" (Kalathuveettil 1992, 245).

24. *India Today*, 7 February 2004.

25. One recruitment poster used prominently in Kolkata features a photograph of Rajiv Gandhi donating his blood, with the caption "A country is great when its leaders are great."

26. We are grateful to an anonymous reviewer for whom this story of the politician's daughter whose weight becomes the measure of blood donation brings to mind the story of King Shibi, whose kingdom, and then his flesh, and then his entire body, become the counterweight to a bird who seeks his protection from a predator. Rather than our (the authors') apparent acceptance of the doctor's description of this event as *tamasha*, might it not—in light of the story of King Shibi—also be read as *yajna*, and in particular, the kind of sacrifice that consecrates a king (or in this case, a politician)? In responding to this we offer several points: The politician in question is a local "strong man" leader of a small Muslim party that is molded in the image of the Shiv Sena. This does not in the least invalidate the points about King Shibi and the *yajna*-like nature of the spectacle (instances that are clearly from the Hindu canon). Indeed, we would agree that the template in which a politician is weighed—usually against cash but here against blood—does take its lead from the ritual consecration of the king, and that from the point of view of those political devotees who participated in the event it probably did form such a consecration (see Copeman [2004] on the conjunction of the king, the politician, and blood donation). We think, however, that most members of the public would ally with the doctor's point of view of the event as a *tamasha*. The weighing of politicians against money, and more recently blood, is an established component of the political rally. At a "May Day Blood Donation Camp" in Rajasthan, 104 Congress workers are reported to have donated blood equivalent to the body weight of Shri B. D. Kalla, president of the Rajasthan Pradesh Congress Committee (http://www.congressandesh.com/june- 2005/june2005.pdf). On the other hand, gurus and temple idols may also be weighed in this way. Gujarat blood donor recruiters related to us the practice of weighing idols of Krishna against donated blood. "A 6-foot Krishna might be 200 units," said one of them. Also in Gujarat, a blood donation event called "*Rakt Tula*" was staged in 2005 at the sixtieth birthday celebrations of the guru Swami Adhyatmananda. Finally, see Jonathan Parry (1989) on the mode of gift called *tula-dan*, which involves the weighing of the donor against the gift to be given.

27. The reference here is to Hansen's (2001) schema.

28. We drew on Gell (1993, 3–20).

29. *Times of India*, 2 September 2009.

30. As the Indian Red Cross website puts it: "Whenever [paid donors] run short of money for drink, drugs or gambling they sell their blood. They care little for their health and suffer from various ailments and disabilities. They are often carriers of blood borne diseases like malaria, hepatitis, syphilis and AIDS. It matters little to them whether the recipient suffers or dies because of poor quality of blood" (http://www.indianredcross .org/blood-bank.htm).

31. *The Telegraph*, 27 March 2007.

32. See *Mainstream* 1994, 27. *India Today* (30 April 1989) reported skeptically, "The CPI(M), the leading partner in the Left Front Government, is going all out to raise funds. It has termed Bakreswar a 'people's project': plans a 'film-star-studded musical evening' on April 14, the Bengali New Year's Day, which is expected to fetch Rs 40 lakh: party MPs have donated a month's salary: and donations have been sought from the people, and even from schoolchildren. The front organizations of the party—the Students' Federation of India and the Democratic Youth Federation of India—organized blood donation camps to raise money by selling blood. There was a flood of donors but, typically, blood preservation facilities were insufficient, and a lot of blood literally went down the drain. All this has earned the party a lot of newspaper headlines, but little money. So most of the funds will have to come from other sources."

33. http://www.cpimwb.org.in/current_topic_details.php?topic_id=911.

34. For a modern equivalent, see the campaign rhetoric of a Samajwadi Party candidate in Uttar Pradesh recorded by Mukulika Banerjee (2014, 65): "Friends, I would rather be beheaded than let you down. I will save your honor and respect at any cost, even if that means I have to give my life and blood for you."

35. *Millennium Post*, 14 March 2016. See also the discussion in chapter 3 of the Samajwadi Party's blood donation camps conducted during an election.

36. Consider, for example, the 2010 "red shirt" protests in Bangkok. See Erik Cohen's (2012) insightful examination of these.

37. A much-cited paraphrase of Carl Schmitt's: "All significant concepts of the modern theory of the state are secularized theological concepts" (2006, 36).

38. Cristóbal Bonelli (2014) has questioned the analytical separation of the material reality of blood and its symbolism; even analyses that posit their intimacy or merger do so from a starting point in which the "reality" of blood and its "symbolic function" are distinct. Among the Pehuenche of southern Chile, however, these categories never were differentiated. Connecting "different entities of Pehuenche life in intersubjective participation" (121), Bonelli sees Pehuenche blood's transcendence of the material/symbolic binary as sounding a warning to anthropologists to avoid imposing their own systems of thought on the substances they encounter during fieldwork. Connected with this has been the accusation that anthropological characterizations of blood are too culturally determined— that is, that blood is portrayed as having significance only insofar as it is entangled in webs of culture and attributed with meaning by humans, rendering the substance itself powerless (Fontein and Harries 2013). That said, recent studies, influenced by the anthropology of material culture, have given prominence to the physical properties of blood: its color, susceptibility to fading, and motility.

39. See, in this respect, Pinney (2004, 202), and Copeman and Quack (2015).

40. *The Hindu*, 25 September 2000; *The Telegraph*, 26 February 2006; *Daily Excelsior*, 2 May 2005.

41. *The Gift of Blood* (newsletter published in Kolkata by the Association of Voluntary Blood Donors, West Bengal), April 2008.

42. "Feudal rot" is after L. Cohen (2007, 108).

43. *The Guardian*, 14 July 2005.

44. As we explain in chapters 4 and 7, it is with respect to the technoscientific aspiration to substitute blood with a synthetic, artificially manufactured variety that the world of blood donation and transfusion comes closest to the biocapitalized and optimized futures so frequently discussed in anthropological (and other) accounts of biomedicine.

45. This is not to say that a concern with semen and its conservation has vanished. As Stefan Ecks (2014, 89) notes, "Across India, Ayurvedic advertising talks of 'vigor,' but what

is really meant is the distillation of the most powerful *dhatu*. The squandering of semen, digestion's finest product, causes a plethora of diseases." See also the insightful discussion by Vicziany and Hardikar (2018).

46. See Copeman (2008).

47. We have discussed elsewhere (Copeman 2009a, chap. 2) a second way in which donated blood is capable of obviating the distinction between sustaining and engendering life, which is connected to prevalent understandings of the intergenerational effects of life-sustaining transfusion. For example, in saving the life of someone yet to produce offspring, donated blood acts as proximate "cause" of otherwise precluded future fecundity.

48. See Copeman (2009a, 26).

49. As Berger (2013, 39) also insightfully notes in a discussion of Marriott's work, "Ayurvedic flows as identified in Indological medical works served as foundational points of reference in . . . arguments [that Marriott and others] expounded on the fallacy of rigid individualism [in the region]." See also Theweleit (1987, 461), who briefly and intriguingly points toward a (European) genealogy of "attempts to envision the internal functioning of human beings as something flowing." He continues: "Consider that the four temperaments of the Greeks were thought of as fluid mixtures. And the fluids were external: 'We enter the same streams and enter them not; they are us, and are not us' (Heraclitus . . .). See [also] Leonardo da Vinci's idea that 'the sea of blood around the heart is the ocean.' . . . Somewhat different . . . is Oswald Spengler, to whom life seems 'an ineffable mystery made up of cosmic currents.'"

50. These gendered implications of blood donation intersect with class and relative socioeconomic statuses. The urban poor often express their reluctance to donate by connecting their poverty with having "less blood." What they see as their deficient blood quantum is likely linked to the sorts of work they perform: "I'm a laborer; I have no blood." Similarly, in a study of a Delhi slum, respondents said that "they already felt weak and that they did not have 'even a drop of blood in their bodies'" (Bir Singh et al. 2002).

51. https://www.facebook.com/Dr-BR-Ambedkar-Blood-Donors-Association-Jalandhar PunjabIndia-1828140684104953/.

52. See the discussion of the expurgation of "senile blood" in Copeman (2009a, 22–26).

53. See Copeman (2015), Deshpande and John (2010), and Jodhka and Shah (2010).

54. See Copeman (2009a, 20–21).

55. See Bentley and Griffiths (2003), and Kaur (2014).

56. *Times of India*, 12 June 2011.

57. Bharat Venkat (2017) also points to the ways in which ethnosociology might be deployed as a present-day analytic. At the same time, he reminds us of the important work done to pry apart the troubling intertwining of morality and biology in the subcontinent, particularly in domains such as the anticaste movements in South India, *bhakti* devotional movements, and the Tamil Self-Respect Movement. See also Rachel Berger's (2013, 37–42) insightful discussion and Cohen's (1998, 155) suggestive remark that accounts such as Marriott's "offer not so much models of social life as models for (and against) it."

58. Cohen also traces the "ethnosociological cinematic" into post-liberalization India in which the trope that now emerges is that of the poor family under duress that must sacrifice body organs in order to keep alive familial kinship bonds. The early postcolonial biosociality of blood transfusion allowing for the imagination of a broad, cohesive citizenry is replaced by a new neoliberal configuration of sacrifice and debt under enormous economic constraint (Cohen 2001).

59. See also Venkat (2017).

60. Replacement donation, meanwhile, is thought to pressurize patients' relatives unduly, pushing many to seek paid donors to donate in their stead and threatening those who cannot arrange for this kind of donation with denial of life-saving treatment; moreover,

that the blood donated does not flow directly to one's own relative but rather releases "other" blood for them is again seen to provide an incentive for the replacement donor to conceal disqualifying factors such as HIV/AIDS.

61. India's Supreme Court banned paid donation from 1 January 1998 and directed the government to begin actively encouraging voluntary, non-remunerated blood donation. The government's subsequent National Blood Policy (2002) additionally required the phasing out of the family-based replacement system within five years. As a recent assessment notes, "The Blood Safety Programme in India began to take shape in 1992 with the establishment of the National AIDS Control Organization (NACO) with three major focus areas that were, surveillance; health education & information; and screening of blood and blood products" (NACO 2014, 18).

62. Copeman (2009a, chap. 1).

63. On NACO's larger function see Venkat (2017, 97).

64. *Times of India*, 7 December 2011.

65. http://www.sankalpindia.net/book/when-voluntary-blood-donation-percentages -go-beserk.

66. Copeman (2009a), D. Banerjee (2011).

67. See Levine (2016) and Strathern (2011, 90).

68. See also Corsín Jiménez's (2004, 15) suggestive hematic-proportional reflection: "Proportions are relations of magnitude. Magnitude, or size, or weight, is inherent to what proportions bring to their connections—recall the saying 'blood is *thicker* than water.' . . . Proportions do not therefore simply set up links between entities or orders of knowledge that had hitherto remained separate, but they actually 'measure up' those links by positing their degree of commensurability, and by emerging in the shape of a new proportional field."

69. Of course, blood flows across other community distinctions besides those of caste, but we bracket these other communal distinctions for now, turning to them more fully in chapters 2 and 4.

70. See also Jennifer Robertson's (2012) important work on blood, race, and nationalism in Japan. Japanese blood donation guidelines portray a "tacit belief in the value and desirability of blood from 'pure' Japanese" (106).

71. Politically charged examples of discrimination and exclusion communicated through a blood idiom include the threats reported in Indian newspapers made by telephone to the Hindu admiral Vishnu Bhagwat for having married a woman of "Muslim blood" (*Frontline*, 16–29 January 1999), and the political party Shiv Sena's call that "only those Hindus who have unadulterated blood in them [i.e., the higher castes] should join this *morcha* [demonstration]" (cited in Hansen 2001, 84). Specifically in terms of Indian kinship reckoning, blood is a highly significant idiom and ideational symbol. To take one example, in Tamil Nadu blood purity is held to be transmitted from parent to child. Condensed, it becomes semen in the man and breast milk in the woman (Fruzzetti, Östör, and Barnett 1982, 13). At marriage, the male aspect of the woman's blood (*utampu*), which derives from her ancestors, transforms into the *utampu* of her husband, the female aspect of her blood (*uyir*) remaining unchanged. In Bengal the category of blood is used to exclude persons from the circle of marriageable partners (Fruzzetti and Östör 1982, 51).

72. The doubling of blood in Ambedkar's writing remains an accurate descriptor of the substance's ambivalent imagination in contemporary anticaste activism. T. K. Oommen describes the difficulty the relation poses for anticaste activists (2002). On the one hand, scholars of caste have come to understand caste and race as both socially constructed categories (not rooted in biological fact), and they also understand the violence inherent in thinking of caste as race in ignorance of a history of intermixing. On the other hand, precisely because the British colonizers used—and upper-caste Hindu nationalists

continue to use—caste, race, and blood interchangeably, anticaste activists must reckon with caste alongside the category of race. Current anticaste mobilizations, sometimes in conjunction with antiracist groups elsewhere in the world, use the discourse of race in recognition of caste and race as comparable systems of oppression, rather than as socio-biological facts (Reddy 2005).

73. See Copeman (2009a, chaps. 4 and 7); and L. Cohen (2001). Whatever the imbalances and asymmetries of actual provision by blood banks to recipients (the Red Cross does not charge for patients in government hospitals and certainly does not discriminate along caste or gender lines, so it can thus make a good claim to universal provision), from the point of view of the donor, the anonymous conditions of voluntary donation produce a universal directionality.

74. See Copeman (2009a, 169–70).

75. See *Inter Press Service News Agency*, 24 June 2002; *Indian Express*, 19 August 2016; *News 18*, 19 August 2016; and *The Hindu*, 20 August 2016. We discuss this Twitter controversy in chapter 7.

76. *Hindustan Times*, 7 November 2016.

2. SOVEREIGNTY AND BLOOD

1. For a recent study of transactions between blood and finance, see Weston (2013a).

2. See Copeman (2009a, chap. 8).

3. *First Post*, 6 October 2016.

4. This work is henceforth cited throughout the text as CWG (*Collected Works of Mahatma Gandhi*), followed by volume number and page number (e.g., CWG 1:423).

5. Our work on Gandhi here is indebted to Alter's insistence on placing bodies and biology at the center of any analysis of Gandhi's politics. However, our work departs from Alter's in making distinctions between the body politic and the biological body. Our argument hinges on the insight that while the individual body and the national body are related, the relation is one of allegory rather than analogy. In contrast, Alter's analysis draws a direct relation between personal bodily practice and public politics.

6. It is worth noting Shahid Amin's (1984) work here on how Gandhi's thinking and writing found themselves translated variedly and beyond recognition in subaltern consciousness. For example, it intersected in fascinating and unpredictable ways with Hindu ecologies of purity and pollution in respect of bodily effluvia.

7. The Bhagavad Gita is a seven-hundred-verse scripture in Sanskrit that is part of the Hindu epic Mahabharata, composed and compiled from about the ninth century BCE to the fourth century CE.

8. It is worth reminding ourselves here that blood is not the only or even the paramount bodily substance of concern but one among others, including semen. But while Gandhi's fixation with celibacy has attracted significant scholarly attention, his concern with blood and its flows has hardly been considered.

9. References to blood sisters tellingly occur much more rarely, and even then, often in relation to women as referents of morality—for example, in a letter to a male correspondent advising him against infidelity, in a speech defending prostitutes (CWG 40:97), and so on. Often the metaphor of blood sister worked to desexualize women, removing the threat of sexual promiscuity and reminding of sexual vigilance. After 1927, forced to acknowledge caste by a growing movement led by Dr. Ambedkar, Gandhi began to refer to untouchables too as blood brothers, while seemingly unable to recognize the violence inflicted by the hypocrisy of such a recognition (CWG 40:487).

10. This was consistent with his lifelong support for the inheritance of social position and the hereditary division of labor; he only opposed the perception of certain kinds of

labor as higher or lower than others. While he famously opposed the practice of caste-based untouchability, his reformist vision was built on the idea of *varnavyavastha*: the organization of Hindu social life through the inherited division of professions.

11. In this, our work joins a growing body of scholarship that contests the association of Gandhian nonviolence with passivity; instead, such scholarship highlights the intense activity demanded of the *satyagrahi*, where the practice of *ahimsa* is much more than the negative of violence, but a politics of directed activity (Iyer 1978; L. Gandhi 1996; Bhrigupati Singh 2010; Skaria 2014). While the scholarship agrees on this broad characterization of *ahimsa*, points of difference emerge in relation to the locus, vector, and purpose of the activity of the *satyagraha*. Our rendition of Gandhi's hemo-politics most closely resembles Ajay Skaria's characterization of the Gandhian *satyagrahi*—a figure whose fundamental aim is to relinquish the very notion of sovereignty and mastery, both over one's own self and toward others.

12. *Indian Express*, 23 June 2011.

13. *Mid-Day*, 25 January 2008.

14. *Rediff*, 3 January 2006, http://www.rediff.com/news/2006/jan/03martyrs.htm.

15. http://jaago—india—jaago.blogspot.co.uk/2008/10/blood-donation-camp-at-jallian walla_03.html.

16. See Bynum (2007, 4) on multifarious imitations of Christ's bleeding.

17. *Indian Express*, 3 October 2001.

18. *Indian Express*, 9 September 2015.

19. *Vrindavan Today*, 21 October 2010.

20. *Rediff*, 3 January 2006.

3. SUBSTANTIAL ACTIVISMS

1. The phrase "rituals of verification" is borrowed from the subtitle of Power's (1997) book on practices of audit and accountancy, and the connection with accountancy is apt.

2. Our use of "promissory matter" follows Charis Thompson (2000) and Brown, Kraft, and Martin (2006).

3. See Copeman (2009a). In almost all *bhakti* traditions, *guru-seva* is ideally performed without self-interest, either for the devotee or for the guru. Officially, this is also the case for the Sant Nirankaris. In practice, however, devotees were explicit and unabashed in speaking to us about the blessings and other spiritual fruits that their devotional blood giving would result in.

4. On the background to this violence, see Copeman (2009a, chap. 4).

5. See in particular Marriott (1976; 1989), and also Parry (1994) for important comments on Marriott's undertaking. See Copeman (2011) and again Parry (1994) on gift-giving as imperiling contact.

6. *DNA*, 30 April 2010.

7. *DNA*, 30 April 2010.

8. *The Hindu*, 2 February 2002.

9. *Deccan Chronicle*, 9 December 2013.

10. *Deccan Chronicle*, 9 December 2013.

11. A medical doctor, the founder of the main rationalist society in Maharashtra, and a staunch secular campaigner, Narendra Dabholkar was murdered in 2013. The murder was reported internationally.

12. See http://news.bbc.co.uk/2/hi/south_asia/3484992.stm.

13. http://www.searchindia.com/2008/08/29/why-do-tamils-burn-themselves/.

14. *Daily Telegraph*, 12 January 2012.

15. See Copeman (2013a).

16. In this, the concept of "biosociality" (Rabinow 1992) to describe new kinds of willed somatic groups in Europe and North America comes under stress. For more on this, see D. Banerjee (2011).

17. The popularity of the "ketogenic diet" draws from the dramatic loss of fat and weight that occurs through the process of ketosis.

18. https://rupikaur.com/period/.

19. *International Business Times*, 16 November 2015.

4. HEMO ECONOMICUS

1. This is a reference to the churning of the ocean (*samudra manthan*) as recounted in many Hindu texts, such as the Vishnu Purana and the Bhagavata Purana. The churning created not only the nectar of immortality, or *amrith*, but also *halahala*, a lethal poison. Shiva is depicted as swallowing the poison to protect all of creation from destruction.

2. Parents, in general, do not encourage their offspring to donate blood, fearing that it risks their health. See Jerstad (2016, 38, chap. 2) on relations between illness, family, work, and the household in a North Indian context.

3. Many other reasons exist for the persistence of low voluntary blood donation figures, some of which we discuss in the following chapter—for instance, blood banks' frequent failure to honor the voluntary blood donor card, which in theory entitles voluntary donors in the future to receive for themselves, or their close family members, a quantity of blood equivalent to that which they have donated. This understandably breeds generalized hostility toward hospitals and blood banks. However, it is the lamentable inability of ordinary Indians to overcome "irrational" fears rather than infrastructural or financial inadequacy that blood banks and civil society groups usually hold responsible for low voluntary blood donation figures. It is difficult to quantify the impacts of these different factors, but the fact that blood donation is understood to be damaging to health is hardly beneficial to campaigns to promote it.

4. Also highly significant is the West Bengal Voluntary Blood Donors' Forum (see http://www.wbvbdf.org/home.php), which conducts a similar program of activities. Our fieldwork, however, was focused on the AVBDWB.

5. See Copeman (2009a, chap. 1).

6. See also Copeman 2011.

7. See also Partha Chatterjee on the split between the domains of "properly constituted" *civil* society and the more ill-defined *political* society (2004), the latter being located "neither within the constitutional limits of the state nor in the orderly transactions of bourgeois civil society" (1999, 117), and the work of Sandria Freitag (1996), which has shown how politics and religion were conceptually and ideationally separated from one another via a number of legal and bureaucratic processes of colonial rule.

8. See chapters 1–3 on the rhetorical force of blood donation in explicitly political contexts in India.

9. http://www.bloodbanksdelhi.com/content/FAQ.htm.

10. Given that the time meant to elapse between donations is three months in most parts of the world, not just in India, this claim should be treated with skepticism.

11. We have discussed elsewhere the demand for special recognition of blood donors by the state. See Copeman (2004) on rhetoric of specialness with respect to blood donors, and Copeman (2009a, 166) on the idea that there ought to be a quota of job reservations for voluntary blood donors.

12. The book famously put forward an evolutionary model of social development based upon replication of cultural information and ideas. Though AVBDWB members hail from a cross-section of society and the organization pursues a conscious strategy of

inclusiveness, the most actively visible members are mostly well read, educated to a high level, and so are familiar with landmark scientific texts such as Dawkins's.

13. At the same time, Dawkins acknowledges that some of his work might be read in such a way: "I do with hindsight notice lapses of my own on the very same subject. These are to be found especially in chapter 1, epitomized by the sentence 'Let us try to teach generosity and altruism because we are born selfish.' There is nothing wrong with teaching generosity and altruism, but 'born selfish' is misleading. . . . Given the dangers of that style of error, I can readily see how the title could be misunderstood, and this is one reason why I should perhaps have gone for *The Immortal Gene*. *The Altruistic Vehicle* would have been another possibility" (Dawkins 2006, ix).

14. See Bataille (1985, 251): "Men assembling for a sacrifice and for a festival, satisfy their need to expend a vital excess. The sacrificial laceration that opens the festival is a liberating laceration. The individual who participates in loss is obscurely aware that this loss engenders the community that supports him."

15. Notwithstanding it can also do precisely the opposite (see Copeman 2011).

16. The mythic sage Dadhichi has in particular been mobilized as a template for nurturing campaigns to promote blood and body donation. See Copeman (2006).

17. See Copeman (2009a, chap. 4).

18. In Latourian parlance, the official classification performs the prototypical modernist work of purification (conceptual separation).

19. The slogan accompanied an international colloquium for the promotion of voluntary blood donation staged in Beijing in 2004.

20. See Copeman (2008, 291–92).

21. The AVBDWB organizes blood donation camps deliberately composed of members of different religious and caste communities annually on the occasion of the *raksha bandhan* festival, "widely celebrated in north India when sisters tie a thread (*rakhi*) on their brothers' wrists to affirm bonds of protection and nurturance. There is a long history of fictive kin relations being established between women and men, even across Hindu-Muslim lines, through the tying of the *rakhi*" (Vanita 2002, 157–58).

22. What Starr (2002) called "the 9/11 blood disaster" is perhaps the most well-known example of dramatically wasteful overcollection. But see also Copeman (2009a, chap. 5) on overcollection in Indian contexts of mass devotional blood giving.

23. This is an adaptation of Willerslev's (2004) "not animal, not not-animal."

5. THE BROKEN WORLD OF TRANSFUSION

1. The details here are drawn from the following sources: *Dainik Jagran*, 12 October 2007; *Times of India*, 11 October 2007; *Times of India*, 12 October 2007; CNN-IBN Online, http://ibnlive.in.com/news/agency/CNN-IBN/, 11 October 2007; http://ibnlive.in.com/videos/50372/10_2007/face_nation1110_2/face-the-nation-superstition-winning-over-science.html (video channel); *Dainik Bhaskar*, 11 October 2007; http://www.canadiandesi.ca/read.php?TID=18894; http://news.webindia123.com/news/ar_show details.asp?id=710110088&cat=&n_date=20071011; http://uberdesi.com/blog/2007/10/15/blood-transfusions-gone-wild-a-case-of-blood-sucking-desi-parents/.

2. See Parry (1994) on susceptibility to spirit possession as a local measure of superstition in Banaras.

3. Related incidents of self-killings by Dalit students at institutes of higher education are too significant to be done justice to within the scope of this chapter. For more on issues of caste-discrimination and suicide in Indian higher education, refer to Praveen Donthi's excellent reporting on the subject: http://www.caravanmagazine.in/reportage/from-shadows-to-the-stars-rohith-vemula.

4. *Hindustan Times*, 28 April 2017.

5. See V. Saria, *The Fallen Idol* (2016), on medical entrance-exam cheating scandals.

6. See, for instance, Appadurai (1981) and C. Bayly (1986). For a recent and particularly vivid publicly reported case involving a convicted murderer's attempt to donate his organs, see Copeman and Reddy (2012).

7. See Copeman (2009a, chap. 4).

8. The literature on the matrix of colonial and contemporary state attempts to inculcate "discipline" both within the medical sphere and without is too vast to even begin to give an account of. A recent fresh and novel perspective is Ajay Gandhi's essay "Standing Still and Cutting in Line: The Culture of the Queue in India" (2013), which can stand here synecdochically for the larger literature on this topic.

9. See Copeman and Reddy (2012), Copeman and Quack (2015), and Copeman (2015). A recent controversy concerns doctors' performance of caesarean sections at dates and times thought by expectant parents—on the advice of astrologers—to be auspicious: "Delhi-based rationalist Sanal Edamaruku said it was 'unethical' for doctors to heed the demands of superstitious mothers. 'Medical ethics clearly define that medical intervention should be done only if it is medically required. . . . [It] is absolutely baseless thinking. How could a star or time influence someone's life favorably? . . . It is an unethical practice and the doctors are promoting superstition,' he added" (*Shillong Times*, 19 August 2008).

10. We underscore, however, that it is not only due to scarcity that such prescriptions become excessive (though, of course, overprescription does exacerbate existing scarcity). It is important to recognize that the whole- or single-unit transfusion, from the clinical activist point of view, is also *qualitatively* unnecessary.

11. Doctors known to requisition single units for transfusion nevertheless tend to deny doing so when confronted by clinical activists. Similarly, when we broached the subject in interviews, the practice was scarcely admitted to, and it is not hard to understand why given the rhetoric of unreason attached to the practice. Very rarely, however, did we encounter medics willing to explain why single-unit transfusions can still be justified on occasion, or why the everyday reality of scarcity can make them inevitable. We quote a particularly eloquent physician employed at a prestigious North Indian government hospital: "There are still indications for only one unit of blood. For example, if a clinician asks for two units of blood, the blood bank might be in a position not to give two, only one. At the end of the year you may look and see how many people have received only one unit, and you may think—so many! But you have not seen that this doctor had asked him for two but had been given only one. Or sometimes a surgery happens. . . . Say there is a tumor in the brain. We have said that this surgery needs three units. So the surgeon arranges three units. But the surgeon is good, so good and meticulous, and the cauteries were sewn so carefully, that he uses only one unit. I cannot tell this doctor, 'Oh no! No! You have wasted! Why have you taken only one unit?' He is good. He asked for three units. But he has been so good that he has consumed only one unit! I should not scold this doctor, 'Oh why are you using only one unit of blood?'" At this the medic leaned across his desk, eyeball to eyeball with us, before continuing slowly, almost in a whisper, emphasizing each syllable: "It should not get *reflected* as a single-unit transfusion. . . . That, also, one has to keep in mind."

12. A central figure in the history of blood donation and transfusion, Karl Landsteiner discovered blood groups in 1900, thereby increasing the safety of transfusion and enabling it to become a major component of modern medical treatment.

13. On the widely held suspicion that this has to do with drug companies making it in medics' interests to prescribe their drugs even when it is medically unnecessary for them to do so, see Ecks (2016) and Saria (2016). For discussion concerning potential conflicts of interest on the part of medics and the impact of inducements on prescribing practices beyond South Asia per se, see Kirmayer and Raikhel (2009).

14. This can lead to accusations of profiteering, as we shall see below.

15. Platelets are disklike structures that are the foundation of clots. Plasma is the colorless coagulable part of blood in which the fat globules float; usually frozen after extraction and centrifuge, it becomes known as fresh frozen plasma (FFP). Red cells contain hemoglobin, which helps carry oxygen from the lungs to other parts of the body. Red cells also collect carbon dioxide waste, moving it to the lungs for expulsion.

16. In the 1950s the key pioneer of modern blood management practices, Edwin Cohn, conducted research on blood and proteins at Harvard Medical School and came to the conclusion, crucial for future developments in transfusion medicine, that it was wasteful to administer blood to patients in its whole form (Starr 1998, 211). A far greater "use-value" could be yielded by isolating the different cellular constituents of the undifferentiated liquid. He called this new approach "component therapy" or "blood economy." Starr explains that the situation up until Cohn's work had been that if one had four units of blood, four people could be treated (assuming that they each needed one unit). If a division is performed (via a centrifuge machine) into red cells and plasma, it becomes possible to treat four people with the red cells and two with the plasma. Plasma can similarly be subdivided (fractionated) by separation into albumin, gamma globulin, and another component identified as Fraction 1 (212). Starr concludes that, by the late 1950s, the efficiency of blood usage had risen by 600 percent relative to the previous decade. A colleague of Cohn's, Charles Janeway, stated at the time that "for the first time real economy in the use of blood becomes possible" (Starr 1998, 212). In India, government blood banks are less likely to possess the technology than private or NGO blood banks, though the biggest government hospitals in Delhi and Kolkata do practice separation techniques. The technology requires a linked set of three blood bags (called triple bags) for the components to be separated into. Indian blood banks, however, only began to move beyond crude glass bottles and introduce PVC collection bags in the early 1980s. It has been estimated that 25 percent of donated blood in the country is now separated into components. In Delhi the percentage is much higher. Blood banks that do not possess this technology invariably plan to acquire it as soon as sufficient funds become available to them. Possessing it is an important mark of modernity for clinics.

17. Compare this with the "whole [cannabis] plant approach" of some parents of epileptic children in the United States. These parents advocate the use of the whole marijuana plant, rather than specific isolated compounds extracted from it, in order for their children to benefit, as they see it, from the synergistic potency of the chemicals in relation to one another: what is known as the "entourage effect" (Sobo 2016).

18. See Copeman (2009a, 39) on the transfusion of whole blood as theft.

19. If one donates only one component—as in apheresis, a form of donation in which only one component of donors' blood is removed, the remaining volume being returned to them even as they donate—then one can give more than four times per year.

20. Its accuracy is questionable on several fronts: though there is a massive shortage of blood in terms of stock levels adequate for a conventional voluntary system, since the system in practice is mixed—comprising voluntary, replacement, paid, and even directed donations—it is difficult to determine how often patients die for want of blood. Moreover, as we have seen, many doctors ask blood banks for whole blood rather than components, so the trainer's assumption that donations are "tripled" is more a counterfactual rhetorical device than an objective calculation of opportunity costs. And as we have seen, each transfusion, at least in theory, should be made up of more than a single unit—so in a double sense, then, it is rarely if ever a case of one donated unit saving one life. Finally, many transfusions form just a part of larger treatment regimes and so are often not obviously isolable as "life saving" in a discrete sense.

21. http://isbti.com/components.html.

22. See Copeman (2009a, chap. 2).

23. See also Cecilia Van Hollen's (2018) excellent paper on debates about disclosure of cancer diagnoses in South India.

24. One can debate whether or not such an entitlement compromises the "voluntary" nature of blood donation. We would suggest that it shows how replacement and voluntary donation are not opposites but very similar to each other; voluntary blood donation comes to appear like a preemptive, or a differently temporally organized, mode of replacement. We also would suggest that the card simply makes explicit that feature of non-remunerated systems in most Euro-American countries whereby we may expect, in case of future need, to draw on for our own purposes what we also share with others (cf. Bird-David 1992).

25. Indeed, this is what really brings the system into disrepute in the eyes of many blood donors who subsequently require blood for themselves or their relatives. Blood banks often are not disposed to honor cards and hand out units of blood in return for blood donations that had been made to different blood banks, an attitude that is symptomatic of the fragmentation of a system that frequently appears to be stacked against *both* donors and recipients.

26. The transmutation of "altruism" into profits for recipient institutions is a feature of numerous systems of biological exchange. Hayden (2007, 730) has noted how "altruistically" given tissue, blood, or gene samples in the United States and Europe can cause disquiet among ethicists, for "such gifts may well enable quite a lot of profit for those on the receiving end of such transactions." Or as Waldby and Mitchell (2006, 24) put it, the norm of altruism in tissue donation "has simply rendered the body an open source of free biological material for commercial use." Familiar with such charges, all varieties of blood banks (government, NGO, and commercial) protest that the fee they demand from recipients and their families is merely a "processing charge" that barely covers the costs of testing, storing, and matching donated blood. Similar to what we find in Sharp's (2006) work on organ transplantation in the United States, a lot of cultural effort goes into downplaying the monetary value of units of blood.

27. See discussion of labor and time in chapter 6.

28. See Copeman (2009a, chap. 2).

29. Bärnreuther (2018b) reports something very similar for reproductive clinics in Delhi where "the notion of *dan* . . . aids in facilitating anonymity and temporary-ness by eclipsing the future trajectory of egg cells in the few cases when donors wonder about possible children resulting from their oocytes. An agent explained that similar to situations where people give to religious institutions, donors should not mind what eventually happens to donated gametes: 'If we give to churches or temples, and give money, we don't worry where the money is gone, whether it is gone for books or paint. We donate, and it is gone.' This reasoning bolsters the practice of donors relinquishing their rights to the donated substances when they sign informed consent forms."

30. On recent important qualitative and quantitative shifts in North Indian dowry practices, see Jeffery (2014b) and Chaudry (2016).

31. Arnold's (1993) work on the reception of Western medicine introduced to India by the British colonialists demonstrates the longstanding nature of such attitudes toward needles and extraction of bodily substance. Rather than places of healing, Western-style medical institutions were perceived as places of cutting and substance-extraction from which people would rarely emerge alive. Rumors of substance-extraction and inappropriate mixing abounded in times of plague. Some of these resulted from the enforced hospitalization of suspected sufferers; in hospital they were held to be intentionally bled to death by staff, a machine then squeezing the oil out of their bodies—oil that was then "transfused" into others who then contracted the disease (Arnold 1993, 220; and see

C. Bayly 1996, 269–71). Treated as "secular objects," exposed to the touch of Western doctors or members of "separate" communities, bodies were held to be put in severe danger by these "foreign" practices.

6. BLOOD IN THE TIME OF THE CIVIC

1. This contrasts with Walter Benjamin's messianic model of time characterized by transcendental discontinuities and ruptures.

2. The breakdown of a major agreement between the government of West Bengal and the global TATA company to build its iconic Nano car at Singur. TATA withdrew, making clear its plan to instead build a new plant in Gujarat.

3. Let us reassert, however, that this is voluntary donation as an ideal type. The data we present in this chapter reveals both the ambivalence of repetition in Indian blood donation and transfusion contexts and the layered temporal reckonings that go into achieving it.

4. With certain types of donation—such as apheresis—it is possible to donate more regularly.

5. Usually this is the case, though not always, since colleagues and friends may also be called upon to donate blood in replacement.

6. See also Parmasad (2016) for similar responses to requests to donate voluntarily in Trinidad.

7. These examples are from NACO (2007).

8. See Copeman (2009a, 31).

9. See Copeman (2009a, 142).

10. As we explain elsewhere (Copeman 2009a, chap. 2), these are highly gendered expressions, for one's *vansh* can be passed on only through the male line. If your blood saves a providing male at a certain point, the assumption is that his whole family will be saved, not only in the present but generatively speaking also.

11. The difference is that in one case the family ties are known, while in the other they are unknown.

12. In the following chapter, we examine a further way in which astrological time reckoning features in the Indian blood donation and transfusion field, focusing on how blood donation may be employed in order to manipulate the future events allotted to a person according to their *bhagya* (fortune, allotted share).

13. In the game of cricket, a person who has scored one hundred runs or more is often referred to as a centurion.

14. The biodata asked for by Mahesh included not just the veteran blood donors' dates, times, and places of birth but also the dates of their first, eleventh, twenty-fifth, fiftieth, seventy-fifth, one-hundredth, and final donations. Details of their academic qualifications and the dates of their marriages and retirement were also requested.

15. Udupa (2016) suggests that the presence of astrology on TV channels shores up and re-entrenches conservative Brahminical orthodoxies in both the Hindi and Anglophone public spheres, which similarly may be a consequence of the recruitment techniques we have been discussing here.

16. http://www.flonnet.com/fl1915/19150130.htm.

17. See Copeman (2009a, chap. 4).

18. Two Sikh members of her security guard shot Indira Gandhi dead on 31 October 1984. She had estranged a large part of the Sikh community after government troops had stormed their most holy site, the Golden Temple in Punjab, in an effort to flush out militant separatists that the temple was apparently harboring. She was succeeded by her son Rajiv, who was ousted from office in 1989 after allegations of corruption. He was killed on 21 May 1991 by a suicide bomber who approached him under the guise of offering him a garland of flowers. The assassination is believed to have been orchestrated by the Liberation

Tigers of Tamil Eelam (LTTE) in retaliation for Rajiv's decision in 1987 to send Indian troops to Sri Lanka to help the Colombo government crush the LTTE.

19. See Copeman (2004).

20. A *kalash* is a brass or copper urn that is sometimes adorned with vermilion or mango leaves and is worshipped as the embodiment of Vishnu.

21. http://www.rss.org/rss-ksmr.htm.

22. http://jaago—india—jaago.blogspot.co.uk/2008/10/blood-donation-camp-at-jallian walla_03.html.

23. http://www.shreedarshan.com/saint-sadguru-aniruddha-bapu.htm. See also Sathya Sai Baba devotees' sensuous imitation of their guru's ascetic body (T. Srinivas 2012, 191). Both devotees (with respect to their guru) and gurus (with respect to other gurus), then, are mimetically inclined.

24. See Copeman (2012). For additional background on the events described here, see Baixas and Simon (2008).

25. Prior to the DSS controversy, the most notorious case of "impostor" guru-ship in recent times concerned the Sant Nirankari Mandal in the late 1970s (though see also Meeta and Rajivlochan [2007] on Baba Bhaniara's alleged crafting of a new "Granth"). Any devotional movement with links to Sikhism and a *dehdari* (i.e., living) guru is problematic from an orthodox Sikh perspective. However, as the example of the Radhasoamis indicates, judicious avoidance of direct associative claims can forestall serious tensions (Juergensmeyer 1996, 86).

26. Rooh Afza is a drink from concentrate containing fruits and herbs that is frequently served to guests throughout northern areas of the subcontinent and sometimes is used for breaking the Ramadan fast.

27. http://www.sepiamutiny.com/sepia/archives/004461.html.

28. http://www.youtube.com/comment_servlet?all_comments=1&v=tH0ZIBeEJvQ.

29. See Copeman (2009a, 130).

30. See Copeman (2009b, 18–19).

31. See Copeman (2009a, 86–87).

32. See Corsín Jiménez (2008, 186).

33. *Oxford Dictionary of English* (2016).

34. http://www.sikhisms.com/2009/03/worlds-largest-blood-donation-camp.html.

35. *DNA*, 14 March 2009.

36. http://www.sikhchic.com/article-detail.php?cat=12&id=750.

7. HEMATIC FUTURES

1. Former RSS leader K. S. Sudarshan, cited in *Times of India*, 19 October 2000.

2. Cf. Bryant (2002, 521–23), who found similar attitudes to be held by Greek Cypriots: "Many Greek Cypriots expressed the belief to me that Turkish Cypriots are Greeks 'by blood,' but that they had converted to Islam in the early years of Ottoman rule. Or as one young professional expressed it to me, 'Even if my brother goes astray [i.e., becomes a Muslim], he's still my brother.'"

3. http://siafdu.tripod.com/fernandes.html.

4. Banguru Laxman, quoted in *The Week*, 10 September 2000. "Respect" afforded to Muslims due to their supposed blood-tie with Hindus is additionally problematic because it is a "respect" that exists "not because they are Muslims and believe in Islam but because, in a more fundamental sense, they are not Muslims!" (Vanaik 1997, 309).

5. *Outlook*, 22 November 2002.

6. It is in part because of prior separations (e.g., based on blood and/or state practices of enumeration) that promissory images of "holding together" or mixing become possi-

ble. Blood, as a site of distinction, contains dual tendencies toward fissiparity and promissory holdings together (Copeman 2009c, 83).

7. The Ganesh portrait is antinomian insofar as it performs what in Marriott's schema is the antipurificatory action of mixing outside an exclusively Hindu world.

8. *Milli Gazette* 3, no. 20 (16–31 October 2002), emphasis added.

9. http://timesofindia.indiatimes.com/cms.dll/html/uncomp/articleshow?msid=47112107. There is a long history of youth organizations in India acting as dynamic vanguard "fronts" for political parties and other organizations. A notorious example is the Bajrang Dal, the militant youth wing of the Hindu supremacist organization Vishwa Hindu Parishad (World Hindu Council).

10. http://timesofindia.indiatimes.com/cms.dll/html/uncomp/articleshow?msid=47617357.

11. *The Hindu*, 20 May 2003.

12. http://timesofindia.indiatimes.com/cms.dll/html/uncomp/articleshow?msid=47208507.

13. *The Hindu*, 24 May 2003.

14. *The Hindu*, 24 May 2003; http://timesofindia.indiatimes.com/cms.dll/html/uncomp/articleshow?msid=47208507.

15. This sentence paraphrases Howe (2000, 77).

16. See also Hoeyer's (2013, 7) caveat that of course he "cannot change the fact that when we talk about materials flowing through bodies, we tend to talk about something already conceptualized as entities."

17. See Fraser and Valentine (2006) for reflections on blood's fluid motility, and Mayblin's (2013) rich account from northeastern Brazil, in which she suggests that "both the metaphorical and the literal capacities of blood are dependent upon the capacity of liquids in general, which are given inherently to movement, or which seem to travel outwards by their own volition, unless actively contained. Possibly there is something to be said about the molecular structure of liquid—perhaps of fluid forms in general—and their tendencies to travel. Rain, sweat, blood, tears, and broth are all substances that travel and, as with water in the Gospel of John, can expand both literally and figuratively" (54).

18. See Henley (1977, 45) on how "time is asymmetrically distributed between nonequals: the powerful share as little of their time as possible with the powerless while the powerless must give up time as the powerful demand it."

19. *The Tribune*, 1 February 2003.

20. http://jeevan.org/mainframe.htm.

21. The different time representations—one of disproportionate transfer, the other of saving family time—converge in narratives of the "extra" time received by way of transfusions that enable "precious family time" (Copeman 2005).

22. Recall that partonomies are hierarchies of part-whole relationships. Elaborating Davis's (1992) work on partonomies in and out of balance in material exchanges, Corsín Jiménez (2008, 186) foregrounds gift-giving as "an expression and effect of proportionality."

23. *Dainik Bhaskar*, 5 January 2010.

24. The specific episode of the show ("Sitare Humare" [Our Stars]) was broadcast on 9 February 2016. IBC24 (Indian Broadcast Channel 24) was known formerly as Zee 24 Ghante Chhattisgarh before separating from the Zee networks in 2013 and becoming IBC24.

25. We do not go into depth here since we have done so elsewhere (Copeman 2009a, chap. 6). Suffice it to say that Bapu is a media-savvy avatar guru whose devotees hold him to be, in their words, the "highest percentage" incarnation of Vishnu since Krishna. Having committed himself fully to spiritual activities in 1996, central to his teaching is his

prophecy of forthcoming untold natural and manmade disasters (*appatti*), brought on by man's wretched moral decline. The world will be seriously threatened but will not end; in 2025 the calamities will cease and *ramrajya*, Bapu's heavenly kingdom on earth, will appear.

26. This is a paraphrasing of Bear (2017, 147).

27. It is also, if we follow Nicholson Baker, a technology of time. The protagonist of Baker's *The Fermata* (1994) seeks more and more ways to pause time so he can pursue his dubious erotics with figures frozen in time. He has to keep finding new ways, since the tricks he discovers only work temporarily. Some of these involve his own bodily substances. He speculates about getting blood work done, for he is fascinated by the blood centrifuge machine, which displays words such as "speed" and "time" on it (115). Were his own blood spun in it, surely this would cause time to pause: a "temporal hematocrit" (112). His "perky little cells" would be spun into "alternative world orders, and that trickster knowledge would power [him] into raptures of self-knowledge" (114).

28. *Times of India*, 19 August 2011.

29. We first came across this poem on the alternative Indian news and commentary website Kafila.org (https://kafila.online/2009/02/18/castegender-in-a-poem-by-varavara -rao/).

30. *The Hindu*, 30 November 2007.

References

Adams, Vincanne, Kathleen Erwin, and Phuoc V. Le. 2010. "Governing through Blood: Biology, Donation, and Exchange in Urban China." In *Asian Biotech: Ethics and Communities of Fate*, edited by Aihwa Ong and Nancy N. Chen, 167–89. Durham, NC: Duke University Press.

Adams, Vincanne, Michelle Murphy, and Adele E. Clarke. 2009. "Anticipation: Technoscience, Life, Affect, Temporality." *Subjectivity* 28 (1): 246–65.

Ager, Sheila L. 2006. "The Power of Excess: Royal Incest and the Ptolemaic Dynasty." *Anthropologica* 48 (2): 165–86.

Alter, Joseph S. 1992. *The Wrestler's Body: Identity and Ideology in North India*. Berkeley: University of California Press.

——. 1993. "The Body of One Color: Indian Wrestling, the Indian State, and Utopian Somatics." *Cultural Anthropology* 8 (1): 49–72.

——. 1994a. "Celibacy, Sexuality, and the Transformation of Gender into Nationalism in North India." *Journal of Asian Studies* 53 (1): 45–66.

——. 1994b. "Somatic Nationalism: Indian Wrestling and Militant Hinduism." *Modern Asian Studies* 28 (3): 557–88.

——. 1996. "Gandhi's Body, Gandhi's Truth: Nonviolence and the Biomoral Imperative of Public Health." *Journal of Asian Studies* 55 (2): 301–22.

——. 1997. "Seminal Truth: A Modern Science of Male Celibacy in North India." *Medical Anthropology Quarterly* 11 (3): 275–98.

——. 2000. *Gandhi's Body: Sex, Diet, and the Politics of Nationalism*. Philadelphia: University of Pennsylvania Press.

——. 2008a. "Ayurveda and Sexuality: Sex Therapy and the 'Paradox of Virility.'" In *Modern and Global Ayurveda: Pluralism and Paradigms*, edited by Dagmar Wujastyk and Frederick M. Smith, 177–200. Albany: State University of New York Press.

——. 2008b. "Yoga *Shivir*: Performativity and the Study of Modern Yoga." In *Yoga in the Modern World*, edited by Mark Singleton and Jean Byrne, 36–48. New York: Routledge.

Ambedkar, B. R. 2014. *Annihilation of Caste*. Edited by S. Anand. London: Verso.

Amin, Shahid. 1984. "Gandhi as Mahatma: Gorakhpur District, Eastern UP, 1921–2." *Subaltern Studies* 3:1–61.

Amsterdam, Anthony G., and Jerome Bruner. 2000. *Minding the Law*. Cambridge, MA: Harvard University Press.

Anagnost, Ann S. 2006. "Strange Circulations: The Blood Economy in Rural China." *Economy and Society* 35 (4): 509–29.

Anand, Nikhil. 2017. *Hydraulic City: Water and the Infrastructures of Citizenship in Mumbai*. Durham, NC: Duke University Press.

Anidjar, Gil. 2011. "Blood." *Political Concepts: A Critical Lexicon* 1 (1). http://www.politicalconcepts.org/blood-gil-anidjar/.

——. 2014. *Blood: A Critique of Christianity*. New York: Columbia University Press.

Anker, Suzanne, and Sarah Franklin. 2011. "Specimens as Spectacles: Reframing Fetal Remains." *Social Text* 29 (1): 103–25.

Appadurai, Arjun. 1981. "Gastro-Politics in Hindu South Asia." *American Ethnologist* 8 (3): 494–511.

Arendt, Hannah. 1959. *The Human Condition: A Study of the Central Dilemmas Facing Modern Man*. New York: Doubleday.

——. 1977. "Public Rights and Private Interests." In *Small Comforts for Hard Times: Humanists on Public Policy*, edited by Michael Mooney and Florian Stuber, 103–8. New York: Columbia University Press.

Arnold, David. 1993. *Colonizing the Body: State Medicine and Epidemic Disease in Nineteenth-Century India*. Berkeley: University of California Press.

——. 2001. *Gandhi*. Harlow, UK: Pearson Education.

Asad, Talal. 2007. *On Suicide Bombing*. New York: Columbia University Press.

AVBDWB. 2015. *Gift of Blood: Official Organ of Association of Voluntary Blood Donors, West Bengal* (119).

Babb, Lawrence A. 2004. *Alchemies of Violence: Myths of Identity and the Life of Trade in Western India*. New Delhi: Sage.

Bairy T. S., Ramesh. 2009. "Brahmins in the Modern World: Association as Enunciation." *Contributions to Indian Sociology* 43: 89–120.

Baixas, Lionel, and Charlène Simon. 2008. "From Protesters to Martyrs: How to Become a 'True' Sikh." *South Asia Multidisciplinary Academic Journal*, para. 2.

Baker, Nicholson. 1994. *The Fermata*. New York: Vintage.

Banerjee, Dwaipayan. 2011. "No Biosociality in India." *BioSocieties* 6 (4): 488–92.

——. 2013. "Writing the Disaster: Substance Activism after Bhopal." *Contemporary South Asia* 21 (3): 230–42.

Banerjee, Dwaipayan, and Jacob Copeman. 2018. "Ungiven: Philanthropy as Critique." *Modern Asian Studies* 52 (1): 325–50.

Banerjee, Mukulika. 2014. *Why India Votes?* New Delhi: Routledge.

Banerjee, Prathama. 2013. "Time and Knowledge." In *Indian Political Thought*, edited by Pradip K. Datta and Sanjay Palshikar. *Political Science*, Vol. 3, edited by Achin Vanaik, 28–62. Delhi: Oxford University Press.

Banerjee, Sukanya. 2010. *Becoming Imperial Citizens: Indians in the Late-Victorian Empire*. Durham, NC: Duke University Press.

Barber, Karin. 2005. "Text and Performance in Africa." *Oral Tradition* 20 (2): 264–77.

——. 2007. *The Anthropology of Texts, Persons, and Publics: Oral and Written Culture in Africa and Beyond*. Cambridge: Cambridge University Press.

Barnett, Joshua Trey. 2015. "Toxic Portraits: Resisting Multiple Invisibilities in the Environmental Justice Movement." *Quarterly Journal of Speech* 101 (2): 405–25.

Bärnreuther, Sandra. 2015. "(Re-)production: An Ethnography of In Vitro Fertilization in India." PhD diss., University of Heidelberg.

——. 2018a. "Suitable Substances: How Biobanks (Re)Store Biologicals." *New Genetics and Society* 37 (4): 319–37.

——. 2018b. "Traders of Gametes, Brokers of Values: Middlemen's Mediations of Commercial Gamete Transactions in Delhi" (draft).

Barthes, Roland. 1972. *Mythologies*. Translated by Annette Lavers. New York: Hill and Wang.

Bataille, Georges. 1985. "The Notion of Expenditure." In *Visions of Excess: Selected Writings, 1927–1939*, edited and with an introduction by Allan Stoekl, 116–29. Translated by Allan Stoekl, with Carl R. Lovitt and Donald M. Leslie Jr. Manchester, UK: Manchester University Press.

——. 1988. *The Accursed Share: An Essay on General Economy*. Vol. 1, *Consumption*. Translated by Robert Hurley. New York: Zone.

Bate, Bernard. 2002. "Political Praise in Tamil Newspapers: The Poetry and Iconography of Democratic Power." In *Everyday Life in South Asia*, edited by Diane P. Mines and Sarah Lamb, 308–25. Bloomington: Indiana University Press.

———. 2009. *Tamil Oratory and the Dravidian Aesthetic: Democratic Practice in South India*. New York: Columbia University Press.

Bauman, Zygmunt. 2007. *Consuming Life*. Cambridge: Polity Press.

Bayly, Christopher A. 1986. "The Origins of Swadeshi (Home Industry): Cloth and Indian Society." In *The Social Life of Things: Commodities in Cultural Perspective*, edited by Arjun Appadurai, 285–322. Cambridge: Cambridge University Press.

———. 1996. *Empire and Information: Intelligence Gathering and Social Communication in India, 1780–1870*. Cambridge: Cambridge University Press.

Bayly, Christopher A., and Tim Harper. 2007. *Forgotten Wars: Freedom and Revolution in Southeast Asia*. Cambridge, MA: Belknap Press of Harvard University Press.

Bayly, Susan. 1999. *Caste, Society, and Politics in India from the Eighteenth-Century to the Modern Age*. Cambridge: Cambridge University Press.

Bear, Laura. 2012. "Sympathy and Its Boundaries: Necropolitics, Labour, and Waste on the Hooghly River." In *Economies of Recycling: The Global Transformation of Materials, Values, and Social Relations*, edited by Catherine Alexander and Joshua Reno, 185–203. London: Zed Books.

———. 2014a. "Doubt, Conflict, Mediation: The Anthropology of Modern Time." In "Doubt, Conflict, Mediation: The Anthropology of Modern Time," edited by Laura Bear, special issue, *Journal of the Royal Anthropological Institute* (N.S.) 20 (S1): 3–30.

———. 2014b. "For Labour: Ajeet's Accident and the Ethics of Technological Fixes in Time." In "Doubt, Conflict, Mediation: The Anthropology of Modern Time," edited by Laura Bear, special issue, *Journal of the Royal Anthropological Institute* (N.S.) 20 (S1): 71–88.

———. 2016a. "Time as Technique." *Annual Review of Anthropology* 45:487–502.

———. 2016b. "Afterword: For a New Materialist Analytics of Time." *Cambridge Journal of Anthropology* 34 (1): 125–29.

———. 2017. "Anthropological Futures: For a Critical Political Economy of Capitalist Time." *Social Anthropology* 25 (2): 142–58.

Belleau, Marie-Claire, and Rebecca Johnson. 2008. "I Beg to Differ: Interdisciplinary Questions about Law, Language, and Dissent." In *Law, Mystery, and the Humanities: Collected Essays*, edited by Logan Atkinson and Diana Majury, 145–66. Toronto: University of Toronto Press.

Bentley, M. E., and P. L. Griffiths. 2003. "The Burden of Anemia among Women in India." *European Journal of Clinical Nutrition* 57 (1): 52–60.

Berger, John. 2007. *Berger on Drawing*. London: Occasional Press.

Berger, Rachel. 2013. *Ayurveda Made Modern: Political Histories of Indigenous Medicine in North India, 1900–1955*. London: Palgrave Macmillan.

Berner, Boel. 2010. "(Dis)connecting Bodies: Blood Donation and Technical Change, Sweden 1915–1950." In *Technology and Medical Practice: Blood, Guts, and Machines*, edited by Ericka Johnson and Boel Berner, 179–201. London: Routledge.

Berner, Boel, and Maria Björkman. 2017. "Modernizing the Flow of Blood: Biomedical Technicians, Working Knowledge, and the Transformation of Swedish Blood Centre Practices." *Social Studies of Science* 47 (4): 485–510.

Beteille, Andre. 1991. "The Reproduction of Inequality: Occupation, Caste, and Family." *Contributions to Indian Sociology* 25 (1): 3–28.

Bhana, Surendra. 1975. "The Tolstoy Farm: Gandhi's Experiment in 'Co-operative Commonwealth.'" *South African Historical Journal* 7 (1): 88–100.

Bharadwaj, Aditya. 2003. "Why Adoption Is Not an Option in India: The Visibility of Infertility, the Secrecy of Donor Insemination, and Other Cultural Complexities." *Social Science and Medicine* 56 (9): 1867–80.

Bharadwaj, Aditya, and Peter Glasner. 2008. *Local Cells, Global Science: The Rise of Embryonic Stem Cell Research in India*. London: Routledge.

Bhatt, Chetan. 2001. *Hindu Nationalism: Origins, Ideologies, and Modern Myths*. Oxford: Berg.

Bhaṭṭācārya, Buddhadeba, Anila Biśvāsa, and Mihira Bhaṭṭācārya. 1997. *People's Power in Practice: 20 Years of Left Front in West Bengal*. Calcutta: National Book Agency.

Biehl, João Guilherme. 2005. *Vita: Life in a Zone of Social Abandonment*. Berkeley: University of California Press.

Biehl, João Guilherme, and Torben Eskerod. 2007. *Will to Live: AIDS Therapies and the Politics of Survival*. Princeton, NJ: Princeton University Press.

Bildhauer, Bettina. 2013. "Medieval European Conceptions of Blood: Truth and Human Integrity." In "Blood Will Out: Essays on Liquid Transfers and Flows," edited by Janet Carsten, special issue, *Journal of the Royal Anthropological Institute* (N.S.) 19 (S1): S57–S76.

Bird-David, Nurit. 1992. "Beyond 'The Original Affluent Society': A Culturalist Reformulation [and Comments and Reply]." *Current Anthropology* 33 (1): 25–47.

Bobel, Chris. 2010. *New Blood: Third-Wave Feminism and the Politics of Menstruation*. New Brunswick, NJ: Rutgers University Press.

Bode, Maarten. 2012. "Ayurveda in the Twenty-First Century: Logic, Practice, and Ethics." In *Medical Pluralism in Contemporary India*, edited by V. Sujatha and Leena Abraham, 59–76. New Delhi: Orient Blackswan.

Boland, Tom. 2013. "Towards an Anthropology of Critique: The Modern Experience of Liminality and Crisis." *Anthropological Theory* 13 (3): 222–39.

Bonelli, Cristóbal. 2014. "What Pehuenche Blood Does: Hemic Feasting, Intersubjective Participation, and Witchcraft in Southern Chile." *HAU: Journal of Ethnographic Theory* 4 (1): 105–27.

Bornstein, Erica. 2009. "The Impulse of Philanthropy." *Cultural Anthropology* 24 (4): 622–51.

Bose, Sugata. 2011. *His Majesty's Opponent: Subhas Chandra Bose and India's Struggle against Empire*. Cambridge, MA: Belknap Press of Harvard University Press.

Bray, Timothy John. 2001. "The Rational Use of Blood in India: Intervention to Promote Good Transfusion Practice." PhD diss., University of London.

Bray, Timothy John, and K. Prabhakar. 2002. "Editorial: Blood Policy and Transfusion Practice–India." *Tropical Medicine and International Health* 7 (6): 477–78.

Brhlikova, Petra, Patricia Jeffery, Gitanjali Priti Bhatia, and Sakshi Khurana. 2009. "Intrapartum Oxytocin (Mis) Use in South Asia." *Journal of Health Studies* 2:33–50.

Brown, Nik, Alison Kraft, and Paul Martin. 2006. "The Promissory Pasts of Blood Stem Cells." *BioSocieties* 1 (3): 329–48.

Bruner, Jerome S. 1986. *Actual Minds, Possible Worlds*. Cambridge, MA: Harvard University Press.

Bryant, Rebecca. 2002. "The Purity of Spirit and the Power of Blood: A Comparative Perspective on Nation, Gender, and Kinship in Cyprus." *Journal of the Royal Anthropological Institute* (N.S.) 8 (3): 509–30.

Buck-Morss, Susan. 1995. "Envisioning Capital: Political Economy on Display." *Critical Inquiry* 21 (2): 434–67.

Buckley, Thomas, and Alma Gottlieb. 1988. *Blood Magic: The Anthropology of Menstruation*. Berkeley: University of California Press.

Butler, Judith. 1993. *Bodies That Matter: On the Discursive Limits of Sex*. London: Routledge.

———. 1998. "Imitation and Gender Insubordination." In *Literary Theory: An Anthology*, edited by Julie Rivkin and Michael Ryan, 722–30. Oxford: Blackwell.

———. 2009. "Non-Thinking in the Name of the Normative." *Frames of War: When Is Life Grievable*, 137–63. London: Verso.

Bynum, Caroline Walker. 2007. *Wonderful Blood: Theology and Practice in Late Medieval Northern Germany and Beyond.* Philadelphia: University of Pennsylvania Press.

Calvino, Italo. (1967) 2014. "Blood, Sea." In *Vapor.* Vol. 2, *Textures of the Anthropocene,* edited by Katrin Klingan, Ashkan Sepahvand, Christoph Rosol, and Bernd M. Scherer, 43–59. Berlin: Revolver.

Camporesi, Piero. 1995. *Juice of Life: Symbolic and Magic Significance of Blood.* New York: Continuum.

Candea, Matei, and Giovanni Da Col. 2012. "The Return to Hospitality." In "The Return to Hospitality: Strangers, Guests, and Ambiguous Encounters," edited by Matei Candea and Giovanni Da Col, special issue, *Journal of the Royal Anthropological Institute* (N.S.) 18 (S1): S1–S19.

Caple James, Erica. 2012. "Witchcraft, Bureaucraft, and the Social Life of (US) Aid in Haiti." *Cultural Anthropology* 27 (1): 50–75.

Carney, Scott. 2011. *The Red Market: On the Trail of the World's Organ Brokers, Bone Thieves, Blood Farmers, and Child Traffickers.* London: HarperCollins.

Carrithers, Michael. 2005. "Why Anthropologists Should Study Rhetoric." *Journal of the Royal Anthropological Institute* (N.S.) 11 (3): 577–83.

———. 2010. "A Social Form and Its Craft-y Use." *Contemporary South Asia* 18 (3): 253–65.

Carsten, Janet. 2004. *After Kinship.* Cambridge: Cambridge University Press.

———. 2007. "Testing the Limits of Kinship and Biomedical Knowledge in Malaysia and Britain." Paper presented at the American Anthropological Association annual meeting, November 2007.

———. 2011. "Substance and Relationality: Blood in Contexts." *Annual Review of Anthropology* 40:19–35.

———. 2013. "Introduction: Blood Will Out." In "Blood Will Out: Essays on Liquid Transfers and Flows," edited by Janet Carsten, special issue, *Journal of the Royal Anthropological Institute* (N.S.) 19 (S1): S1–S23.

Chakrabarty, Dipesh. 2000. "Subaltern Studies and Postcolonial Historiography." *Nepantla: Views from South* 1 (1): 9–32.

Charbonneau, Johanne, and André Smith, eds. 2016. *Giving Blood: The Institutional Making of Altruism.* London: Routledge.

Chatterjee, Partha. 1997. *Our Modernity.* Rotterdam: South-South Exchange Programme for Research on the History of Development and the Council for the Development of Social Science Research in Africa.

———. 1998. "Beyond the Nation? Or Within?" *Social Text* (56): 57–69.

———. 1999. "Modernity, Democracy, and a Political Negotiation of Death." *South Asia Research* 19 (2): 103–19.

———. 2004. *The Politics of the Governed: Reflections on Political Society in Most of the World.* New York: Columbia University Press.

Chaudry, Shruti. 2016. "Lived Experiences of Marriage: Regional and Cross-Regional Brides in Rural North India." PhD diss., University of Edinburgh.

Chidester, David. 2005. *Authentic Fakes: Religion and American Popular Culture.* Berkeley: University of California Press.

Chowdhury, Indira. 2001. *The Frail Hero and Virile History: Gender and the Politics of Culture in Colonial Bengal.* Delhi: Oxford University Press.

Chozinski, Brittany Anne. 2016. "Science Fiction as Critique of Science: Organ Transplantation and the Body." *Bulletin of Science, Technology, and Society* 36 (1): 58–66.

Chua, Jocelyn Lim. 2011. "Making Time for the Children: Self-Temporalization and the Cultivation of the Antisuicidal Subject in South India." *Cultural Anthropology* 26 (1): 112–37.

Clifford, James, and George E. Marcus, eds. 1986. *Writing Culture: The Poetics and Politics of Ethnography.* Berkeley: University of California Press.

Cohen, Erik. 2012. "Contesting Discourses of Blood in the 'Red Shirts' Protests in Bangkok." *Journal of Southeast Asian Studies* 43 (2): 216–33.

Cohen, Gillian. 1989. *Memory in the Real World.* Hove: Lawrence Erlbaum.

Cohen, Lawrence. 1995a. "Holi in Banaras and the Mahaland of Modernity." In "Inqueery/Intheory/Indeed," edited by Geeta Patel and Kevin Kopelson, special issue, *GLQ* 2 (4): 399–424.

———. 1995b. "The Epistemological Carnival: Meditations on Disciplinary Intentionality and Ayurveda." In *Knowledge and the Scholarly Medical Traditions,* edited by Don Bates, 320–43. Cambridge: Cambridge University Press.

———. 1997. "Semen, Irony and the Atom Bomb." *Medical Anthropology Quarterly* 11 (3): 301–3.

———. 1998. *No Aging in India: Alzheimer's, the Bad Family, and Other Modern Things.* Berkeley: University of California Press.

———. 1999. "Where It Hurts: Indian Material for an Ethics of Organ Transplantation." *Daedalus* 128 (4): 135–65.

———. 2001. "The Other Kidney: Biopolitics beyond Recognition." *Body and Society* 7 (2–3): 9–29.

———. 2003. "Senility and Irony's Age." *Social Analysis* 47 (2): 122–34.

———. 2004. "Operability: Surgery at the Margin of the State." In *Anthropology in the Margins of the State,* edited by Veena Das and Deborah Poole, 165–90. Santa Fe, NM: School of American Research Press.

———. 2005. "Operability, Bioavailability, and Exception." In *Global Assemblages: Technology, Politics, and Ethics as Anthropological Problems,* edited by Aihwa Ong and Stephen Collier, 79–90. Oxford: Blackwell Publishing.

———. 2007. "Song for Pushkin." *Daedalus* 136 (2): 103–15.

———. 2008. "Science, Politics, and Dancing Boys: Propositions and Accounts." *Parallax* 14 (3): 35–47.

———. 2011a. "Migrant Supplementarity: Remaking Biological Relatedness in Chinese Military and Indian Five-Star Hospitals." *Body and Society* 17 (2–3): 31–54.

———. 2011b. "Accusations of Illiteracy and the Medicine of the Organ." *Social Research* 78 (1): 123–42.

———. 2012. "The Gay Guru: Fallibility, Unworldliness, and the Scene of Instruction." In *The Guru in South Asia,* edited by Jacob Copeman and Aya Ikegame, 97–112. London: Routledge.

———. 2013. "Given Over to Demand: Excorporation as Commitment." *Contemporary South Asia* 21 (3): 318–32.

———. 2017. "Duplicate." *South Asia: Journal of South Asian Studies* 40 (2): 301–4.

Colebrook, Claire. 2010. *Deleuze and the Meaning of Life.* London: Continuum.

Comaroff, Jean, and John L. Comaroff. 1999. "Occult Economies and the Violence of Abstraction: Notes from the South African Postcolony." *American Ethnologist* 26 (2): 279–303.

Cooper, Melinda. 2006. "Pre-empting Emergence: The Biological Turn in the War on Terror." *Theory, Culture, and Society* 23 (4): 113–35.

Copeman, Jacob. 2004. "'Blood Will Have Blood': A Study in Indian Political Ritual." *Social Analysis* 48 (3): 126–48.

———. 2005. "Veinglory: Exploring Processes of Blood Transfer between Persons." *Journal of the Royal Anthropological Institute* (N.S.) 11 (3): 465–85.

———. 2006. "Cadaver Donation as Ascetic Practice in India." *Social Analysis* 50 (1): 103–26.

———. 2008. "Violence, Non-violence, and Blood Donation in India." *Journal of the Royal Anthropological Institute* (N.S.) 14 (2): 278–96.

———. 2009a. *Veins of Devotion: Blood Donation and Religious Experience in North India.* New Brunswick, NJ: Rutgers University Press.

———. 2009b. "Introduction: Blood Donation, Bioeconomy, Culture." In "Blood Donation, Bioeconomy, Culture," edited by Jacob Copeman, special issue, *Body and Society* 15 (2): 1–28.

———. 2009c. "Gathering Points: Blood Donation and the Scenography of 'National Integration' in India." In "Blood Donation, Bioeconomy, Culture," edited by Jacob Copeman, special issue, *Body and Society* 15 (2): 71–99.

———. 2011. "The Gift and Its Forms of Life in Contemporary India." *Modern Asian Studies* 45 (5): 1051–94.

———. 2012. "The Mimetic Guru: Tracing the Real in Sikh-Dera Sacha Sauda Relations." In *The Guru in South Asia: New Interdisciplinary Perspectives*, edited by Jacob Copeman and Aya Ikegame, 156–80. London: Routledge.

———. 2013a. "The Art of Bleeding: Memory, Martyrdom, and Portraits in Blood." In "Blood Will Out: Essays on Liquid Transfers and Flows," edited by Janet Carsten, special issue, *Journal of the Royal Anthropological Institute* (N.S.) 19 (S1): S149–S171.

———. 2013b. "Portraits of Substance: Image, Text, and Intervention in India's Sanguinary Politics." *Contemporary South Asia* 21 (3): 243–59.

———. 2015. "Secularism's Names: Commitment to Confusion and the Pedagogy of the Name." *South Asia Multidisciplinary Academic Journal* (12).

Copeman, Jacob, and Johannes Quack. 2015. "Godless People and Dead Bodies: Materiality and the Morality of Atheist Materialism." *Social Analysis* 59 (2): 40–61.

———. 2018. "Contemporary Religiosities." In *Critical Themes in Indian Sociology*, edited by Sanjay Srivastava, Janaki Abraham, and Yasmeen Arif, 44–61. Delhi: Sage.

Copeman, Jacob, and Deepa S. Reddy. 2012. "The Didactic Death: Publicity, Instruction, and Body Donation." *HAU: Journal of Ethnographic Theory* 2 (2): 59–83.

Corsín Jiménez, Alberto. 2004. "The Form of the Relation, or Anthropology's Enchantment with the Algebraic Imagination." Unpublished manuscript.

———. 2008. "Well-Being in Anthropological Balance: Remarks on Proportionality as Political Imagination." In *Culture and Well-Being: Anthropological Approaches to Freedom and Political Ethics*, edited by Alberto Corsín Jiménez, 180–97. London: Pluto Press.

———. 2013. *An Anthropological Trompe L'Oeil for a Common World: An Essay on the Economy of Knowledge.* Oxford: Berghahn Books.

Corsín Jiménez, Alberto, and Adolfo Estalella. 2016. "Ethnography: A Prototype." *Ethnos.* DOI: 10.1080/00141844.2015.1133688, 1–21.

Cronon, William, ed. 1995. *Uncommon Ground: Toward Reinventing Nature.* New York: W. W. Norton.

Dalrymple, William. 1993. *City of Djinns: A Year in Delhi.* New York: Penguin.

Das, Nabina. 2015. "Blood, Period." *Economic and Political Weekly* 50 (16): 95–96.

Das, Veena. 1988. "Femininity and the Orientation to the Body." In *Socialisation, Education, and Women: Explorations in Gender Identity*, edited by Karuna Chanana, 193–207. New Delhi: Orient Longman.

———. 2004. "The Signature of the State: The Paradox of Illegibility." In *Anthropology in the Margins of the State*, edited by Veena Das and Deborah Poole, 225–52. Santa Fe, NM: School of American Research Press.

———. 2007. *Life and Words: Violence and the Descent into the Ordinary.* Berkeley: University of California Press.

——. 2010. "Engaging the Life of the Other: Love and Everyday Life." In *Ordinary Ethics: Anthropology, Language, and Action*, edited by Michael Lambek, 376–99. New York: Fordham University Press.

——. 2012. "The Dreamed Guru: The Entangled Lives of the Amil and the Anthropologist." In *The Guru in South Asia: New Interdisciplinary Perspectives*, edited by Jacob Copeman and Aya Ikegame, 133–55. London: Routledge.

——. 2015a. "What Does Ordinary Ethics Look Like?" In *Four Lectures on Ethics: Anthropological Perspectives*, edited by Michael Lambek, Veena Das, Didier Fassin, and Webb Keane, 53–125. Chicago: HAU Books.

——. 2015b. *Affliction: Health, Disease, Poverty*. New York: Fordham University Press.

Davidson, Arnold. 2008. "In Praise of Counter-Conduct." In "Foucault across the Disciplines," edited by Colin Koopman, special issue, *History of the Human Sciences* 24 (4): 25–41.

Davis, John. 1992. *Exchange*. Minneapolis: University of Minnesota Press.

Davis, K. 1941. "Intermarriage in Caste Societies." *American Anthropologist* 43 (3): 376–95.

Davis, R. H. 1993. "Indian Art Objects as Loot." *Journal of Asian Studies* 52 (1): 22–48.

Dawkins, Richard. 2006. *The Selfish Gene*, 30th anniversary ed. New York: Oxford University Press.

Derrida, Jacques. 1992. *Given Time: I. Counterfeit Money*. Translated by Peggy Kamuf. Chicago: University of Chicago Press.

——. 1997. "The Time of the King." In *The Logic of the Gift: Towards an Ethic of Generosity*, edited by Alan D. Schrift, 121–47. London: Routledge.

Deshpande, Satish, and Mary E. John. 2010. "The Politics of Not Counting Caste." *Economic and Political Weekly* 45:39–42.

Devji, Faisal. 2004. "Globalization and Apocalypse." *Yale Politic* 5 (4): 22–24.

Dixon-Woods, Mary, Duncan Wilson, Clare Jackson, Debbie Cavers, and Kathy Pritchard-Jones. 2008. "Human Tissue and 'The Public': The Case of Childhood Cancer Tumour Banking." *BioSocieties* 3 (1): 57–80.

Doniger, Wendy. 1976. *The Origins of Evil in Hindu Mythology*. Berkeley: University of California Press.

Douglas, Mary. 1967. "Primitive Rationing: A Study in Controlled Exchange." In *Themes in Economic Anthropology*, edited by Raymond Firth, 119–45. London: Tavistock.

——. (1966) 2002. *Purity and Danger: An Analysis of Concepts of Pollution and Taboo*. London: Routledge.

——. (1970) 2003. *Natural Symbols: Explorations in Cosmology*. London: Routledge.

Dumit, Joseph. 2012. *Drugs for Life: How Pharmaceutical Companies Define Our Health*. Durham, NC: Duke University Press.

Durkheim, Emile. 1951. *Suicide: A Study in Sociology*. Glencoe: Free Press.

——. (1895) 1964. *The Rules of Sociological Method*. New York: Free Press.

Duschinski, Haley. 2010. "Reproducing Regimes of Impunity: Fake Encounters and the Informalization of Everyday Violence in Kashmir Valley." *Cultural Studies* 24 (1): 110–32.

Ecks, Stefan. 2014. *Eating Drugs: Psychopharmaceutical Pluralism in India*. New York: New York University Press.

——. 2016. "Ethnographic Critiques of Global Mental Health." *Transcultural Psychiatry* 53 (6): 804–8.

Egorova, Yulia. 2011. "Castes of Genes? Representing Human Genetic Diversity in India." *Genomics, Society, and Policy* 6 (3): 1–18.

Engelke, Matthew. 2007. *A Problem of Presence: Beyond Scripture in an African Christian Church*. Berkeley: University of California Press.

Erwin, Kathleen. 2006. "The Circulatory System: Blood Procurement, AIDS, and the Social Body in China." *Medical Anthropology Quarterly* 20 (2): 139–59.

Erwin, Kathleen, Vincanne Adams, and Phuoc Le. 2009. "Glorious Deeds: Work Unit Blood Donation and Postsocialist Desires in Urban China." In "Blood Donation, Bioeconomy, Culture," edited by Jacob Copeman, special issue, *Body and Society* 15 (2): 51–70.

Evens, T. M. S. 2008. *Anthropology as Ethics: Nondualism and the Conduct of Sacrifice.* Oxford: Berghahn Books.

Faber, Jean Claude. 2004. "Quality Management of Blood Donors and the Impact on Donor Recruitment." Lecture given at the ninth International Colloquium on the Recruitment of Voluntary, Non-remunerated Blood Donors, April 3–7, Beijing.

Feldman, Allen. 1991. *Formations of Violence: The Narrative of the Body and Political Terror in Northern Ireland.* Chicago: University of Chicago Press.

Finkler, Kaja. 2001. "The Kin of the Gene: The Medicalization of Family and Kinship in American Society." *Current Anthropology* 42 (2): 235–63.

Fischer, Michael M. J. 2009. *Anthropological Futures.* Durham, NC: Duke University Press.

Fleming, Chris, and John O'Carroll. 2010. "The Art of the Hoax." *Parallax* 16 (4): 45–59.

Fontein, Joost, and John Harries. 2013. "The Vitality and Efficacy of Human Substances." *Critical African Studies* 5 (3): 115–26.

Foucault, Michel. 1977. "Nietzsche, Genealogy, History." In *Language, Counter-Memory, Practice: Selected Essays and Interviews*, edited and with an introduction by Donald F. Bouchard, translated by Donald F. Bouchard and Sherry Simon, 139–64. Ithaca, NY: Cornell University Press.

———. 1978. *The History of Sexuality.* Translated by Robert Hurley. New York: Pantheon Books.

———. 1991. "What Is Enlightenment?" In *The Foucault Reader*, edited by Paul Rabinow, translated by Catherine Porter, 32–50. London: Penguin.

———. 1996. "The Simplest of Pleasures." In *Foucault Live (Interviews, 1961–1984)*, edited by Sylvère Lotringer, translated by Lysa Hochroth and John Johnston, 295–96. New York: Semiotext(e).

———. 2007. *Security, Territory, Population: Lectures at the Collège de France, 1977–78.* Edited by Arnold I. Davidson and translated by Graham Burchell. Basingstoke: Palgrave Macmillan.

Franklin, Sarah. 2013. "From Blood to Genes? Rethinking Consanguinity in the Context of Geneticization." In *Blood and Kinship: Matter for Metaphor from Ancient Rome to the Present*, edited by Christopher H. Johnson, Bernhard Jussen, David Warren Sabean, and Simon Teuscher, 285–306. Oxford: Berghahn Books.

———. 2014. "Analogic Return: The Reproductive Life of Conceptuality." In "Social Theory after Strathern," edited by Alice Street and Jacob Copeman, special issue, *Theory, Culture, and Society* 31 (2–3): 243–61.

Fraser, Suzanne, and Kylie Valentine. 2006. "'Making Blood Flow': Materializing Blood in Body Modification and Blood-borne Virus Prevention." *Body and Society* 12 (1): 97–119.

Freitag, Sandria. 1996. "Contesting in Public: Colonial Legacies and Contemporary Communalism." In *Making India Hindu: Religion, Community, and the Politics of Democracy in India*, edited by David Ludden, 211–34. Delhi: Oxford University Press.

Fruzzetti, Lina, and Ákos Östör. 1982. "Bad Blood in Bengal: Category and Affect in the Study of Kinship, Caste, and Marriage." In *Concepts of Person: Kinship, Caste, and Marriage in India*, edited by Lina Fruzzetti, Ákos Östör, and Steve Barnett, 31–55. Delhi: Oxford University Press.

Fruzzetti, Lina, Ákos Östör, and Steve Barnett. 1982. "The Cultural Construction of the Person in Bengal and Tamil Nadu." In *Concepts of Person: Kinship, Caste, and Marriage in India*, edited by Lina Fruzzetti, Ákos Östör, and Steve Barnett, 8–30. Delhi: Oxford University Press.

Fry, Tony. 1999. *A New Design Philosophy: An Introduction to Defuturing*. Sydney: University of New South Wales Press.

Fuller, Christopher John. 1992. "India through Hindu Categories. Edited by McKim Marriott. New Delhi: Sage Publications, 1990. xvi, 209 pp. $32.00." *Journal of Asian Studies* 51 (2): 432–33.

——. 2004. *The Camphor Flame: Popular Hinduism and Society in India*. Princeton, NJ: Princeton University Press.

Gambetta, Diego. 2005. *Making Sense of Suicide Missions*. Oxford: Oxford University Press.

Gandhi, Ajay. 2013. "Standing Still and Cutting in Line: The Culture of the Queue in India." *South Asia Multidisciplinary Academic Journal*.

Gandhi, Leela. 1996. "Concerning Violence: The Limits and Circulations of Gandhian 'Ahimsa' or Passive Resistance." *Cultural Critique* (35): 105–47.

Gandhi, Mohandas K. 1946a. *Hind Swaraj*. Ahmedabad: Navajivan Publishing House.

——. 1946b. *The Gospel of Selfless Action: Or, The Gita according to Gandhi*. Ahmedabad: Navajivan Publishing House.

——. 1999. *The Collected Works of Mahatma Gandhi (Electronic Book)*, 98 vols. (CWG). New Delhi: Publications Division Government of India.

Gandhi, Mohandas, and Mahadev Haribhai Desai. 1949. *Gandhi, an Autobiography: The Story of My Experiments with Truth*. London: Phoenix Press.

Gane, Mike. 1998. "Canguilhem and the Problem of Pathology." *Economy and Society* 27 (2–3): 298–312.

Garro, Linda C. 1988. "Explaining High Blood Pressure: Variation in Knowledge about Illness." *American Ethnologist* 15 (1): 98–119.

Gell, Alfred. 1992. *The Anthropology of Time: Cultural Constructions of Temporal Maps and Images*. Oxford: Berg.

——. 1993. *Wrapping in Images: Tattooing in Polynesia*. Oxford: Clarendon Press.

——. 1998. *Art and Agency: An Anthropological Theory*. Oxford: Clarendon Press.

——. 1999. "The Technology of Enchantment and the Enchantment of Technology." In Alfred Gell, *The Art of Anthropology: Essays and Diagrams*, edited by Eric Hirsch, 159–86. London: Athlone Press.

Godelier, Maurice. 1999. *The Enigma of the Gift*. Translated by Nora Scott. Cambridge: Polity.

Gold, Daniel. 1987. *The Lord as Guru: Hindi Sants in the North Indian Tradition*. Oxford: Oxford University Press.

——. 2012. "Continuities as Gurus Change." In *The Guru in South Asia: New Interdisciplinary Perspectives*, edited by Jacob Copeman and Aya Ikegame, 243–54. London: Routledge.

Gould, William. 2011. *Religion and Conflict in Modern South Asia*. Cambridge: Cambridge University Press.

Guenzi, Caterina. 2012. "The Allotted Share: Managing Fortune in Astrological Counseling in Contemporary India." *Social Analysis* 56 (2): 39–55.

Han, Clara, and Veena Das. 2015. "Introduction: A Concept Note." In *Living and Dying in the Contemporary World: A Compendium*, edited by Veena Das and Clara Han, 1–37. Oakland: University of California Press.

Handler, Richard. 1986. "Authenticity." *Anthropology Today* 2 (1): 2–4.

Hanna, Bridget, Ward Morehouse, and Satinath Sarangi, eds. 2005. *The Bhopal Reader: Remembering Twenty Years of the World's Worst Industrial Disaster*. Goa: Other India Press.

Hansen, Thomas Blom. 1999. *The Saffron Wave: Democracy and Hindu Nationalism in Modern India*. Princeton, NJ: Princeton University Press.

——. 2001. *Wages of Violence: Naming and Identity in Postcolonial Bombay*. Princeton, NJ: Princeton University Press.

Haraway, Donna J. 1985. "A Manifesto for Cyborgs: Science, Technology, and Socialist Feminism in the 1980s." *Socialist Review* 15 (2): 65–107.

——. 1995. "Universal Donors in a Vampire Culture: It's All in the Family: Biological Kinship Categories in the Twentieth-Century United States." In *Uncommon Ground: Toward Reinventing Nature*, edited by William Cronon, 321–66. New York: W. W. Norton.

Harrison, Simon. 1992. "Ritual as Intellectual Property." *Man* (N.S.) 27 (2): 225–44.

Harvey, David. 1989. *The Condition of Postmodernity: An Enquiry into the Origins of Cultural Change*. Oxford: Blackwell.

——. 2005. *A Brief History of Neoliberalism*. Oxford: Oxford University Press.

Hayden, Corinne P. 1995. "Gender, Genetics, and Generation: Reformulating Biology in Lesbian Kinship." *Cultural Anthropology* 10 (1): 41–63.

——. 2007. "Taking as Giving: Bioscience, Exchange, and the Politics of Benefit-Sharing." *Social Studies of Science* 37 (5): 729–58.

Healy, Kieran. 2006. *Last Best Gifts: Altruism and the Market for Human Blood and Organs*. Chicago: University of Chicago Press.

Heesterman, Johannes Cornelius. 1985. *The Inner Conflict of Tradition: Essays in Indian Ritual, Kinship, and Society*. Chicago: University of Chicago Press.

Helmreich, Stefan. 2009. *Alien Ocean: Anthropological Voyages in Microbial Seas*. Berkeley: University of California Press.

——. 2014. "Blood, Waves: On Italo Calvino's 'Blood, Sea.'" In *Vapor*. Vol. 2, *Textures of the Anthropocene*, edited by Katrin Klingan, Ashkan Sepahvand, Christoph Rosol, and Bernd M. Scherer, 49–53. Berlin: Revolver.

Henley, Nancy M. 1977. *Body Politics: Power, Sex, and Nonverbal Communication*. Englewood Cliffs, NJ: Prentice-Hall.

Heuzé, Gerard. 1992. "Shiv Sena and 'National' Hinduism." *Economic and Political Weekly* 27 (41): 2253–63.

Hirschkind, Charles. 2001. "Civic Virtue and Religious Reason: An Islamic Counterpublic." *Cultural Anthropology* 16 (1): 3–34.

Hodges, Sarah. 2006. "Indian Eugenics in an Age of Reform." In *Reproductive Health in India: History, Politics, Controversies*, edited by Sarah Hodges, 115–38. New Delhi: Orient Longman.

——. 2010. "South Asia's Eugenic Past." In *The Oxford Handbook of the History of Eugenics*, edited by Alison Bashford and Philippa Levine, 228–42. Oxford: Oxford University Press.

——. 2013. "Umbilical Cord Blood Banking and Its Interruptions: Notes from Chennai, India." *Economy and Society* 42 (4): 651–70.

——. 2017. *Contraception, Colonialism, and Commerce: Birth Control in South India, 1920–1940*. London: Routledge.

Hoeyer, Klaus. 2009. "Tradable Body Parts? How Bone and Recycled Prosthetic Devices Acquire a Price without Forming a 'Market.'" *BioSocieties* 4 (2–3): 239–56.

——. 2013. *Exchanging Human Bodily Material: Rethinking Bodies and Markets*. Dordrecht: Springer Science & Business Media.

Holmes, Douglas R., and George E. Marcus. 2008. "Para-ethnography." In *The SAGE Encyclopedia of Qualitative Research Methods*, edited by Lisa M. Given, 595–97. London: SAGE Publications.

Howe, Leo. 2000. "Risk, Ritual and Performance." *Journal of the Royal Anthropological Institute* (N.S.) 6 (1): 63–79.

Inden, Ronald B., and Ralph W. Nicholas. 2005. *Kinship in Bengali Culture*. New Delhi: Chronicle Books.

Indian Ministry of Health and Family Welfare. 2003. "National Blood Policy." In *The Blood Bankers' Legal Handbook*, by M. L. Sarin, 44–53. Chandigarh: Sarin Memorial Legal Aid Foundation.

Ingold, Tim. 2007. "Materials against Materiality." *Archaeological Dialogues* 14 (1): 1–16.

Iyer, Raghavan. 1978. *The Moral and Political Thought of Gandhi*. New Delhi: Oxford University Press.

Jacob, Preminda. 2009. *Celluloid Deities: The Visual Culture of Cinema and Politics in South India*. Lanham, MD: Lexington Books.

Jalal, Ayesha. 1985. *The Sole Spokesman: Jinnah, the Muslim League, and the Demand for Pakistan*. Cambridge: Cambridge University Press.

Jeffery, Patricia. 2014a. "Underserved and Overdosed? Muslims and the Pulse Polio Initiative in Rural North India." In *Development Failure and Identity Politics in Uttar Pradesh*, edited by Roger Jeffery, Craig Jeffrey, and Jens Lerche, 46–74. Delhi: Sage.

——. 2014b. "Supply-and-Demand Demographics: Dowry, Daughter Aversion, and Marriage Markets in Contemporary North India." *Contemporary South Asia* 22 (2): 171–88.

Jeffrey, Robin. 1976. "Temple-Entry Movement in Travancore, 1860–1940." *Social Scientist* 4 (8): 3–27.

Jerstad, Heid. 2016. "Weathering Relationships: The Intra-action of People with Climate in Himalayan India." PhD diss., University of Edinburgh.

Jodhka, Surinder S., and Ghanshyam Shah. 2010. "Comparative Contexts of Discrimination: Caste and Untouchability in South Asia." *Economic and Political Weekly* 45 (48): 99–106.

Johnson, Christopher D. 2010. *Hyperboles: The Rhetoric of Excess in Baroque Literature and Thought*. Cambridge, MA: Harvard University Press.

Johnson, Christopher H., Bernhard Jussen, David Warren Sabean, and Simon Teuscher, eds. 2013. *Blood and Kinship: Matter for Metaphor from Ancient Rome to the Present*. Oxford: Berghahn Books.

Juergensmeyer, Mark. 1996. *Radhasoami Reality: The Logic of a Modern Faith*. Corrected ed. Princeton, NJ: Princeton University Press.

Kalathuveettil, Thomas, ed. 1992. *Serving Youth Today in India: Papers, Reports, and Final Statement of the All India Research Seminar on Youth, Kristu Jyoti College, Bangalore 560036, Oct. 28–Nov. 1, 1992*. Bangalore: Kristu Jyoti Publications.

Kapferer, Bruce, ed. 1976. *Transaction and Meaning: Directions in the Anthropology of Exchange and Symbolic Behavior*. Philadelphia: Institute for the Study of Human Issues.

Kaur, Kawaljit. 2014. "Anaemia 'A Silent Killer' among Women in India: Present Scenario." *European Journal of Zoological Research* 3 (1): 32–36.

Kaur, Raminder. 2001. "Rethinking the Public Sphere: The Ganapati Festival and Media Competitions in Mumbai." *South Asia Research* 21 (1): 23–50.

Kavuri-Bauer, Santhi. 2011. *Monumental Matters: The Power, Subjectivity, and Space of India's Mughal Architecture*. Durham, NC: Duke University Press.

Kelty, Christopher M. 2008. *Two Bits: The Cultural Significance of Free Software*. Durham, NC: Duke University Press.

Kent, Julie. 2008. "The Fetal Tissue Economy: From the Abortion Clinic to the Stem Cell Laboratory." *Social Science and Medicine* 67 (11): 1747–56.

Khilnani, Sunil. 1997. *The Idea of India*. New Delhi: Penguin Books India.

Kierkegaard, Søren. 1983. *Repetition: A Venture in Experimenting Psychology, by Constantin Constantius*. In *Fear and Trembling; Repetition*, edited and translated by Howard V. Hong and Edna H. Hong. Vol. 6, *Kierkegaard's Writings*, 129–231. Princeton, NJ: Princeton University Press.

Kirmayer, Laurence J., and Eugene Raikhel. 2009. "From *Amrita* to Substance D: Psychopharmacology, Political Economy, and Technologies of the Self." *Transcultural Psychiatry* 46 (5): 5–15.

Kockelman, Paul, and Anya Bernstein. 2012. "Semiotic Technologies, Temporal Reckoning, and the Portability of Meaning, or Modern Modes of Temporality—Just How Abstract Are They?" *Anthropological Theory* 12 (3): 320–48.

Konrad, Monica. 2005. *Nameless Relations: Anonymity, Melanesia, and Reproductive Gift Exchange between British Ova Donors and Recipients*. Oxford: Berghahn Books.

Krause, Inga-Britt. 1989. "Sinking Heart: A Punjabi Communication of Distress." *Social Science and Medicine* 29 (4): 563–75.

Krishnamurthy, Mathangi. 2018. *1800-Worlds: The Making of the Indian Call Centre Economy*. Delhi: Oxford University Press.

Kumar, Ravinder. 1971. *Essays on Gandhian Politics: The Rowlatt Satyagraha of 1919*. Oxford: Clarendon Press.

Laidlaw, James. 1995. *Riches and Renunciation: Religion, Economy, and Society among the Jains*. Oxford: Clarendon Press.

——. 2004. "Introduction." In *Ritual and Memory: Toward a Comparative Anthropology of Religion*, edited by James Laidlaw and Harvey Whitehouse, 89–109. Walnut Creek, CA: Altamira Press.

Lallemand-Stempak, Jean-Paul. 2016. "What Flows between Us: Blood Donation and Transfusion in the United States (Nineteenth to Twentieth Centuries)." In *Giving Blood: The Institutional Making of Altruism*, edited by Johanne Charbonneau and André Smith, 21–32. London: Routledge.

Lamb, Sarah. 2005. "The Politics of Dirt and Gender: Body Techniques in Bengali India." In *Dirt, Undress, and Difference: Critical Perspectives on the Body's Surface*, edited by Adeline Masquelier, 350–83. Bloomington: Indiana University Press.

Lambek, Michael. 2008. "Value and Virtue." *Anthropological Theory* 8 (2): 133–57.

——, ed. 2010. *Ordinary Ethics: Anthropology, Language, and Action*. New York: Fordham University Press.

Lambert, Helen. 2000. "Sentiment and Substance in North Indian Forms of Relatedness." In *Cultures of Relatedness: New Approaches to the Study of Kinship*, edited by Janet Carsten, 73–89. Cambridge: Cambridge University Press.

Landecker, Hannah. 2007. *Culturing Life: How Cells Became Technologies*. Cambridge, MA: Harvard University Press.

Langford, Jean. 2002. *Fluent Bodies: Ayurvedic Remedies for Postcolonial Imbalance*. Durham, NC: Duke University Press.

Lash, Scott. 2006. "Life (Vitalism)." *Theory, Culture, and Society* 23 (2–3): 323–29.

Latour, Bruno, and Michel Callon. 1997. "'Thou Shall Not Calculate!' Or How to Symmetricalize Gift and Capital." Unpublished manuscript. Translated by Javier Krauel from "Tu ne calculeras pas!" http://www.bruno-latour.fr/sites/default/files/downloads/P-71%20CAPITALISME-MAUSS-GB.pdf.

Law, John. 2004. *After Method: Mess in Social Science Research*. London: Routledge.

Leder, Drew. 1990. *The Absent Body*. Chicago: University of Chicago Press.

Lemley, Mark A., and Brett M. Frischmann. 2007. "Spillovers." *Columbia Law Review* 107 (1): 257–301.

Leslie, Julia I., trans. 1989. *The Perfect Wife: The Orthodox Hindu Woman according to the Strīdharmapaddhati of Tryambakayajvan*. New Delhi: Oxford University Press.

Levine, Amy. 2016. *South Korean Civil Movement Organisations: Hope, Crisis, and Pragmatism in Democratic Transition.* Manchester: Manchester University Press.

Lévi-Strauss, Claude. 1966. *The Savage Mind.* Chicago: University of Chicago Press.

Li, Tania Murray. 2010. "To Make Live or Let Die? Rural Dispossession and the Protection of Surplus Populations." *Antipode* 41 (s1): 66–93.

Lock, Margaret. 1996. "Death in Technological Time: Locating the End of Meaningful Life." *Medical Anthropology Quarterly* 10 (4): 575–600.

Longmore, Murray, Ian Wilkinson, Andrew Baldwin, and Elizabeth Wallin. 2014. *Oxford Handbook of Clinical Medicine.* 9th ed. Oxford: Oxford University Press.

Lorenzen, David. 1995. "The Historical Vicissitudes of Bhakti Religion." In *Bhakti Religion in North India: Community Identity and Political Action*, edited by David N. Lorenzen, 1–32. Albany: State University of New York Press.

MacKenzie, Donald. 2017. "A Material Political Economy: Automated Trading Desk and Price Prediction in High-Frequency Trading." *Social Studies of Science* 47 (2): 172–94.

Mahmood, Saba. 2005. *Politics of Piety: The Islamic Revival and the Feminist Subject.* Princeton, NJ: Princeton University Press.

Manica, Daniela Tonelli, and Clarice Rios. 2017. "(In)visible Blood: Menstrual Performances and Body Art." *Vibrant: Virtual Brazilian Anthropology* 14 (1): 1–25.

Mann, Thomas. 1981. "Freud and the Future." In *Freud: A Collection of Critical Essays*, edited by Perry Meisel, 37–54. Englewood Cliffs, NJ: Prentice-Hall.

Marglin, Frédérique Apffel. 1977. "Power, Purity, and Pollution: Aspects of the Caste System Reconsidered." *Contributions to Indian Sociology* 11 (2): 245–70.

Marrati, Paola. 2011. "The Novelty of Life." *Constellations* 18 (1): 46–52.

Marriott, McKim. 1976. "Hindu Transactions: Diversity without Dualism." In *Transaction and Meaning: Directions in The Anthropology of Exchange and Symbolic Behavior*, edited by Bruce Kapferer, 109–42. Philadelphia: Institute for the Study of Human Issues.

——. 1989. "Constructing an Indian Ethnosociology." *Contributions to Indian Sociology* 23 (1): 1–39.

——, ed. 1990. *India through Hindu Categories.* New Delhi: Sage Publications.

Marsland, Rebecca, and Ruth Prince. 2012. "What Is Life Worth? Exploring Biomedical Interventions, Survival, and the Politics of Life." *Medical Anthropology Quarterly* 26 (4): 453–69.

Martin, Emily. 1994. *Flexible Bodies: Tracking Immunity in American Culture: From the Days of Polio to the Age of AIDS.* Boston: Beacon Press.

——. 2007. *Bipolar Expeditions: Mania and Depression in American Culture.* Princeton, NJ: Princeton University Press.

Marx, Karl. (1867) 1990. *Capital: A Critique of Political Economy.* Vol. 1. Translated by Ben Fowkes. London: Penguin Books, in association with New Left Review.

Maurer, Bill. 2003. "Uncanny Exchanges: The Possibilities and Failures of 'Making Change' with Alternative Monetary Forms." *Environment and Planning D: Society and Space* 21 (3): 317–40.

Mauss, Marcel. (1925) 2016. *The Gift.* Expanded ed. Selected, annotated, and translated by Jane I. Guyer. Chicago: HAU Books.

Mayblin, Maya. 2013. "The Way Blood Flows: The Sacrificial Value of Intravenous Drip Use in Northeast Brazil." In "Blood Will Out: Essays on Liquid Transfers and Flows," edited by Janet Carsten, special issue, *Journal of the Royal Anthropological Institute* (N.S.) 19 (S1): S42–S56.

Mayer, Adrian C. 1981. "Public Service and Individual Merit in a Town of Central India." In *Culture and Morality: Essays in Honor of Christoph von Furer-Haimendorf*, edited by Adrian C. Mayer, 153–73. Delhi: Oxford University Press.

Mazzarella, William. 2003. *Shoveling Smoke: Advertising and Globalization in Contemporary India*. Durham, NC: Duke University Press.

———. 2009. "A Torn Performative Dispensation: The Affective Politics of British Second World War Propaganda in India and the Problem of Legitimation in an Age of Mass Publics." *South Asian History and Culture* 1 (1): 1–24.

———. 2010. "The Myth of the Multitude, or Who's Afraid of the Crowd?" *Critical Inquiry* 36 (4): 697–727.

Mazzarella, William, and Raminder Kaur, eds. 2009. *Censorship in South Asia: Cultural Regulation from Sedition to Seduction*. Bloomington: Indiana University Press.

Mbembé, Achille. 2003. "Necropolitics." Translated by Libby Meintjes. *Public Culture* 15 (1): 11–40.

McCormack, Donna. 2012. "Intimate Borders: The Ethics of Human Organ Transplantation in Contemporary Film." *Review of Education, Pedagogy, and Cultural Studies* 34 (3–4): 170–83.

Meeta, and Rajivlochan. 2007. "Caste and Religion in Punjab: Case of the Bhaniarawala Phenomenon." *Economic and Political Weekly* 42 (21): 1909–13.

Mehta, Deepak. 2000. "Circumcision, Body, Masculinity: The Ritual Wound and Collective Violence." In *Violence and Subjectivity*, edited by Veena Das, Mamphela Ramphele, Arthur Kleinman, and Pamela Reynolds. Berkeley: University of California Press.

Mines, Diane P. 2002. "Hindu Nationalism, Untouchable Reform, and the Ritual Production of a South Indian Village." *American Ethnologist* 29 (1): 58–85.

Moffatt, Michael. 1990. "Deconstructing McKim Marriott's Ethnosociology: An Outcaste's Critique." *Contributions to Indian Sociology* 24 (2): 215–36.

Mol, Annemarie. 1998. "Lived Reality and the Multiplicity of Norms: A Critical Tribute to George Canguilhem." *Economy and Society* 27 (2–3): 274–84.

Moroşanu, Roxana, and Felix Ringel. 2016. "Time-Tricking: A General Introduction." *Cambridge Journal of Anthropology* 34 (1): 17–21.

Mudur, Ganapati. 1998. "Ban on Payment to Donors Causes Blood Shortage in India." *British Medical Journal* 316 (January 17): 167.

Mukharji, Projit Bihari. 2014. "From Serosocial to Sanguinary Identities: Caste, Transnational Race Science, and the Shifting Metonymies of Blood Group B, India c. 1918–1960." *Indian Economic and Social History Review* 51 (2): 143–76.

———. 2016. *Doctoring Traditions: Ayurveda, Small Technologies, and Braided Sciences*. Chicago: University of Chicago Press.

Mumtaz, Zubia, and Adrienne Levay. 2013. "Forbidden Exchanges and Gender: Implications for Blood Donation during a Maternal Health Emergency in Punjab, Pakistan." *Contemporary South Asia* 21 (3): 260–74.

Mumtaz, Zubia, Sarah Bowen, and Rubina Mumtaz. 2012. "Meanings of Blood, Bleeding, and Blood Donations in Pakistan: Implications for National vs. Global Safe Blood Supply Policies." *Health Policy and Planning* 27 (2): 147–55.

Murray, Stuart J. 2006. "Thanatopolitics: On the Use of Death for Mobilizing Political Life." *Polygraph: An International Journal of Politics and Culture* 18:191–215.

Naipaul, Vidiadhar Surajprasad. 1964. *An Area of Darkness*. New York: Vintage.

Nandy, Ashis. 1970. "The Culture of Indian Politics: A Stock Taking." *Journal of Asian Studies* 30 (1): 57–79.

———. 1983. *The Intimate Enemy: Loss and Recovery of Self under Colonialism*. Delhi: Oxford University Press.

Nanu, Ambika, S. P. Sharma, Kabita Chatterjee, and P. Jyoti. 1997. "Markers for Transfusion-Transmissible Infections in North Indian Voluntary and Replacement Blood Donors: Prevalence and Trends 1989–1996." *Vox Sanguinis* 73 (2): 70–73.

Naoroji, Dadabhai. 1901. *Poverty and Un-British Rule in India*. London: Swan Sonnen-schein & Co.

National AIDS Control Organisation (NACO). 2007. *Voluntary Blood Donation Programme: An Operational Guideline*. Delhi: National AIDS Control Organisation.

Neocleous, Mark. 2003. "The Political Economy of the Dead: Marx's Vampires." *History of Political Thought* 24 (4): 668–84.

Ong, Aihwa, and Nancy N. Chen, eds. 2010. *Asian Biotech: Ethics and Communities of Fate*. Durham, NC: Duke University Press.

Ong, Aihwa, and Stephen J. Collier, eds. 2005. *Global Assemblages: Technology, Politics, and Ethics as Anthropological Problems*. Oxford: Blackwell Publishing.

Oommen, T. K. 2002. "Race, Religion, and Caste: Anthropological and Sociological Perspectives." *Comparative Sociology* 1 (2): 115–26.

Openshaw, Jeanne. 2002. *Seeking Bāuls of Bengal*. Cambridge: Cambridge University Press.

Osella, Caroline. 2008. "Introduction." *South Asia: Journal of South Asian Studies* 31 (1): 1–9.

Osella, Caroline, and Filippo Osella. 2003. "Migration and the Commoditisation of Ritual: Sacrifice, Spectacle, and Contestations in Kerala, India." *Contributions to Indian Sociology* 37 (1–2): 109–39.

Osella, Filippo. 2018. "Charity and Philanthropy in South Asia: An Introduction," edited by Filippo Osella and Sumathi Ramaswamy, special issue, *Modern Asian Studies* 52 (1): 4–34.

Osella, Filippo, and Caroline Osella. 2003. "'Ayyappan Saranam': Masculinity and the Sabarimala Pilgrimage in Kerala." *Journal of the Royal Anthropological Institute* (N.S.) 9 (4): 729–54.

Osella, Filippo, and Sumathi Ramaswamy, eds. 2018. "Charity and Philanthropy in South Asia." Special issue, *Modern Asian Studies* 52 (1).

Palladino, Paolo. 2010. "Picturing the Messianic Agamben and Titian's 'The Nymph' and 'The Shepherd.'" *Theory, Culture, and Society* 27 (1): 94–109.

Pande, Amrita. 2009. "'It May Be Her Eggs but It's My Blood': Surrogates and Everyday Forms of Kinship in India." *Qualitative Sociology* 32 (4): 379–97.

——. 2014. *Wombs in Labor: Transnational Commercial Surrogacy in India*. New York: Columbia University Press.

Parmasad, Vishala. 2016. "She Is My Blood: Donation and Reciprocity in Trinidad." In *Giving Blood: The Institutional Making of Altruism*, edited by Johanne Charbonneau and André Smith, 199–218. London: Routledge.

Parry, Jonathan. 1986. "The Gift, the Indian Gift, and the 'Indian Gift.'" *Man* (N.S.) 21 (3): 453–73.

——. 1989. "On the Moral Perils of Exchange." In *Money and the Morality of Exchange*, edited by Jonathan Parry and Maurice Bloch, 64–93. Cambridge: Cambridge University Press.

——. 1994. *Death in Banaras*. Cambridge: Cambridge University Press.

——. 2015. "The Sacrifices of Modernity in a Soviet-Built Steel Town in Central India." *Anthropology of This Century* (12), January 2015. http://aotcpress.com/articles/sacrifices/.

Parry, Jonathan, and Maurice Bloch, eds. 1989. *Money and the Morality of Exchange*. Cambridge: Cambridge University Press.

Pedersen, Morten Axel, and Morten Nielsen. 2013. "Trans-temporal Hinges: Reflections on an Ethnographic Study of Chinese Infrastructural Projects in Mozambique and Mongolia." *Social Analysis* 57 (1): 122–42.

Petryna, Adriana. 2002. *Life Exposed: Biological Citizens after Chernobyl*. Princeton, NJ: Princeton University Press.

Petryna, Adriana, Andrew Lakoff, and Arthur Kleinman, eds. 2006. *Global Pharmaceuticals: Ethics, Markets, Practices*. Durham, NC: Duke University Press.

Pinney, Christopher. 2004. *"Photos of the Gods": The Printed Image and Political Struggle in India*. London: Reaktion Books.

———. 2011. *Photography and Anthropology*. London: Reaktion Books.

Pocock, David. 1973. *Mind, Body, and Wealth: A Study of Belief and Practice in an Indian Village*. Oxford: Basil Blackwell.

Polsky, Allyson D. 2002. "Blood, Race, and National Identity: Scientific and Popular Discourses." *Journal of Medical Humanities* 23 (3–4): 171–86.

Poole, Ross. 1991. *Modernity and Morality*. London: Routledge.

Power, Michael. 1997. *The Audit Society: Rituals of Verification*. Oxford: Oxford University Press.

Prasad, Amit. 2009. "Capitalizing Disease: Biopolitics of Drug Trials in India." *Theory, Culture, and Society* 26 (5): 1–29.

Prasanna, Chitra Karunakaran. 2016. "Claiming the Public Sphere: Menstrual Taboos and the Rising Dissent in India." *Agenda* 30 (3): 91–95.

Qureshi, Ayaz. 2018. *AIDS in Pakistan: Bureaucracy, Public Goods, and NGOs*. Basingstoke: Palgrave Macmillan.

Rabinow, Paul. 1992. "Artificiality and Enlightenment: From Sociobiology to Biosociality." In *Zone 6: Incorporations*, edited by Jonathan Crary and Sanford Kwinter, 234–52. New York: Zone Books.

Raheja, Gloria Goodwin. 1989. "Centrality, Mutuality, and Hierarchy: Shifting Aspects of Inter-caste Relationships in North India." *Contributions to Indian Sociology* 23 (1): 79–101.

Ramaswamy, Sumathi. 1997. *Passions of the Tongue: Language Devotion in Tamil India, 1891–1970*. Berkeley: University of California Press.

———. 2008. "Maps, Mother/Goddesses, and Martyrdom in Modern India." *Journal of Asian Studies* 67 (3): 819–53.

———. 2009. *The Goddess and the Nation: Mapping Mother India*. Durham, NC: Duke University Press.

Rao, Anupama. 2009. *The Caste Question: Dalits and the Politics of Modern India*. Berkeley: University of California Press.

Rao, Aparna. 2000. "Blood, Milk, and Mountains: Marriage Practice and Concepts of Predictability among the Bakkarwal of Jammu and Kashmir." In *Culture, Creation, and Procreation: Concepts of Kinship in South Asian Practice*, edited by Monica Böck and Aparna Rao, 101–34. Oxford: Berghahn.

Reddy, Deepa S. 2005. "The Ethnicity of Caste." *Anthropological Quarterly* 78 (3): 543–84.

Reed, Adam. 2017. "An Office of Ethics: Meetings, Roles, and Moral Enthusiasm in Animal Protection." In "Meetings: Ethnographies of Organizational Process, Bureaucracy, and Assembly," edited by Hannah Brown, Adam Reed, and Thomas Yarrow, special issue, *Journal of the Royal Anthropological Institute* (N.S.) 23 (S1): 166–81.

Ricoeur, Paul. 1966. *Freedom and Nature: The Voluntary and the Involuntary*. Translated and with an introduction by Erazim V. Kohák. Evanston, IL: Northwestern University Press.

Robertson, Jennifer. 2012. "Hemato-nationalism: The Past, Present, and Future of 'Japanese Blood.'" *Medical Anthropology* 31 (2): 93–112.

Rose, Nikolas S. 1998. "Life, Reason, and History: Reading Georges Canguilhem Today." *Economy and Society* 28 (2–3): 154–70.

———. 2007. *The Politics of Life Itself: Biomedicine, Power, and Subjectivity in the Twenty-First Century*. Princeton, NJ: Princeton University Press.

Rose, Nikolas, and Carlos Novas. 2005. "Biological Citizenship." In *Global Assemblages: Technology, Politics, and Ethics as Anthropological Problems*, edited by Aihwa Ong and Stephen J. Collier, 439–63. Oxford: Blackwell Publishing.

Roychowdhury, Poulami. 2015. "Over the Law: Rape and the Seduction of Popular Politics." *Gender and Society* 30 (1): 80–94.

Säävälä, Minna. 2001. "Low Caste but Middle-Class: Some Religious Strategies for Middle-Class Identification in Hyderabad." *Contributions to Indian Sociology* 35 (3): 293–318.

Sadana, Rashmi. 2010. "On the Delhi Metro: An Ethnographic View." *Economic and Political Weekly* 45 (46): 77–83.

Saha, Ranjana. 2017. "Milk, 'Race,' and Nation: Medical Advice on Breastfeeding in Colonial Bengal." *South Asia Research* 37 (2): 147–65.

Salisbury, L. 1875. *Minute. P. P. 1881* 71 (1): 468–79.

Samanta, Suchitra. 1994. "The 'Self-Animal' and Divine Digestion: Goat Sacrifice to the Goddess Kālī in Bengal." *Journal of Asian Studies* 53 (3): 779–803.

Sanabria, Emilia. 2009. "Alleviative Bleeding: Bloodletting, Menstruation, and the Politics of Ignorance in a Brazilian Blood Donation Centre." In "Blood Donation, Bioeconomy, Culture," edited by Jacob Copeman, special issue, *Body and Society* 15 (2): 123–44.

Sant Nirankari Mandal. 2003. *Sant Nirankari Mission: An Introduction*. Delhi: Sant Nirankari Mandal.

Saria, Vaibhav. 2016. *The Fallen Idol: Corruption, Care, and the Clinic in India* (draft).

Saunders, J. B. de C. M. 1972. "A Conceptual History of Transplantation." In *Transplantation*, edited by J. S. Najarian and R. L. Simmons, 3–25. Philadelphia: Lea and Febiger.

Savarkar, V. D. 2007. "Extract from *Hindutva: Who Is a Hindu?* [1923]." In *Hindu Nationalism: A Reader*, edited by Christophe Jaffrelot, 87–96. Princeton, NJ: Princeton University Press.

Schaffer, Simon. 2005. "Seeing Double: How to Make Up a Phantom Body Politic." In *Making Things Public: Atmospheres of Democracy*, edited by Bruno Latour and Peter Weibel, 196–202. Boston: MIT Press.

Schaller, Joseph. 1996. "Sanskritization, Caste Uplift, and Social Dissidence in the Sant Ravidās Panth." In *Bhakti Religion in North India: Community Identity and Political Action*, edited by David N. Lorenzen, 94–119. Albany: State University of New York.

Scheper-Hughes, Nancy. 2000. "The Global Traffic in Human Organs." *Current Anthropology* 41 (2): 191–224.

Schmitt, Carl. (1922) 2005. *Political Theology: Four Chapters on the Concept of Sovereignty*. Edited and translated by George Schwabb. Chicago: University of Chicago Press.

Schneider, David M. 1980. *American Kinship: A Cultural Account*. 2nd ed. Chicago: University of Chicago Press.

——. 1984. *A Critique of the Study of Kinship*. Ann Arbor: University of Michigan Press.

Schoenberg, Nancy E., and Elaine M. Drew. 2002. "Articulating Silences: Experiential and Biomedical Constructions of Hypertension Symptomatology." *Medical Anthropology Quarterly* 16 (4): 458–75.

Seligman, Adam B., Robert P. Weller, Michael J. Puett, and Bennett Simon. 2008. *Ritual and Its Consequences: An Essay on the Limits of Sincerity*. Oxford: Oxford University Press.

Sennett, Richard. 2006. "Introduction." In Émile Durkheim, *On Suicide*, xi–xxiv. New York: Penguin.

Sharp, Lesley. 2006. *Strange Harvest: Organ Transplants, Denatured Bodies, and the Transformed Self*. Berkeley: University of California Press.

———. 2007. *Bodies, Commodities, and Biotechnologies: Death, Mourning, and Scientific Desire in the Realm of Human Organ Transfer.* New York: Columbia University Press.

Shore, Cris. 1999. "Fictions of Fieldwork: Depicting the 'Self' in Ethnographic Writing (Italy)." In *Being There: Fieldwork in Anthropology*, edited by C. W. Watson, 25–48. London: Pluto Press.

Siddiqui, Ali. 1982. *Son of India.* New Delhi: Siddiqui.

Siebers, Tobin. 2003. "The Return to Ritual: Violence and Art in the Media Age." *Journal for Religious and Cultural Theory* 5 (1): 9–32.

Simpson, Bob. 2009. "'Please Give a Drop of Blood': Blood Donation, Conflict, and the Haemato-Global Assemblage in Contemporary Sri Lanka." In "Blood Donation, Bioeconomy, Culture," edited by Jacob Copeman, special issue, *Body and Society* 15 (2): 101–22.

———. 2011. "Blood Rhetorics: Donor Campaigns and Their Publics in Contemporary Sri Lanka." *Ethnos* 76 (2): 254–75.

Singh, Bhrigupati. 2010. "Asceticism and Eroticism in Gandhi, Thoreau, and Nietzsche: An Essay in Geo-philosophy." *Borderlands* 9 (3): 1–34.

Singh, Bir, R. M. Pandey, N. D'Souza, A. Anushyanthan, Vibhor Krishna, V. Gupta, et al. 2002. "Knowledge, Attitudes, and Socio-Demographic Factors Differentiating Blood Donors from Non-Donors in an Urban Slum of Delhi." *Indian Journal of Community Medicine* 27 (3). http://www.indemedica.com/ journals.php?journalid=7&issueid=41&articleid=519&action=article.

Singh, Jagat. 1977. *Sanjay Gandhi and Awakening of Youth Power.* New Delhi: Pankaj Publications.

Singh, Trishala. 2016. "Women's Right to Access: Seeking Gender Equality in Places of Worship." *Arts and Education International Research Journal* 3 (1): 108–10.

Singha, Radhika. 2011. "The Recruiter's Eye on 'The Primitive': To France—and Back—in the Indian Labour Corps, 1917–1918." In *Other Combatants, Other Fronts: Competing Histories of the First World War*, edited by James E. Kitchen, Alisa Miller, and Laura Rowe, 199–223. Newcastle upon Tyne: Cambridge Scholar Series.

Skaria, Ajay. 2010. "Living by Dying: Gandhi, Satyagraha, and the Warrior." In *Ethical Life in South Asia*, edited by Anand Pandian and Daud Ali, 211–31. Bloomington: Indiana University Press.

———. 2014. "Gandhi's Radical Conservatism." *India Seminar* (662), October 2014. http://www.india-seminar.com/2014/662/662_ajay_skaria.htm.

———. 2016. *Unconditional Equality: Gandhi's Religion of Resistance.* Minneapolis: University of Minnesota Press.

Smith, André, and Johanne Charbonneau. 2016. "Conclusion: Blood Donation in the Social World: Toward a Critical, Contextualized Paradigm of Understanding." In *Giving Blood: The Institutional Making of Altruism*, edited by Johanne Charbonneau and André Smith, 219–37. London: Routledge.

Spencer, Jonathan. 1997. "Post-colonialism and the Political Imagination." *Journal of the Royal Anthropological Institute* (N.S.) 3 (1): 1–19.

———. 2007. *Anthropology, Politics, and the State: Democracy and Violence in South Asia.* Cambridge: Cambridge University Press.

———. 2008. "A Nationalism without Politics? The Illiberal Consequences of Liberal Institutions in Sri Lanka." *Third World Quarterly* 29 (3): 611–29.

Spinosa, Charles, Fernando Flores, and Hubert L. Dreyfus. 1999. *Disclosing New Worlds: Entrepreneurship, Democratic Action, and the Cultivation of Solidarity.* Boston: MIT Press.

Srinivas, Mysore Narasimhachar. 1952. *Religion and Society among the Coorgs of South India.* Bombay: Asia Publishing House.

Srinivas, Smriti. 2016. "Roadside Shrines, Storefront Saints, and Twenty-First Century Life-styles: The Cultural and Spatial Thresholds of Indian Urbanism." In *Place/No-Place in Urban Asian Religiosity*, edited by Joanne Punzo Waghorne, 131–47. Singapore: Springer Science & Business Media.

Srinivas, Tulasi. 2012. "Relics of Faith: Fleshly Desires, Ascetic Disciplines and Devotional Affect in the Transnational Sathya Sai Movement." In *Routledge Handbook of Body Studies*, edited by Bryan S. Turner, 78–91. London: Routledge.

Srivastava, Sanjay. 2001. "Non-Gandhian Sexuality, Commodity Cultures, and a 'Happy Married Life': The Cultures of Masculinity and Heterosexuality in India." *South Asia: Journal of South Asian Studies* 24 (1): 225–49.

——. 2007. *Passionate Modernity: Sexuality, Class and Consumption in India*. Delhi: Oxford University Press.

Ssorin-Chaikov, Nikolai. 2006. "On Heterochrony: Birthday Gifts to Stalin, 1949." *Journal of the Royal Anthropological Institute* (N.S.) 12 (2): 355–75.

——. 2013. "Ethnographic Conceptualism: An Introduction." *Laboratorium* 5 (2): 5–18.

Ssorin-Chaikov, Nikolai, and Olga Sosnina. 2004. "The Faculty of Useless Things: Gifts to Soviet Leaders." In *Personality Cults in Stalinism / Personenkulte im Stalinismus*, edited by Klaus Heller and Jan Plamper, 277–300. Göttingen: Vandenhoeck and Ruprecht.

Starr, Douglas. 1998. *Blood: An Epic History of Medicine and Commerce*. New York: Knopf.

——. 2002. "Bad Blood: The 9/11 Blood-Donation Disaster." *New Republic* 227 (5): 13–16. Stevenson, Lisa. 2012. "The Psychic Life of Biopolitics: Survival, Cooperation, and Inuit Community." *American Ethnologist* 39 (3): 592–613.

Stokes, Eric. 1978. *The Peasant and the Raj: Studies in Agrarian Society and Peasant Rebellion in Colonial India*. Cambridge: Cambridge University Press.

Stoler, Ann Laura. 2016. *Duress: Imperial Durabilities in Our Times*. Durham, NC: Duke University Press.

Strathern, Marilyn. 1990. "Artefacts of History: Events and the Interpretation of Images." In *Culture and History in the Pacific*, edited by Jukka Siikala, 24–44. Helsinki: Finnish Anthropological Society.

——, ed. 1995. *Shifting Contexts: Transformations in Anthropological Knowledge*. London: Psychology Press.

——. 1997. "Double Standards." In *The Ethnography of Moralities*, edited by Signe Howell, 127–51. London: Routledge.

——. 2005. *Kinship, Law, and the Unexpected: Relatives Are Always a Surprise*. Cambridge: Cambridge University Press.

——. 2009. "Comparing Concerns: Some Issues in Organ and Other Donations." *Suomen Antropologi: Journal of the Finnish Anthropological Society* 34 (4): 5–21.

——. 2011. "Binary License." *Common Knowledge* 17 (1): 87–103.

——. 2014. "An Interview with Marilyn Strathern: Kinship and Career." In "Social Theory after Strathern," edited by Alice Street and Jacob Copeman, special issue, *Theory, Culture, and Society* 31 (2–3): 263–81.

——. 2017. "Afterword." In "Meetings: Ethnographies of Organizational Process, Bureaucracy, and Assembly," edited by Hannah Brown, Adam Reed, and Thomas Yarrow, special issue, *Journal of the Royal Anthropological Institute* (N.S.) 23 (S1): 166–81.

Street, Alice. 2009. "Failed Recipients: Extracting Blood in a Papua New Guinean Hospital." In "Blood Donation, Bioeconomy, Culture," edited by Jacob Copeman, special issue, *Body and Society* 15 (2): 193–215.

Strong, Thomas. 2009. "Vital Publics of Pure Blood." In "Blood Donation, Bioeconomy, Culture," edited by Jacob Copeman, special issue, *Body and Society* 15 (2): 169–91.

Sugg, Richard. 2016. *Mummies, Cannibals, and Vampires: The History of Corpse Medicine from the Renaissance to the Victorians*. London: Routledge.

Sujatha, V., 2007. "Pluralism in Indian Medicine: Medical Lore as a Genre of Medical Knowledge." *Contributions to Indian Sociology* 41 (2): 169–202.

Sunder Rajan, Kaushik. 2006. *Biocapital: The Constitution of Postgenomic Life*. Durham, NC: Duke University Press.

Sutton-Smith, Brian. 1997. *The Ambiguity of Play*. Cambridge, MA: Harvard University Press.

Tambiah, Stanley Jeyaraja. 1996. *Leveling Crowds: Ethnonationalist Conflicts and Collective Violence in South Asia*. Berkeley: University of California Press.

Tarlo, Emma. 2003. *Unsettling Memories: Narratives of the Emergency in Delhi*. Berkeley: University of California Press.

Taussig, Michael. 2009. "What Do Drawings Want?" *Culture, Theory, and Critique* 50 (2): 263–74.

Theweleit, Klaus. 1987. *Male Fantasies*. 2 vols. Minneapolis: University of Minnesota Press.

Thompson, Catherine. 1985. "The Power to Pollute and the Power to Preserve: Perceptions of Female Power in a Hindu Village." *Social Science and Medicine* 21 (6): 701–11.

Thompson, Charis. 2000. "The Biotech Mode of Reproduction." Paper prepared for the School of American Research advanced seminar "Animation and Cessation: Anthropological Perspectives on Changing Definitions of Life and Death in the Context of Biomedicine," Santa Fe, New Mexico.

Thrift, Nigel. 2006. "Re-inventing Invention: New Tendencies in Capitalist Commodification." *Economy and Society* 35 (2): 279–306.

———. 2008. *Non-representational Theory: Space, Politics, Affect*. London: Routledge.

Titmuss, Richard M. 1970. *The Gift Relationship: From Human Blood to Social Policy*. London: Allen and Unwin.

Trilling, Lionel. 1971. *Sincerity and Authenticity*. Cambridge, MA: Harvard University Press.

Turner, Victor. 1982. *From Ritual to Theatre: The Human Seriousness of Play*. New York: Paj Publications.

Udupa, Sahana. 2016. "Fast Time Religion: News, Speculation, and Discipline in India." *Critique of Anthropology* 36 (4): 397–418.

Urban, Hugh B. 2008. "Matrix of Power: Tantra, Kingship, and Sacrifice in the Worship of Mother Goddess Kāmākhyā." *South Asia: Journal of South Asian Studies* 31 (3): 500–534.

Urry, John. 2010. "Consuming the Planet to Excess." *Theory, Culture, and Society* 27 (2–3): 191–212.

Vanaik, Achin. 1997. *The Furies of Indian Communalism: Religion, Modernity, and Secularization*. London: Verso Books.

Van Alphen, E. 1997. "The Portrait's Dispersal: Concepts of Representation and Subjectivity in Contemporary Portraiture." In *Portraiture: Facing the Subject*, edited by Joanna Woodall, 239–56. Manchester: Manchester University Press.

Van de Port, Mattijs. 2011. "(Not) Made by the Human Hand: Media Consciousness and Immediacy in the Cultural Production of the Real." *Social Anthropology* 19 (1): 74–89.

van der Veer, Peter. 1989. "The Concept of the Ideal Brahman as an Indological Construct." In *Hinduism Reconsidered*, edited by Günter-Dietz Sontheimer and Hermann Kulke, 67–81. New Delhi: Manohar.

Van Hollen, Cecilia. 2011. "Breast or Bottle? HIV-Positive Women's Responses to Global Health Policy on Infant Feeding in India." *Medical Anthropology Quarterly* 25 (4): 499–518.

———. 2013. *Birth in the Age of AIDS: Women, Reproduction, and HIV/AIDS in India*. Stanford, CA: Stanford University Press.

———. 2018. "Handle with Care: Rethinking the Rights versus Culture Dichotomy in Cancer Disclosure in India." *Medical Anthropology Quarterly* 32 (1): 59–84.

Vanita, Ruth. 2002. "Dosti and Tamanna: Male-Male Love, Difference, and Normativity in Hindi Cinema." In *Everyday Life in South Asia*, edited by Diane P. Mines and Sarah Lamb, 146–58. Bloomington: Indiana University Press.

Venkat, Bharat. 2017. "Scenes of Commitment." *Cultural Anthropology* 32 (1): 93–116.

Vicziany, Marika. 2001. "HIV and AIDS in India: Love, Disease, and Technology Transfer to the Kamasutra Condom." *Contemporary South Asia* 10 (1): 95–129.

Vicziany, Marika, and Jaideep Hardikar. 2018. "Point-of-Care Blood Tests: Do Indian Villagers Have Cultural Objections?" *Frontiers in Chemistry* 6 (505): 1–12.

Viveiros de Castro, Eduardo. 1998. "Cosmological Deixis and Amerindian Perspectivism." *Journal of the Royal Anthropological Institute* (N.S.) 4 (3): 469–88.

Vora, Kalindi. 2015. *Life Support: Biocapital and the New History of Outsourced Labor*. Minneapolis: University of Minnesota Press.

Wagner, Kim A. 2016. "'Calculated to Strike Terror': The Amritsar Massacre and the Spectacle of Colonial Violence." *Past and Present* 233 (1): 185–225.

Wagner, Roy. 1986. *Symbols That Stand for Themselves*. Chicago: University of Chicago Press.

Waldby, Catherine. 2000. *The Visible Human Project: Informatic Bodies and Posthuman Medicine*. London: Routledge.

Waldby, Catherine, and Robert Mitchell. 2006. *Tissue Economies: Blood, Organs, and Cell Lines in Late Capitalism*. Durham, NC: Duke University Press.

Weiermair, Peter. 2001. "Reflections on Blood in Contemporary Art." In *Blood: Art, Power, Politics, and Pathology*, edited by James M. Bradburne, 205–15. Munich: Prestel.

Weiner, James F. 1999. "Psychoanalysis and Anthropology: On the Temporality of Analysis." In *Anthropological Theory Today*, edited by Henrietta Moore, 234–61. Cambridge: Polity.

Weston, Kath. 2013a. "Lifeblood, Liquidity, and Cash Transfusions: Beyond Metaphor in the Cultural Study of Finance." In "Blood Will Out: Essays on Liquid Transfers and Flows," edited by Janet Carsten, special issue, *Journal of the Royal Anthropological Institute* (N.S.) 19 (S1): S24–S41.

———. 2013b. "Biosecuritization: The Quest for Synthetic Blood and the Taming of Kinship." In *Blood and Kinship: Matter for Metaphor from Ancient Rome to the Present*, edited by Christopher H. Johnson, Bernhard Jussen, David Warren Sabean, and Simon Teuscher, 244–65. Oxford: Berghahn Books.

Whitehouse, Harvey. 2000. *Arguments and Icons: Divergent Modes of Religiosity*. Oxford: Oxford University Press.

Whitehouse, Harvey, and James Laidlaw. 2004. *Ritual and Memory: Toward a Comparative Anthropology of Religion*. Walnut Creek, CA: AltaMira Press.

Willerslev, Rane. 2004. "Not Animal, Not Not-Animal: Hunting, Imitation, and Empathetic Knowledge among the Siberian Yukaghirs." *Journal of the Royal Anthropological Institute* (N.S.) 10 (3): 629–52.

Williams, Brackette F. 1995. "Classification Systems Revisited: Kinship, Caste, Race, and Nationality as the Flow of Blood and the Spread of Rights." In *Naturalizing Power: Essays in Feminist Cultural Analysis*, edited by Sylvia J. Yanagisako and Carol L. Delaney, 201–36. London: Routledge.

Winterson, Jeanette. 2006. *Tanglewreck*. New York: Bloomsbury Publishing.

Wollheim, Richard. 1987. "Pictorial Style: Two Views." In *The Concept of Style*, edited by Berel Lang, 183–202. Ithaca, NY: Cornell University Press.

World Health Organization (WHO). 2012. *Blood Donor Selection: Guidelines on Assessing Donor Suitability for Blood Donation*. Geneva: WHO.

Zachariah, Benjamin. 2010. "Rethinking (the Absence of) Fascism in India, c. 1922–45." In *Cosmopolitan Thought Zones: South Asia and the Global Circulation of Ideas*, edited by Sugata Bose and Kris Manjapra, 178–209. Basingstoke: Palgrave Macmillan.

Zelizer, Barbie. 2004. "The Voice of the Visual in Memory." In *Framing Public Memory*, edited by Kendall R. Phillips, 157–86. Tuscaloosa: University of Alabama Press.

NEWS ARTICLES

Anand, Anu. 2015. "Blood for Sale: India's Illegal 'Red Market.'" http://www.bbc.com/news/business-30273994.

Azad, Nikita. 2015. "'A Young Bleeding Woman' Pens an Open Letter to the Keepers of Sabrimala Temple." *Youth Ki Awaaz*, November 20, 2015. https://www.youthkiawaaz.com/2015/11/open-letter-to-devaswom-chief-sabrimala/.

Bellafante, Ginia. 2016. "The Bohemian Capitalist." *New York Times*, February 2016. https://www.nytimes.com/2016/02/28/nyregion/thinx-underwear-underground.html.

Bobel, Chris. 2015. "The Year the Period Went Public." *Gender and Society*, November 12, 2015. https://gendersociety.wordpress.com/2015/11/12/the-year-the-period-went-public/.

Chada, Kumkum. 2011. "Sanjay's Men and Women." *Hindustan Times Blogs*, January 4, 2011. http://archive.is/Ofi1.

Daniyal, Shoaib. 2016. "As Right-Wing BJP Seeks to Appropriate Bose, a Reminder: Congress Expelled Him for Being Too Left." *Scroll.in*, February 5, 2016. https://scroll.in/article/802593/as-right-wing-bjp-seeks-to-appropriate-bose-a-reminder-congress-expelled-him-for-being-too-left.

Gowen, Annie. 2016. "Women Fight for Access to Sacred Places in India." *Washington Post*, January 29, 2016. https://www.washingtonpost.com/news/worldviews/wp/2016/01/29/women-fight-for-access-to-sacred-places-in-india/.

Gupta, Kanchan. 1996. "Subhas Chandra Bose as a Mascot of Hindutva." *BJP Today*, May 1–15, 1996.

International Business Times. 2015. "Kerala Devaswom Chief Wants Machine to Scan Women for Purity at Sabarimala." November 16, 2015. https://www.ibtimes.co.in/kerala-devaswom-chief-wants-machine-scan-women-purity-sabarimala-654925.

Mishra, S. 2009. "Kids Forced to Donate Blood on Rajiv B'day." *Mail Today*, August 23, 2009.

Panigrahi, Saswat. 2017. "Hindutva and Cultural Nationalism: The Missing Chapter in Netaji's Life." *Swarajya*, January 23, 2017. https://swarajyamag.com/culture/hindutva-and-cultural-nationalism-the-missing-chapter-in-netajis-life.

Rajagopal, Krishnadas. 2016. "Why Is Menstruation a Religious Taboo, Students Ask SC." *The Hindu*, February 15, 2016. http://www.thehindu.com/news/national/Why-is-menstruation-a-religious-taboo-students-ask-SC/article15619096.ece.

Ram, Vidya. 2018. "Kerala Girl at Centre of 'Period Poverty' Campaign in London." *The Hindu*, January 13, 2018. http://www.thehindu.com/society/kerala-girl-at-centre-of-period-poverty-campaign-in-london/article22435221.ece.

Sobo, Elisa. 2016. "Language, Power, and Pot: Speaking of Cannabis as Medicine." *Savage Minds*, September 1, 2016. http://savageminds.org/2016/09/01/language-power-and-pot-speaking-of-cannabis-as-medicine.

Index